Cranial Ultrasonography of Infants

Cranial Ultrasonography of Infants

DIANE S. BABCOCK, M.D.
BOKYUNG K. HAN, M.D.
Division of Radiology
Children's Hospital Medical Center
Cincinnati, Ohio

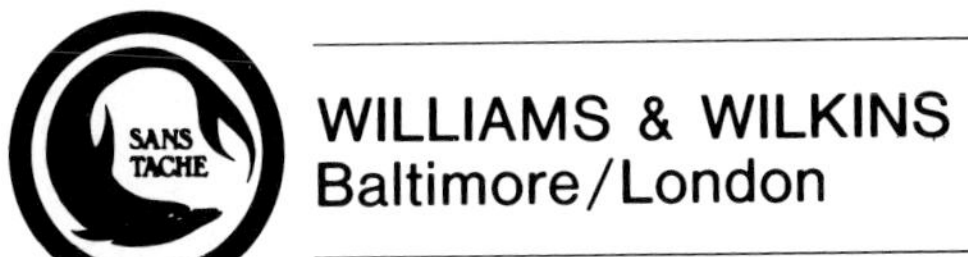

WILLIAMS & WILKINS
Baltimore/London

428 East Preston Street
Baltimore, MD 21202, U.S.A.

Made in the United States of America

Reprinted 1982

Library of Congress Cataloging in Publication Data

Babcock, Diane S.

Cranial ultrasonography of infants.
Includes index.
1. Pediatric neurology—Diagnosis. 2. Ultrasonic encephalography. 3. Infants—Diseases—Diagnosis. I. Han, Bokyung Kim, 1948- II. Title. [DNLM: 1. Brain diseases—Diagnosis. 2. Brain diseases—In infancy and childhood. 3. Ultrasonics—Diagnostic use. WE 705 B112c]
RJ488.5.U47B33 618.92′0975107543 81-10340
ISBN 0-683-00300-3 AACR2

Composed and printed at the
Waverly Press, Inc.
Mt. Royal and Guilford Aves.
Baltimore, MD 21202, U.S.A.

Dedication

To my husband, John, and to our parents, for their continued encouragement and support.

DIANE SCHWEMLEIN BABCOCK, M.D.

To my husband, Donghoon, and our son, Benjamin, for their love, patience, and encouragement.

BOKYUNG KIM HAN, M.D.

Foreword

Serious use of ultrasound as a clinical diagnostic tool began in the late 1960s with A-mode and then B-mode scanning. In Neuroradiology, A-mode scans were used to assess the position of midline structures in the calvaria, but this method had limited success, and indeed fell into some disrepute in the early 1970s because of overutilization and limited reliability. In the meantime, the accuracy, reliability and use of B-mode ultrasound for abdominal diagnosis increased rapidly and indeed spectacularly.

Suddenly, in the 1970s, it became apparent to a number of observers that B-mode ultrasound scanning could be used for head scanning in young infants by passing the ultrasound through the open fontanelle (or fontanelles). Kossoff first detailed the cross-sectional anatomic study of the brain in the neonate in 1974. The value of this imaging technique was widely appreciated, and rapid development in technical equipment, with increased ease of scanning and much improved resolution, led to its being adopted by many centers with newborn intensive care units and nurseries. Dr. Garry LeQuesne in our Department was one of the pioneers in this work, and we owe him recognition and gratitude for his vigorous and productive investigations in 1977 and 1978.

Drs. Babcock and Han, using contact B-mode scans and real time scans have, since 1978, made numerous contributions to the evaluation of intracranial anatomy, particularly in the neonate. Their work has won widespread recognition and acclaim, and this small book summarizes and brings to the interested reader current knowledge of the use of ultrasound scanning techniques in diseases of the infant's brain.

It is no small accomplishment to be able to demonstrate by a simple and noninvasive examination done at the bedside, without disturbing the infant, so much about intracranial structures and whether they are perturbed, particularly by neonatal hemorrhage and its complications.

Drs. Babcock and Han have been able to encompass most of what is known in this rapidly developing field in a concise presentation which loses nothing in clarity and completeness by being brief.

J. S. Dunbar, M.D.

Preface

While the potential usefulness of B-mode ultrasonography for examining the infant's head was demonstrated in images published as early as 1963, it was not until the late 1970s when technical advances in ultrasound equipment resulted in high quality gray scale images that enthusiasm for the technique developed among ultrasonographers and pediatric radiologists. In the past 2 years cranial ultrasonography has developed from a method used only in a few pediatric medical centers around the world to one that has become a routine part of medical care in most newborn centers. The overwhelming popularity of cranial ultrasound has been due to the fact that it avoids harmful ionizing radiation and can be performed portably on very ill infants. This book is written to share our experiences and the knowledge gained over a 3-year period with those radiologists, ultrasonographers, and clinicians just getting into the field of cranial ultrasonography. While there are many texts on A-mode ultrasonography of the infant and adult head, there were no texts or atlases devoted to B-mode imaging at the time we started this project.

This book is written for two particular audiences. For those concerned with imaging procedures, i.e. radiologists and ultrasonographers, we have included sections discussing the various types of ultrasound equipment and their application to head scanning. We have also attempted to describe and illustrate the techniques used to obtain both contact and real-time images. Ultrasonography is a highly operator-dependent imaging modality, and technique is of utmost importance. We found this section the most difficult to write (a little like an artist trying to explain how one paints a picture).

Sections on normal anatomy and examples of abnormal cases were included to show their ultrasound appearance. In many instances, the ultrasound images are very similar to those obtained with cranial computed tomography, but there are several differences. Cranial computed tomography has classically used the axial plane for presentation of the anatomy, whereas ultrasound produces the best images in the coronal and sagittal plane by scanning through the anterior fontanelle.

The book is also written for those clinicians caring for these infants, to acquaint them with the uses, advantages, and capabilities of this modality. A method is only useful if it helps to improve patient care.

Our book is intended as a general text on B-mode gray scale ultrasonography of the infant head and we were not able to include in-depth discussions of the disease processes described. For more detail, the reader is referred to the several excellent general and pediatric neuroradiology texts already available and which are referenced. We have included computed tomographic, pneumoencephalographic, and angiographic correlation when available and helpful, however, the main emphasis in our book is on ultrasonography. The role of cranial ultrasonography vis-à-vis these other modalities is being evaluated at the present time and must be left to future texts for more thorough discussion.

Acknowledgments

We would like to thank the following people for their help in preparing this book: The Professional Staff of the Children's Hospital Medical Center of Cincinnati for their acceptance of ultrasonography which made this book possible; our colleagues in pediatric radiology who have actively encouraged the integration of ultrasonography into the overall diagnostic radiological evaluation of the pediatric patient; Marsha Ellington, Theresa Adams, and Debora Root for performing the sonographic studies and helping prepare the section on scanning technique; Drs. Corning Benton and J. Scott Dunbar for editorial assistance in preparation of the manuscript; Dr. Garry LeQuesne who set up the ultrasound section and introduced head scanning at our institution; Marlena Tyre and Norma Woolum for secretarial assistance in manuscript preparation; Richard Isham for the photography; and Marcia Hartsock for the art work.

We would also like to give special thanks to Drs. Benjamin Felson and J. Scott Dunbar, whose advice and encouragement were instrumental to us in completing this book.

Contributors

Diane S. Babcock, M.D.
Division of Radiology
Children's Hospital Medical Center
Cincinnati, Ohio

Kai Haber, M.D.
Department of Radiology
University of Arizona
Tucson, Arizona

Bokyung K. Han, M.D.
Division of Radiology
Children's Hospital Medical Center
Cincinnati, Ohio

Michael Johnson, M.D.
Department of Radiology
University of Colorado Health Sciences Center
Denver, Colorado

Contents

CHAPTER 1

Introduction

Historical Background

The history of sonography in neuroradiology goes back to 1956 when Leksell[1] described the use of A-mode or one-dimensional ultrasonography (Fig. 1.1) for cranial imaging and recommended its use to determine the position of the midline of the brain. Since that time, many articles and books have been written about this technique for detecting a variety of intracranial abnormalities including shifts of the midline structures due to intracranial masses, dilatation of the ventricles, extra-axial fluid collections, and congenital anomalies.

B-mode or two-dimensional ultrasonography was developed in the middle 1950s and its use for cranial imaging was first reported by Vleiger et al.[2] in 1963 and by Brinker and Taveras[3] in 1966 using a contact scanning technique. In 1965 Makow and Real[4] reported a water-immersion scanning technique for two-dimensional images of the brain which necessitated suspending the patient's head in a water tank which was cumbersome and not really practical. Using these types of equipment, cross-sectional images of the intracranial structures could be produced; however, the thickness of the skull bones in adult patients limited its use. Efforts to increase the role of sonography in neuroradiologic evaluations continued, and there was some progress in the development of apparatus for neurosonics up to 1973 and even later. However, the development of cranial computed tomography (CT) at about that time diverted interest away from sonography to this new, noninvasive technique.

Interest in sonography to study the brain of the infant in whom the fontanelles are large enough to permit scanning between rather than through the cranial bones continued, and in 1974 and 1975 Kossoff, Garrett et al.[5, 6] reported visualization of the normal brain anatomy in the infant as well as visualization of hydrocephalus using contact scanning technique and images obtained with bistable equipment. About this time, equipment producing gray scale images became commercially available, and in 1975 Shkolnik[7] reported demonstration of a brain tumor (craniopharyngioma) by gray scale B-mode ultrasonography and several subsequent authors reported demonstration of hydrocephalus and other abnormalities[8–17] using B-mode gray scale contact scanning techniques.

In the past few years it has become apparent that real-time sonographic instruments are excellent for studying the brain in the infant and have the advantage of allowing portable examinations at the bedside. Many recent articles have reported results using a variety of real-time ultrasound equipment.[18-22] Also, in 1979 and 1980[23] results using an automated water-delay ultrasonic scanner were reported to produce good quality scans easily.

At the present time, all three major types of scanning equipment are being used to obtain cranial images in the infant—contact, real-time, and automated water-delay scanners. Technical details concerning these types of scanners and images obtained will be discussed further in Chapters 2 and 6. Images obtained with the presently available equipment rival those seen with CT, particularly in the newborn infant, and sonography of the head has now replaced CT as the primary mode of investigation in the newborn infant.

Research continues in instrumentation and, although sonographic cross-sectional imaging of the adult brain is limited due to absorption of the sound waves by the bony skull, the use of signal processing by computers may someday overcome this major limitation and allow application of sonographic imaging to the brain of adults.

Basic Principles

Sound waves are mechanical oscillations which are transmitted by particles in a gas, liquid, or solid medium.[24] Diagnostic ultrasonography is an imaging modality using high frequency sound waves beyond the audible range of the human ear to visualize structures within the body. The sound waves are produced in the transducer by the piezoelectric effect. Inside the transducer is a crystal which emits a sound wave with a predetermined frequency when a rapidly alternating electric current is applied across the crystal. The sound waves are projected into the patient's body and the returning sound waves or echoes are picked up by the transducer and cause slight mechanical deformation of the crystal and a resulting electrical pulse as a result of the piezoelectric properties of the crystal. Thus, the transducer emits intermittent brief pulses of sound waves alternately with periods of listening for the returning echoes in a ratio of approximately 1:100. The frequencies most commonly used in head scanning are between 2 and 7.5 megahertz (MHz).

There are several methods of detecting and displaying the returning echoes. A-mode, or amplitude modulation, displays the echoes as vertical spikes along the baseline axis with the spike height related to the amplitude of the echo and the baseline representing distance from the transducer face (Fig. 1.1). This display method was the original one developed and has been used extensively for evaluating intracranial structures in the past.

B-mode, or brightness modulation, is by far the most widely used presentation for ultrasound images at the present time, and it displays the echoes as a spot of light of varying intensity on a two-dimensional screen (Fig. 1.2). The larger the returning echo, the brighter the dot. A B-mode scan is produced from a large series of A-scans. The transducer is moved manually in one plane and the echoes of the original A-scan are held on the screen to build up a two-dimensional image. Other means can be found for mechanically or electronically moving the ultrasound beam, but all these systems, the so-called real-time systems, result in formation of B-scan tomograms.

The term "gray scale" refers to the selective amplification of the low level echoes which originate from within soft tissues and the display of these echoes at the expense of larger echoes. Thus these low level parenchymal echoes, or back scatter echoes, can be displayed in shades of gray depending on their intensities. The current equipment distributes the echoes among 16 to 32 possible levels or shades of gray (Fig. 1.2*B*). The advent of gray scale equipment in 1975 enabled the differentiation between different brain tissues such as cerebrum and cerebellum.

Another important development in ultrasound equipment was the digital scan converter available in 1977 and 1978. The scan converter is a memory tube which stores the image as it is being produced. The original analog scan converters had several advantages; however, there was a gradual drift of the focus and gray scale qualities with temperature and time, which resulted in gradual deterioration to an almost bistable quality image.[25] Also, they had a slow writing speed. Digital scan converters have been introduced wich employ digital memory and circuitry, and there is no drift in digital memory so that the problems with focusing, thermal, and aging drift no longer occur. The digital scan converter is also capable of reading and writing at the same time. Since the information is in a digital format it may be manipulated by the operator during signal processing between the transducer and the memory (pre-signal processing) and further operator manipulation of the data can be carried out between the memory and the display (post-signal processing). Thus, the entire field of image enhancement and data manipulation allows the possible extraction of quantitative information.

Acoustical Properties of Tissue

The intensity of the returning echo is determined by the type of tissue being scanned. Biological tissues have a number of different properties which affect the interaction between them and the ultrasound beam. The sound beam is reflected at tissue interfaces according to the difference in acoustic impedance between the two tissues. Acoustic impedance is the product of the velocity of sound in a medium and the density of that medium. The differences in velocity and density between soft tissues are small and therefore produce low level echoes (back scatter echoes) while differences in acoustic impedance between soft tissue and air and between soft tissue and bone are large, producing substantial reflection of the sound beam at these interfaces (specular echoes).

Recently a property of tissue called the bulk modulus of the medium, which refers to its elasticity or its rigidity, has been found to be important in determining the echogenicity of a tissue. It now appears that there are multiple mechanisms whereby echoes are produced from soft tissues and important among these are the presence in the tissue of collagen and fat particles.

The ultrasound beam is partially attenuated by bone because of the strong interface between soft tissue and bone. This has caused problems in scanning the head, since only a small portion of the beam is transmitted through the bone to image the intracranial structures. The infant skull is thinner and contains less organic material, allowing more of the sound beam to be transmitted than in the adult patient. Also, in the infant, the sound beam can be transmitted through the open sutures and fontanelles where there is little attenuation. This allows the transmission and display of the low energy level echoes that arise from the brain tissue. These low level echoes can then be displayed in shades of gray, thus enabling differentiation between the different brain tissues such as cerebrum and cerebellum. Fissures, the falx cerebri, the tentorium cerebelli, and the septum pellucidum are strongly echogenic and produce specular echoes. The impedance mismatch between brain and cerebrospinal fluid allows demonstration of the walls of any intracranial fluids collection such as the ventricles or cysts. Solid masses such as blood clots or shunt tubes can be identified within the ventricles and within other fluid collections.

Summary

Cranial ultrasonography is not a new technique but, in fact, has been in use for 25 years. Initial scans were performed with A-mode equipment, and with the development of B-mode and then gray scale equipment, two-dimensional images of the head could be obtained. Computed tomography of the head became popular about the same time that diagnostic B-mode ultrasonography became available and for several years CT overshadowed ultrasonography for evaluation of the head. Recent advances in B-mode and real-time equipment have caused renewed interest in cranial ultrasonography in infants, and now ultrasonography has become the preferred modality for evaluating the head in this age group.

References

1. Leksell L. Echoencephalography: detection of the intracranial complications following head injury. Acta Chir Scand 1956; 110:301–315.
2. Vleiger M de, Sterke A, De Molin CE, Van der Ven C. Ultrasound for two-dimensional echoencephalography. Ultrasonics 1963; 1:148–151.
3. Brinker RA, Taveras JM. Ultrasound cross-sectional pictures of the head. Acta Radiol (Diagn) (Stockh) 1966; 5:745–753.
4. Makow DM, Real RR. Emersion ultrasonic brain examination with 360 degree scan. Ultrasonics 1965; 3:75–80.
5. Kossoff G, Garrett WJ, Radavanovich G. Ultrasonic atlas of normal brain of infant. Ultrasound Med Biol 1974; 1:259–266.
6. Garrett WJ, Kossoff G, Jones RFC. Ultrasonic cross-sectional visualization of hydrocephalus in infants. Neuroradiology 1975; 8:279–288.
7. Shkolnik A. B-mode scanning of the infant brain. A new approach. Case report. Craniopharyngioma. JCU 1975; 3:229–231.
8. Lees RF, Harrison RB, Sims TL. Gray scale ultrasonography in the evaluation of hydrocephalus and associated abnormalities in infants. Am J Dis Child 1978; 132:376–378.
9. Skolnick ML, Rosenbaum AE, Matzuk T, Guthkelch AN, Heinz ER. Detection of dilated cerebral ventricles in infants. A correlative study between ultrasound and computed tomography. Radiology 1979; 131:447–451.
10. Morgan CL, Trought WS, Rothman SJ, Jiminez JP. Comparison of gray-scale ultrasonography and computed tomography in the evaluation of macrocrania in infants. Radiology 1979; 132:119–123.
11. Johnson ML, Mack LA, Rumack CM, Frost M, Rashbaum C. B-mode echoencephalography in the normal and high risk infant. AJR 1979; 133:375–381.

12. Dewbury KC, Aluwihare APR. The anterior fontanelle as an ultrasound window for study of the brain: a preliminary report. Br J Radiol 1980; 53:81–84.
13. Ben-Ora A, Eddy L, Hatch G, Solida B. The anterior fontanelle as an acoustic window to the neonatal ventricular system. JCU 1980; 8:65–67.
14. Babcock DS, Han BK, LeQuesne GW. B-mode gray scale ultrasound of the head in the newborn and young infant. AJR 1980; 134:457–468.
15. Johnson ML, Rumack CM. Ultrasonic evaluation of the neonatal brain. Radiol Clin North Am 1980; 18:117–131.
16. Mack LA, Rumack CM, Johnson ML. Ultrasound evaluation of cystic intracranial lesions in the neonate. Radiology 1980; 137:451–455.
17. Babcock DS, Han BK. Cranial sonographic findings in meningomyelocele. AJNR 1980; 1: 493–499 and AJR 1981; 136:563–569.
18. London DA, Carroll BA, Enzmann DR. Sonography of ventricular size and germinal matrix hemorrhage in premature infants. AJR 1980; 135:559–564.
19. Grant EG, Schellinger D, Borts FT, McCullough DC, Friedman GR, Sivasubramanian KN, Smith Y. Real-time sonography of the neonatal and infant head. AJNR 1980; 487–492.
20. Edwards MK, Brown DL, Muller J, Grossman CB, Chua GT. Cribside neurosonography: real-time sonography for intracranial investigation of the neonate. AJNR 1980; 1:501–505.
21. Sauerbrei EE, Harrison PB, Ling E, Cooperberg PL. Neonatal intracranial pathology demonstrated by high-frequency linear array ultrasound. JCU 1981; 9:33–36.
22. Babcock DS, Han BK. The accuracy of high resolution real-time ultrasonography of the head in infancy. Radiology 1981; 139:665–676.
23. Haber K, Wachter RD, Christenson PC, Yaucher Y, Sahn DJ, Smith JR. Ultrasonic evaluation of intracranial pathology in infants: a new technique. Radiology 1980; 134:173–178.
24. Ziskin MC. Basic principles and instrumentation. In: *Diagnostic Uses of Ultrasound.* Goldberg BB, Cotler MN, Ziskin MC, Waxham RD (eds). New York: Grune & Stratton, 1975; 1–69.
25. Taylor KJW. Introduction to basic principles, and real-time instrumentation, automated imaging, and pulsed Doppler devices. In: *Manual of Ultrasonography.* Taylor KJW, Jacobson P, Talmont CA, Winters R (eds). New York: Churchill Livingstone, 1980; 1–34.

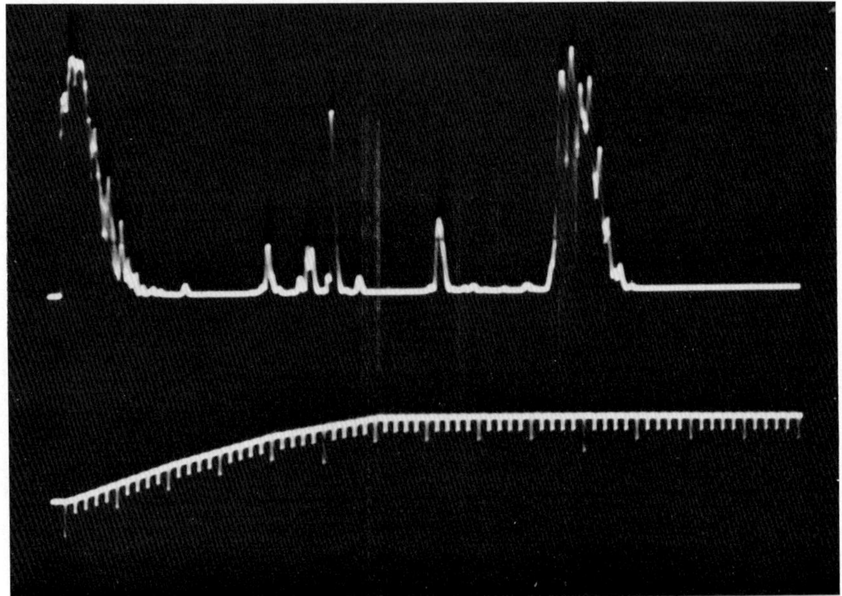

Figure 1.1 A-mode, or amplitude modulation. Each echo displayed as spike; height of spike (*Y* axis) proportional to amplitude of echo. Distance from main bang to spike (*X* axis) porportional to distance from transducer to interface.

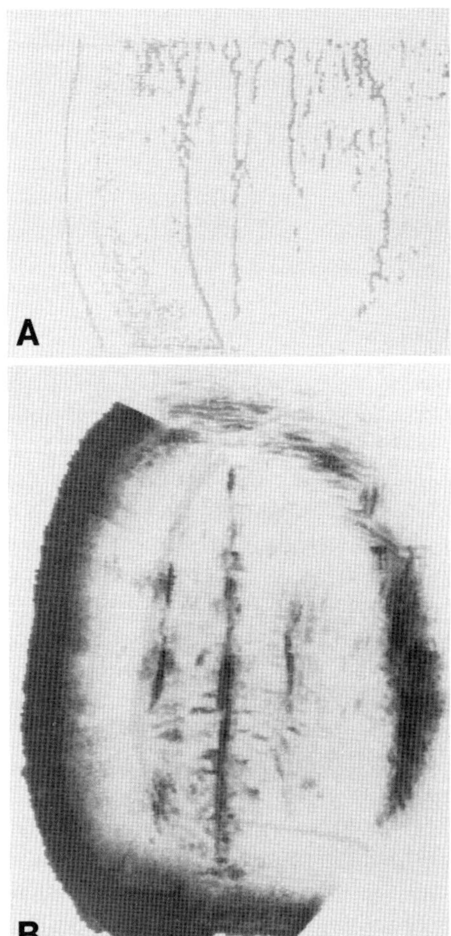

Figure 1.2 B-mode, or brightness modulation. Returning echoes displayed as spot of light of varying intensity on two-dimensional screen. Brightness of dot related to intensity of returning echo. (*A*) Bistable scanning. Echoes at or above threshold displayed as dot. Any echo at or above threshold produces same size and brightness of dot. Final picture has only two shades (black and white). No intermediate gray shade displayed. (*B*) Gray scale scanning. Morphologic details within parenchyma of organs can be displayed in shades of gray depending on their intensities by amplifying low level parenchymal or back scatter echoes.

CHAPTER 2

Instrumentation

Contact Scanners

Three basic types of ultrasound equipment are currently used for head imaging—contact scanners, real-time scanners, and automated water-delay scanners. Contact scanners are now available from several companies and provide excellent images of the infant brain. With contact scanning the transducer (Fig. 2.1) is manually moved over the baby's head, producing the image (Fig. 2.2*A*). Sector scans can be performed through the open sutures and fontanelles where there is little attenuation compared to scanning through the bony skull. Optimal resolution of brain tissue can be obtained with this technique. Digital scan converters now available, provide a constant high quality image and allow for high speed writing of the image. Compared to the other two types of equipment, real-time and water bath delay, it does take the sonographer longer to produce each image and therefore the examinations are longer in duration (about 30 min for the average case). Transducers of varying frequency (Fig. 2.1) are available for these machines and a 5 or 7.5 MHz, 6 mm, short-focused transducer is used for newborns and small infants. The optimal transducer has a small end allowing maximum maneuverability for the sector sweep in the fontanelle. Older infants with larger heads require a lower frequency transducer such as a 3.5 or 5.0 MHz, 13 mm, medium-focused transducer.

The image produced can be recorded either on Polaroid film or on x-ray film using a multiformat camera. We prefer the multiformat camera since the images can be examined on a viewbox as are other radiographic examinations and cameras are available which produce several different size images. In a teaching hospital the multiformat camera with larger pictures is useful when scans are shown in conferences. A camera with a 35 mm slide size format is also useful for making slides for projection for lectures.

The advantages of the contact type scanners include optimal resolution with sector scans through the fontanelle and sutures, and good near-field resolution. Panoramic images of the entire head are obtained (Fig. 2.2, *B* and *C*). Disadvantages include nonportability, longer time necessary for performing an examination, and more technical expertise and experience is required.

Real-Time Scanners

Real-time refers to the dynamic presentation of sequential images, at frame rates of up to 60 per second, which results in a movie of structures as they change position with time. Motion of structures such as pulsating blood vessels can be demonstrated. In real-time the ultrasound beam is moved in space either mechanically or electronically producing automated imaging which is largely independent of the manual skill of the sonographer. Real-time scanning equipment is limited to sector scanners and linear array scanners.

Sector scanners are either mechanical or electronic. With mechanical sectors (Fig. 2.3*A*) a single transducer is moved back and forth or rotates at a high speed and results in a pie-shaped image. The sector arc can be varied from 15° to 90° and at a frame rate of up to 60 per second. This type scanner has been particularly successful in imaging the heart and we have also found it useful for imaging the head. The image is pie-shaped with the apex at the transducer face (Fig. 2.3, *B* and *C*). The widest angle possible (90°) is generally used, so that almost the entire head is viewed on each scan. Sector real-time scanners are preferable to linear array scanners for examining the head because a wide internal axis can be obtained with minimal surface contact on a small fontanelle or suture. Transducers of different frequencies are available and a 5 to 7 MHz medium-focused transducer is used for scanning newborns and small heads, while a 3 MHz transducer is used for older infants when the 5 MHz does not adequately penetrate. Rocking type transducers have the mechanical problem of discomfort produced by the constant oscillation of the rocking transducer on the skin. Rotating transducers (wheel) surmount this problem by smoothly rotating the transducer just off the surface of the skin. We have found that sector scanners are more prone to equipment failure and repairs because of moving parts. Of the different types of real-time scanners now available, the rotating head or wheel type produces the best image by scanning through the fontanelle.

Electronic sector scanners are available in which the electronic beam is steered to an arc or sector scan, and this is achieved rapidly without the limitations imposed by mechanical oscillation of the transducer head. These transducers are known as phased arrays and these systems tend to be more expensive because of the technology involved. The equipment currently available is limited to relatively low frequency transducers (2.25 MHz) and the resolution is decreased compared to the mechanical sector with a 5 MHz transducer.

Linear array real-time equipment (Fig. 2.4*A*) has been successfully utilized in obstetrics and abdominal scanning for the past 5 years. The transducer consists of a block of 64 transducers arranged in a line and fired in series. The size of the transducer varies depending upon the frequency, however, even the smallest high frequency transducer is relatively large measuring about 7 cm in length. The disadvantage of the linear array transducer is that the beam is emitted from a long straight face which forms poor contact with a curved surface such as the infant head and, therefore, a limited sized image is produced by only a small portion of the transducer array (Figs. 2.4 (*B* and

C) and 2.5). The problem may be overcome by a water bath or couplant attached to the transducer and such a device is now being devised.[1] In the past, the resolution has been poor compared to contact scanners; however, the most current equipment has improved resolution and is comparable to sector scanners using similar frequency transducers. Transducers are available in various frequencies from 2.25 to 7 MHz. These scanners are generally less expensive than sector scanners.

The images from the real-time equipment can be recorded on Polaroid film or on x-ray film using a multiformat camera. Scanners with direct video output are available, allowing direct hook-up to the multiformat camera or videotape. Freeze-frame capability is also available thereby eliminating motion artefact. Portable examinations can be recorded first on video tape and then transferred to the multiformat camera and x-ray film, or a multiformat camera can be installed in the cart. Character generators are available for labeling the scans.

The resolution of the new real-time equipment is now adequate for visualizing normal intracranial structures as well as most pathologic conditions, although not as accurate as the articulated arm contact B-scanner or an automated water bath delay scanner. We have noted that near-field artifacts obscure small amounts of fluid in the interhemispheric fissure and therefore extra-axial fluid collections, unless large, could be missed, particularly with the mechanical sector scanner. The resolution in the far-field with this type of equipment falls off as evidenced by larger, more "blobby" echoes. This type of far-field degradation of the image is not seen in images from the contact scanner or the water delay scanning system. In addition, the image produced is an incomplete sector of a portion of the head, and those observers not familiar with the anatomy find the images more difficult to understand.

In many instances the minor decrease in resolution and limited-sized image are outweighed by the advantages of real-time ultrasonography. Since most machines are portable, the machine can be taken to the baby in the intensive care unit and the baby scanned in its Isolette (Fig. 2.3*A*). This is particularly important with unstable premature infants. Real-time scanning is faster and our typical examination with real-time equipment can be performed in 10–15 min, while an exam with similar views obtained using a contact scanner requires 30 min of scanning time. The transducer is easily manipulated so that views in unusual angles can be easily obtained with real-time equipment. An additional advantage is the lower cost of real-time ultrasound equipment compared to the contact and automatic water-delay scanners (except for the phased array type). In our experience, producing a diagnostic scan with real-time equipment requires less technical experience and expertise than does contact scanning. These combined considerations make the newer real-time equipment more universally applicable especially for institutions where this type of examination is not frequently performed.

Mechanized Water-Delay Scanners

This type scanner in current use employs multiple 2.9 MHz transducers in a curved linear array which are mechanically sectored in unison either automatically or manually by remote control. The array can be positioned anywhere within the water bath to obtain the desired anatomical section, while the patient lies on a plastic membrane covering the water tank[2] (Fig. 2.6*A*). This technique has advantages in that generally infants and small children are lulled to sleep on the warm water bed and require no sedation. The images are obtained rapidly, thus decreasing scanning time. Panoramic images of the entire head comparable to CT images are obtained (Fig. 2.6*B*). The images shown are good; however, the resolution is somewhat less than that possible with contact scanners using high frequency transducers, probably because of the relatively low frequency of the transducers (2.9 MHz) and scanning through the bony skull.

Newer models with higher frequency transducers may have improved resolution. For some views, coronal and sagittal especially, the infant must be suspended head down which may be difficult and dangerous for very sick infants. The equipment is significantly more expensive than other types of ultrasound equipment and the water bath makes it a physically large piece of equipment. This type of scanner will be discussed further in Chapter 6.

Summary

The field of ultrasonic instrumentation is changing rapidly, and recommendations concerning equipment now available will be rapidly outdated. At present, contact scanners produce images with the best resolution, but require the most technical expertise. Real-time scanners provide adequate images rapidly with less expertise necessary. We have found that sector scanners allow good contact with the baby's curved head and good quality images by scanning through the open fontanelle and sutures. We feel that an active pediatric ultrasound service requires both types of scanners.

References

1. Smith WL, Franklin TD, Katakura K, Patrick JT, Fry FJ, Eggleton RC. A simple device to couple linear array transducers to neonate heads for ultrasonic scanning of the brain. Radiology 1980; 137:838–839.
2. Haber K, Wachter RD, Christenson PC, Yaucher Y, Sahn DJ, Smith JR. Ultrasonic evaluation of intracranial pathology in infants: a new technique. Radiology 1980; 134:173–178.

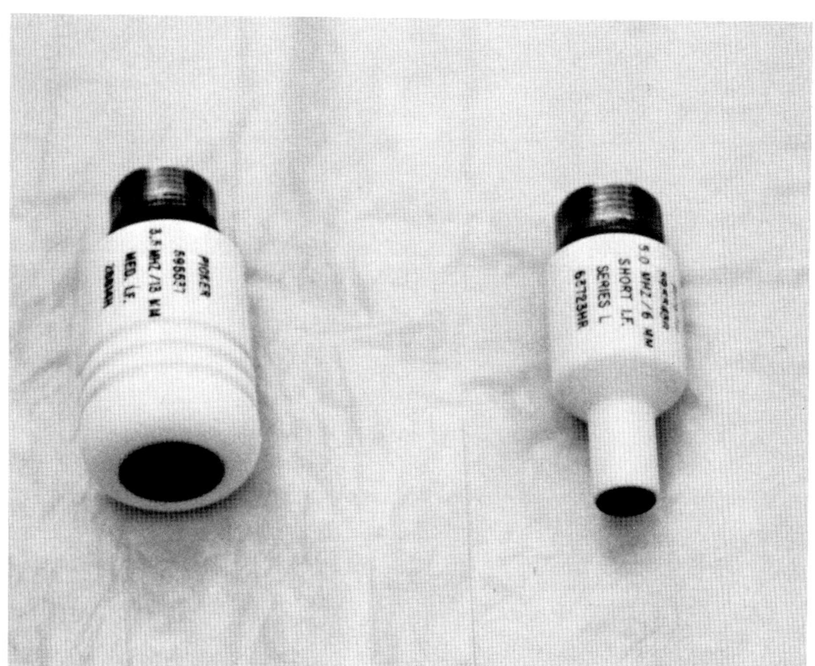

Figure 2.1 Transducers of different frequency. The 5.0 MHz 6 mm short-focused transducer (*right*) is used for newborns and small infants. Small transducer end allows maximum maneuverability for sector sweep in fontanelle. A 3.5 MH 13 mm, medium-focused transducer (*left*) is used for older infants with larger heads.

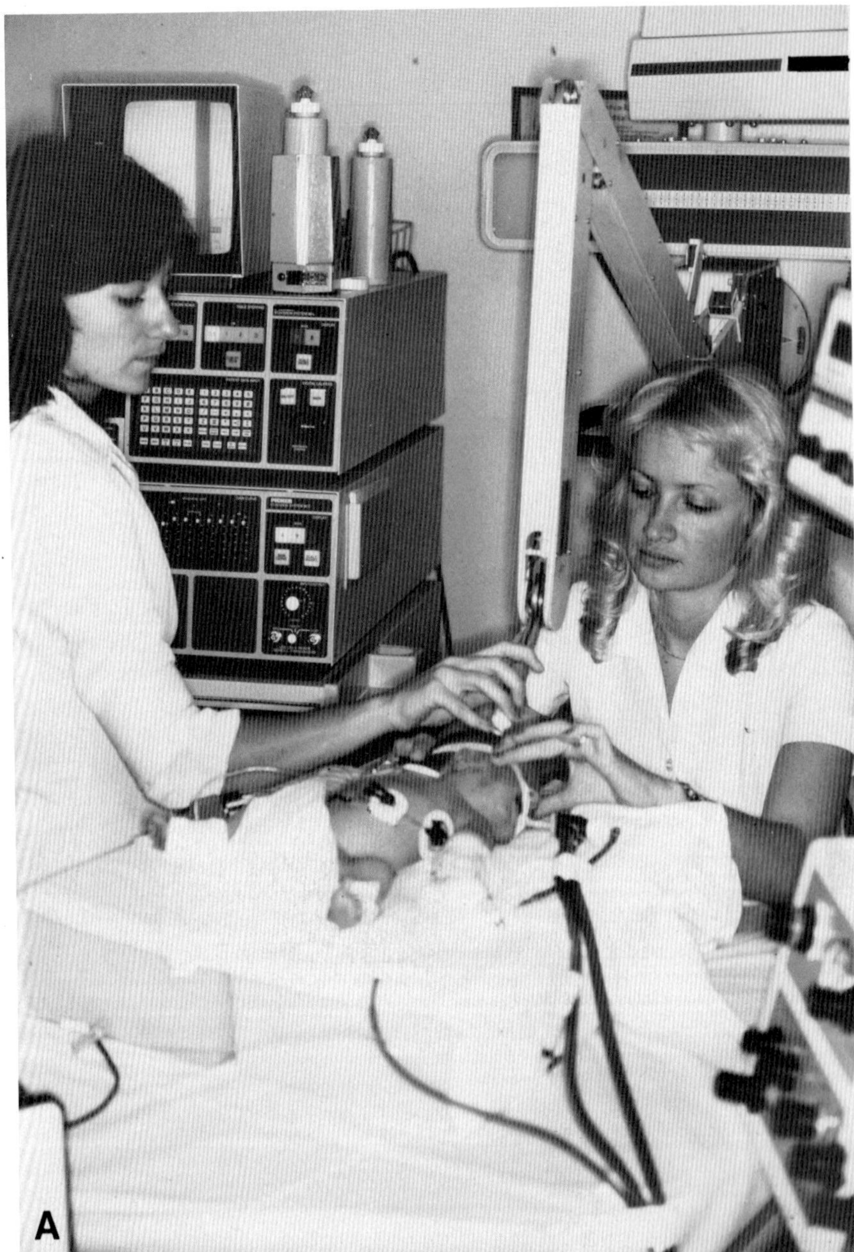

Figure 2.2 Contact scanner. (*A*) Sonographer scanning baby's head with contact scanner. Transducer manually moved over baby's head producing image. Sector scans performed through open sutures and fontanelles. (*B*) Axial and (*C*) coronal images produced showing excellent image of infant brain with moderate hydrocephalus. Good resolution with optimal near-field visualization. Panoramic images of entire head obtained.

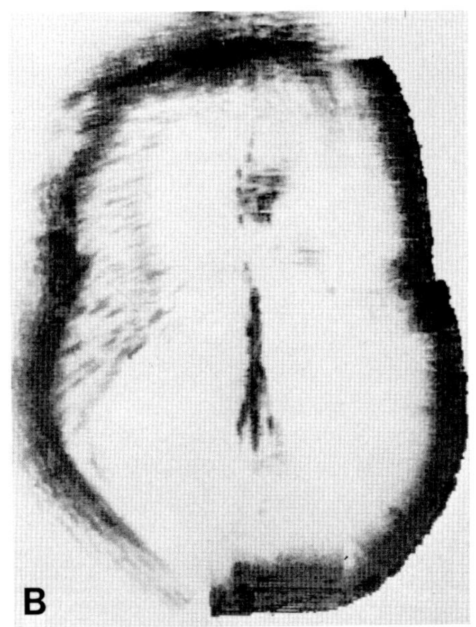
B

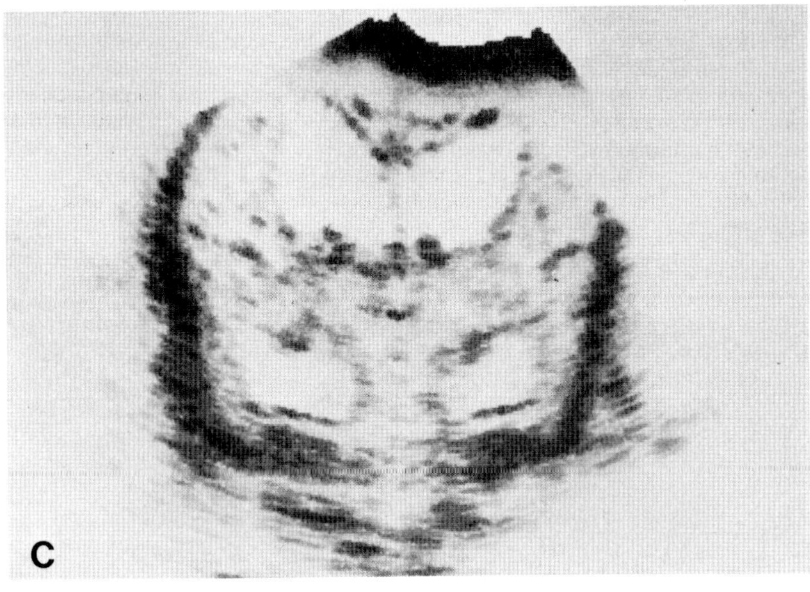
C

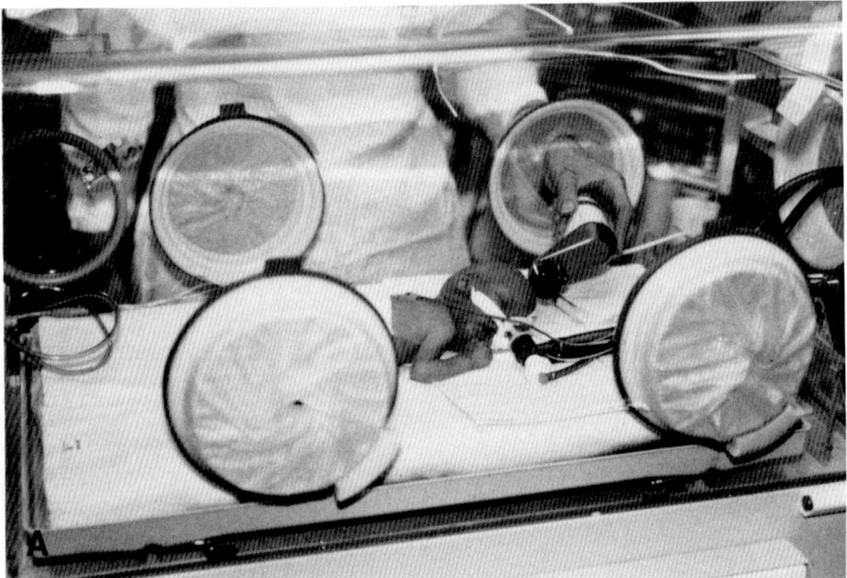

Figure 2.3 Real-time sector scanner. (*A*) Sonographer scanning baby in Isolette with real-time sector scanner. With mechanical sector scanner, single transducer moved back and forth or rotated at high speed producing pie-shaped image. (*B*) Axial and (*C*) coronal images produced showing good image of infant head with moderate hydrocephalus. Near-field artifacts obscure anatomy, slight degradation of image in far-field evidenced by large, more blobby dots, and limited size image are disadvantages; however, overall resolution adequate for imaging head.

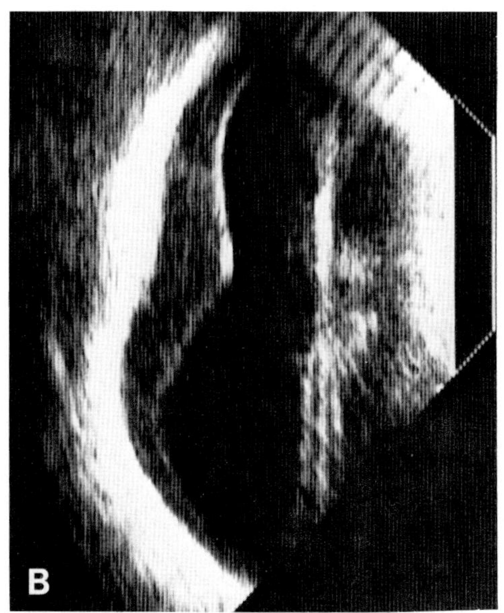
B

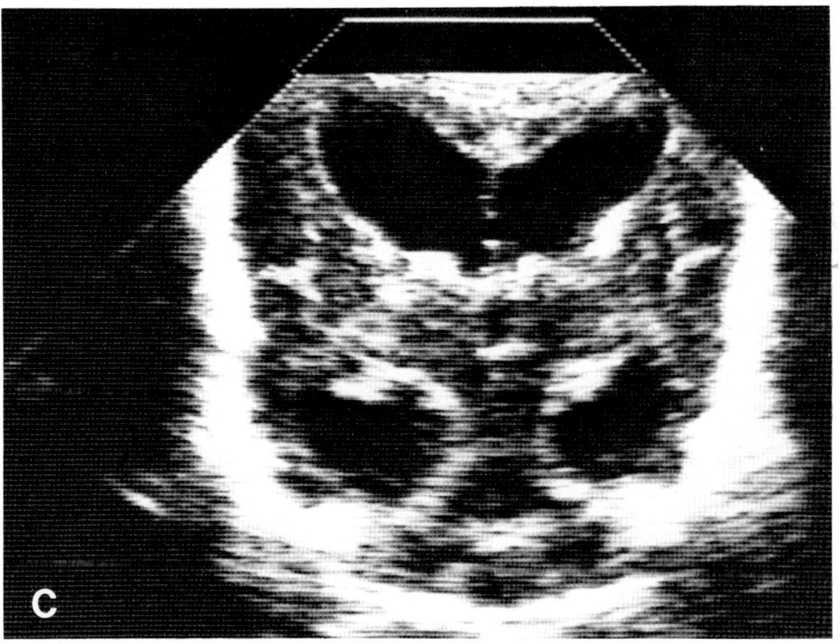
C

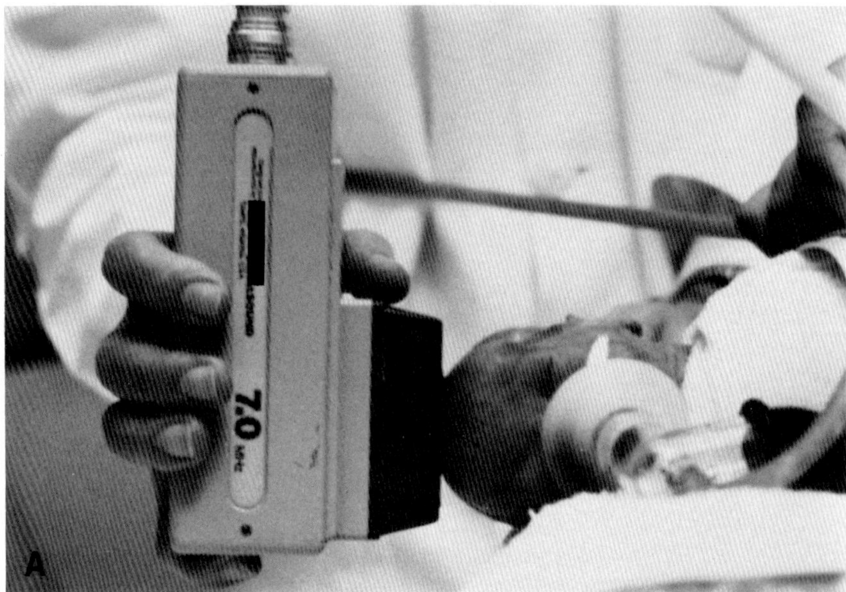

Figure 2.4 Linear array real-time scanner. (*A*) Sonographer scanning baby's head with linear array real-time scanner. Transducer relatively large and consists of block of 64 transducers arrayed in line and fired in series producing rectangular image. (*B*) Axial and (*C*) coronal, images of limited size produced by only small portion of transducer array. Near-field artifacts obscure anatomy. (Courtesy of David Martin, M.D., Toronto, Ontario.)

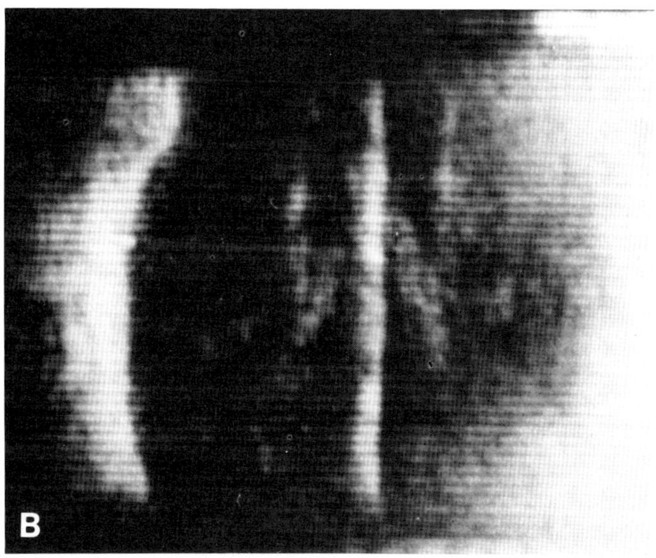

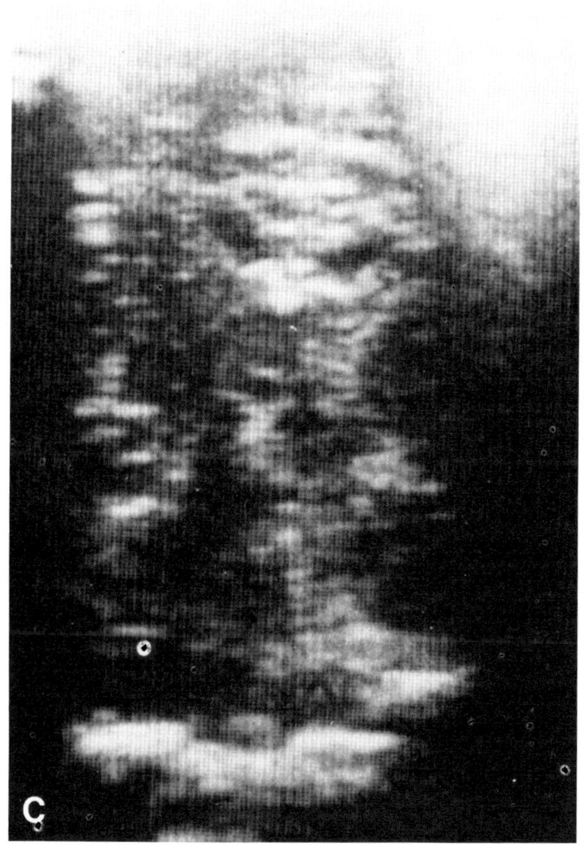

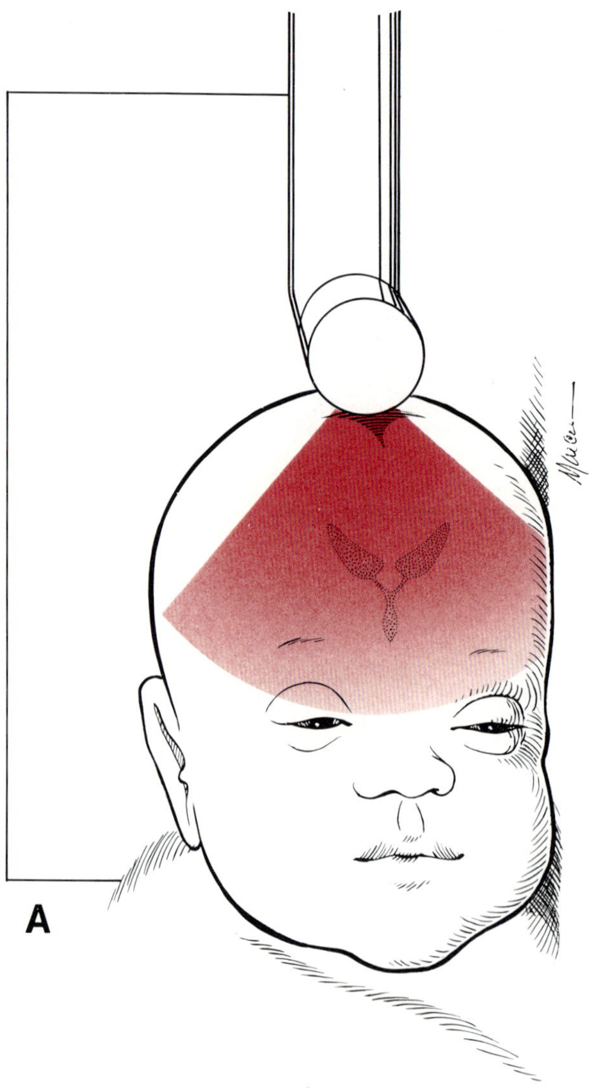

Figure 2.5 Scan plane—sector vs. linear array real-time. (*A*) Sector scanner produces pie-shaped image with apex at transducer face. With widest angle (90°), almost entire head viewed on each scan. (*B*) Linear array scanner produces rectangular image. Only small portion of center of head imaged on each scan.

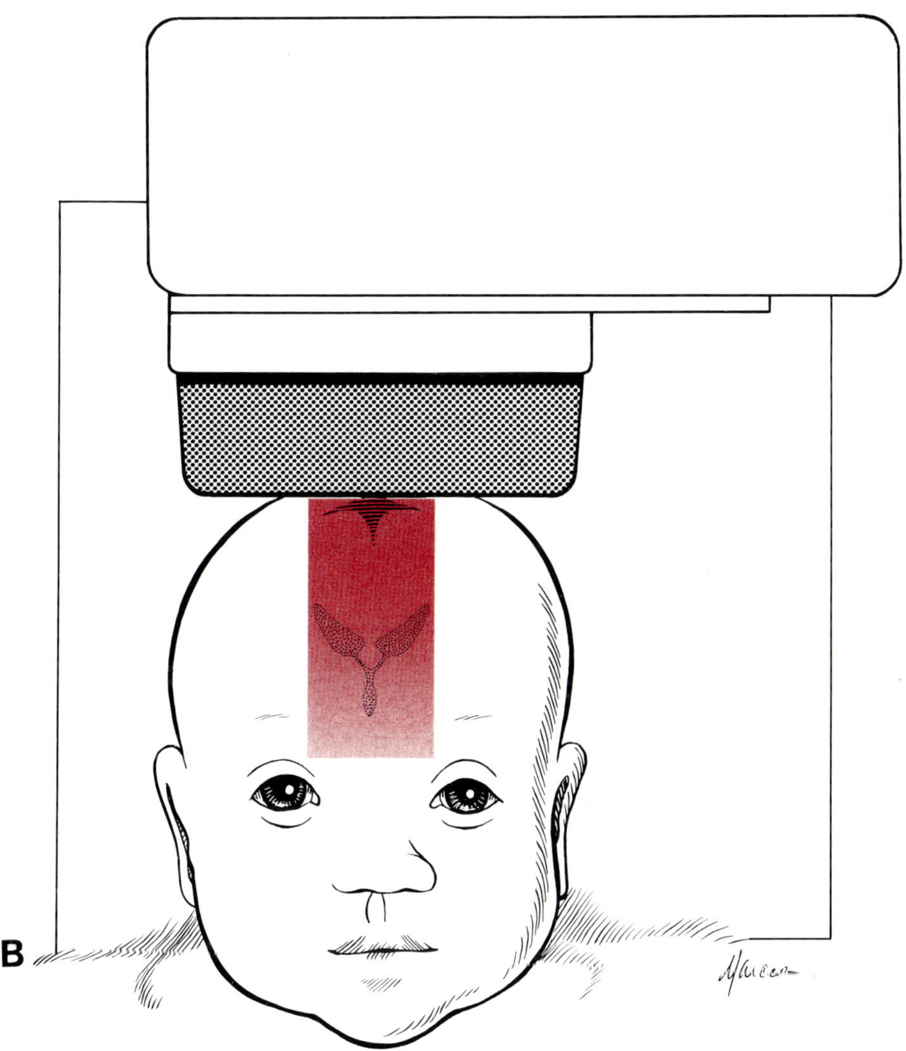
B

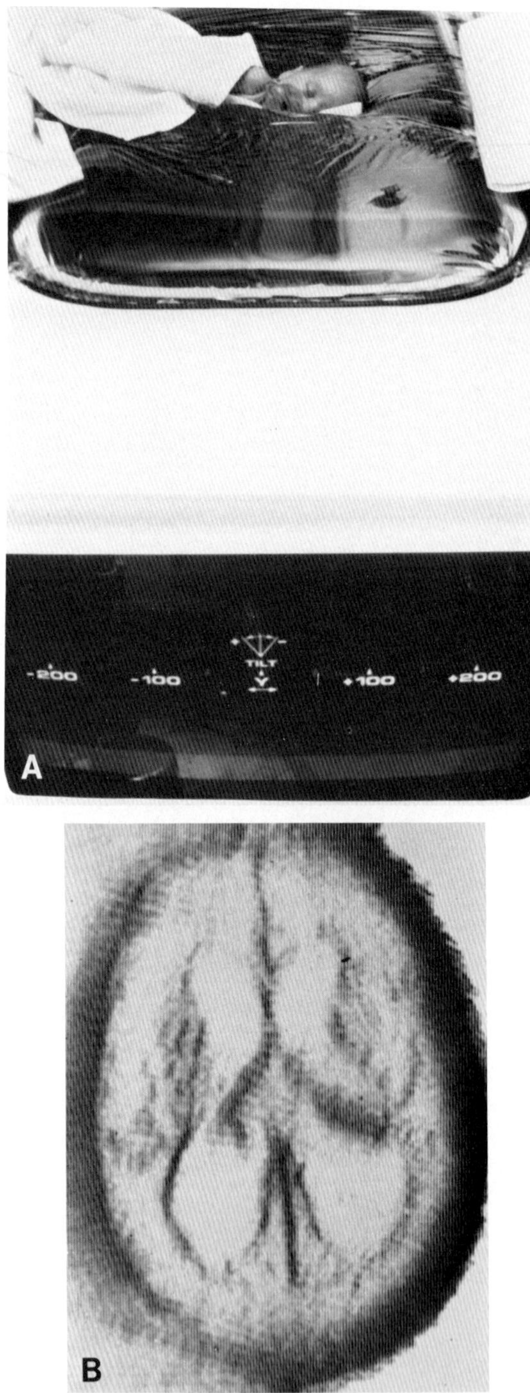

Figure 2.6 Mechanized water delay scanner. (*A*) Baby lying on plastic membrane covering warmed water tank in which multiple 2.9 MHz trandsucers are placed in curved linear array and mechanically sectored in unison either automatically or manually by remote control. Array can be positioned anywhere within water bath to obtain desired anatomic section. (*B*) Axial image produced with mechanized water delay scanner. Panoramic image of entire head possible and comparable to CT image. (Courtesy of Kai Haber, M.D., Tucson, Arizona.)

CHAPTER 3

Scanning Techniques

General Comments

Since the image is obtained by scanning through openings in the bony skull, technically adequate examinations of the head are possible only in children with open sutures and fontanelles, that is, under the age of about 2 years, or in older infants with split sutures. Older patients with craniotomy defects can also be examined with this technique. We have found that long or thick hair occasionally interferes with scanning contact and can cause inadequate examinations.

Indications for head ultrasonography in infants include: increased head size, seizures, abnormal neurological examination, apnea, screening of premature infants at risk for intracranial hemorrhage, meningitis not responding to therapy, congenital anomalies associated with known brain anomalies such as patients with meningomyelocele or facial cleft defects, and trauma.

Immobilization

The child under the age of 2 months rarely needs sedation. The infant is immobilized by wrapping him in a sheet, placing a sandbag on the legs, and providing the infant with a pacifier or feeding during the examination (Fig. 3.1). Also, feeding the infant immediately prior to the examination often induces sleep. Providing a darkened and quiet environment and stroking the infant is helpful.

During the examination a helper should physically hold the infant's head in place thereby maintaining the correct positioning for the various views (Fig. 3.1).

Sedation

Immobilization alone does not usually suffice in infants over 2 months of age and sedation is used. Infants with meningitis or increased intracranial pressure have been noted to be particularly irritable and sometimes difficult to sedate. We routinely use chloral hydrate in an oral dose of 50 mg/kg. The sedation is given in the ultrasound room rather than on the floor, since we have found inadequate doses are sometimes given and timing can be critical. Adequate sedation occurs in 15–45 min and lasts about 1 hr. If sedation is given on the floor, timing may be wrong and the infant is awakened during transport to the radiology department. Occasional patients, particularly with liver disease, do not respond to chloral hydrate, and Nembutal in an intramuscular dose of 6 mg/kg for children up to 15 kg can be used. The child is monitored and observed throughout the sedation by our radiology department nurse. Chloral hydrate has a relatively low incidence of complications even in very ill patients and does not depress the respiratory system. We have had no complications to date using this sedation.

Room Preparation

Maintaining an infant's normal body temperature is very important. Premature infants are particularly unstable, and our room is equipped with an overhead servo-control radiant heater (Solaroid Electric Infrared Heater, Aitken Products Inc., Geneva, Ohio, and Proportional Temperature Controller, Yellow Springs Instrument Co., Yellow Springs, Ohio). The infant's body temperature is monitored with a skin probe and the heater turns on and off automatically to maintain the temperature at a preset level (Fig. 3.2). The ultrasound room is also equipped with air, suction, and oxygen outlets so that critical life support measures can be maintained, including a respirator. The room is also equipped with an alarm button which can be rung if additional help is necessary for resuscitation of a patient. Babies who are clinically unstable or on respirators are not transported to the radiology department, but are examined in the nursery or intensive care unit with our portable real-time equipment.

General Scanning Technique

The baby is positioned either supine or prone with its head turned to the side in a lateral position. Placing the baby on a foam sponge so that the head is up off the table provides improved access for sector scans through the fontanelles and sagittal suture (Fig. 3.1). Aqueous gel is used as the couplant and is warmed in a commercially available gel warmer. Mineral oil can be used, but tends to run down onto the baby's face. After the examination the gel is washed from the hair using baby shampoo.

Scanning Planes

A series of scans is performed at 5-mm intervals across the entire head in several planes (Fig. 3.3). An axial series is performed parallel to a line 10° from the canthomeatal line and is comparable to the usual CT brain scan images. Scans are performed at 5-mm intervals starting at a level 1 cm above the external auditory meatus and working toward the top of the head (Fig. 3.4). Coronal and modified coronal series are performed at angles 90° and 60°, respectively, from the canthomeatal line and often produce our best images. These scans are performed at 5-mm intervals starting as anterior as we can make contact in the anterior fontanelle and working posteriorly scanning through the fontanelle and sagittal suture (Fig. 3.5).

A posterior fossa (150°) series perpendicular to the clivus is performed in selected cases in which posterior fossa abnormalities or a dilated fourth ventricle are suspected (Fig. 3.6). A sagittal series is performed by scanning through the anterior funtanelle in the midline and through each lateral ventricle by angling the transducer to the left and right (Fig. 3.7). A routine examination includes axial, coronal, and sagittal views. The sagittal views are difficult to obtain with a contact scanner and a real-time scanner is usually used.

Machine Set-up and Contact Scanning Techniques

Newborn—Coronal. For a newborn infant a 5 MHz, 6 mm, short internal focus transducer is used (Fig. 3.8). The casing on the transducer should be thin to improve maneuverability in the fontanelle. The time-gain-compensation (TGC) curve is set with a mild slope (3 dB) from 0 to 6 cm depth (Fig. 3.9). The overall gain is set at 51 on our machine, but this may vary depending on the type of equipment. The overall gain and slope are adjusted until the echoes are homogeneous throughout the brain. Coronal and modified coronal images are made by a sector sweep through the anterior fontanelle or sagittal suture (see Figs. 3.10 (*A* and *C*) and 3.11*A*). If the entire brain is not imaged the transducer is moved across the head toward the baseline, thus filling in the outline of the skull (Figs. 3.10 (*B* and *C*) and 3.11*B*).

Newborn—Axial. For axial scans a slightly higher overall gain is necessary (60) and the TGC curve is adjusted with a slightly greater slope from 0 to 6 cm depth (3–3.5 dB) (Fig. 3.12). Axial scans are performed using a compounding technique. The transducer is moved over the parietal, frontal, and occipital bones which are up. As windows such as the coronal and lambdoid sutures are encountered, sector sweeps are made through these areas to fill in portions of the brain (Figs. 3.13–3.15).

Infant—Coronal. With infants 1 months of age and older a 3.5 MHz, 13 mm, medium internal focus transducer is used, particularly on the axial scans (Fig. 3.8). For coronal scans again the TGC curve is set with a slight curve (3 dB) from 0 to 6 cm depth. The overall gain is adjusted until the desired number of echoes are seen within the brain (51 dB overall gain on our machine). On older infants with small fontanelles and sutures a single sector sweep through the fontanelle will give only a narrow angle sweep so that compounding technique is used on this view (Figs. 3.10 and 3.11). Often in older infants a coronal series will be obtained both with the 5 and the 3.5 MHz transducers since the 3.5 MHz visualizes the deeper structures such as the ventricles, and the 5 mHz visualizes the near field structures such as the interhemispheric fissure (Fig. 3.16).

Infant—Axial. Axial scans are performed on older infants using the compounding technique described above (Figs. 3.13–3.15). Again the TGC curve is adjusted with a dB slope from 0 to 6 cm depth. The overall gain with the 3.5 MHz for older infants is almost maximum at 57 dB.

Posterior Fossa. Scans are performed using the same machine settings as for axial scans. A compounding technique is used, and as the transducer is moved over the occipital and posterior temporal bones, sector sweeps are made through windows such as the lambdoid sutures and posterior fontanelle (Fig. 3.17).

Each image is labeled as to view—axial, etc., right or left, and anterior and posterior. The patient's name, date, the transducer used, and the overall gain are also labeled on each scan.

Real-Time Scanning Techniques

For newborn infants a 5 MHz medium-focused transducer is used. The TGC curve is set relatively flat on the real-time unit and the overall gain adjusted as necessary and is usually at the maximum with the 5 MHz transducer. A 3.0 MHz transducer is used on older infants and frequently even on newborn infants for the axial view.

Coronal. The coronal series is performed by scanning through the anterior fontanelle (Figs. 3.18 and 3.19). Scans are made starting anteriorly and working posteriorly, however rather than moving the transducer at 5-mm intervals as with contact scanning, the tranducer is angled to the back of the head for the more posterior scans. Thus, the more anterior pictures are 90° coronals while the more posterior pictures are 60° coronals.

Sagittal. Sagittal scans are easily obtained with the sector real-time transducer by scanning through the anterior fontanelle (Fig. 3.20). A midline scan is obtained to demonstrate the third and fourth ventricles (Fig. 3.20, *A* and *B*). By angling the transducer to right and left the lateral ventricles can be imaged (Fig. 3.20*C*).

Axial. Axial views (Figs. 3.21 and 3.22) are obtained by scanning through the parietal bone at various levels from the external auditory meatus as described for contact scanning. Frequently even in newborn infants a 3.0 MHz transducer is used to penetrate the bone on this view.

For recording images with the portable machine the videotape is set to record throughout the procedure. When appropriate images are obtained they are frozen on the screen for a few seconds. A foot switch connected to the freeze frame facilitates this and allows the procedure to be performed by one sonographer. After the examination the machine is returned to the ultrasound department, and the videotape recorder is hooked up to the multiformat camera. The videotape is replayed, and hard copy images are made of the frozen images. The videotape recording can then either be kept for permanent copy or erased and reused. Recently, small cameras are available that fit on the cart, and the permanent films may be exposed as the examination is performed. As a result of this process we have a hard copy image on x-ray film for the patient's file.

Summary

Performing ultrasonography on infants requires special attention to immobilization or sedation, and to the maintenance of the normal body temperature. These problems can be overcome by having the proper equipment and personnel available at the time of the examination. Our routine examination includes a series of scans in axial, coronal, and sagittal planes. If both a contact and real-time machine are available, a routine examination includes contact axial and coronal scans and real-time coronal and sagittal scans. Posterior fossa and modified coronal views are obtained in occasional cases, especially those with posterior fossa pathology.

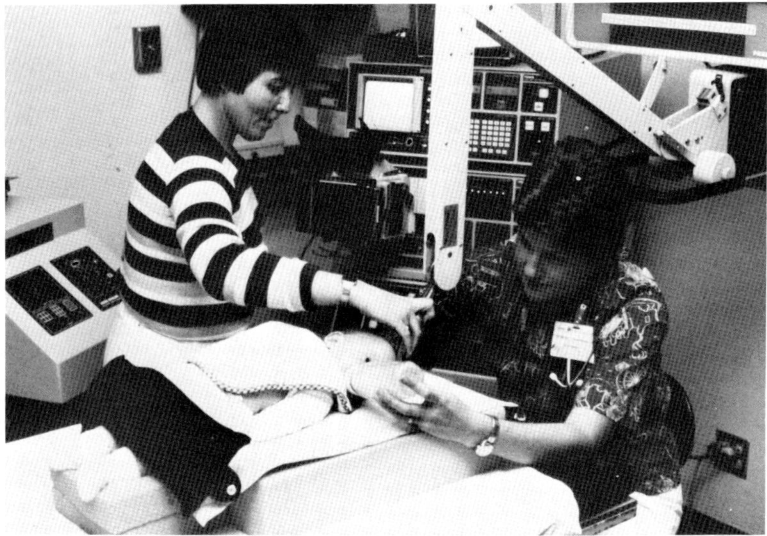

Figure 3.1 Immobilization. Infant immobilized by wrapping him in sheet and placing sandbag on legs. Department nurse holds infant's head in place and feeds during examination.

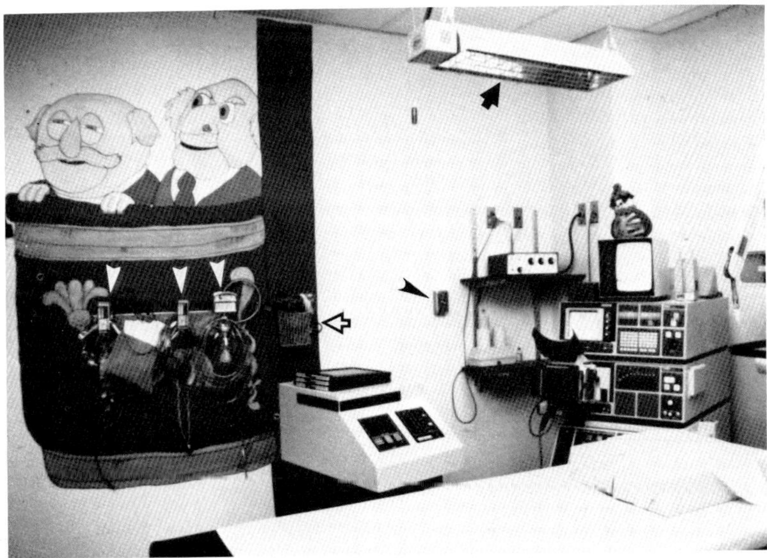

Figure 3.2 Ultrasound scanning room. Room equipped with servo-control radiant heater suspended over table (*arrow*), air, suction, and oxygen outlets (*white arrowheads*), emergency alarm button (*black arrowhead*), and blood pressure cuff (*open arrow*). Decorations and toys make room less frightening for older infants and children.

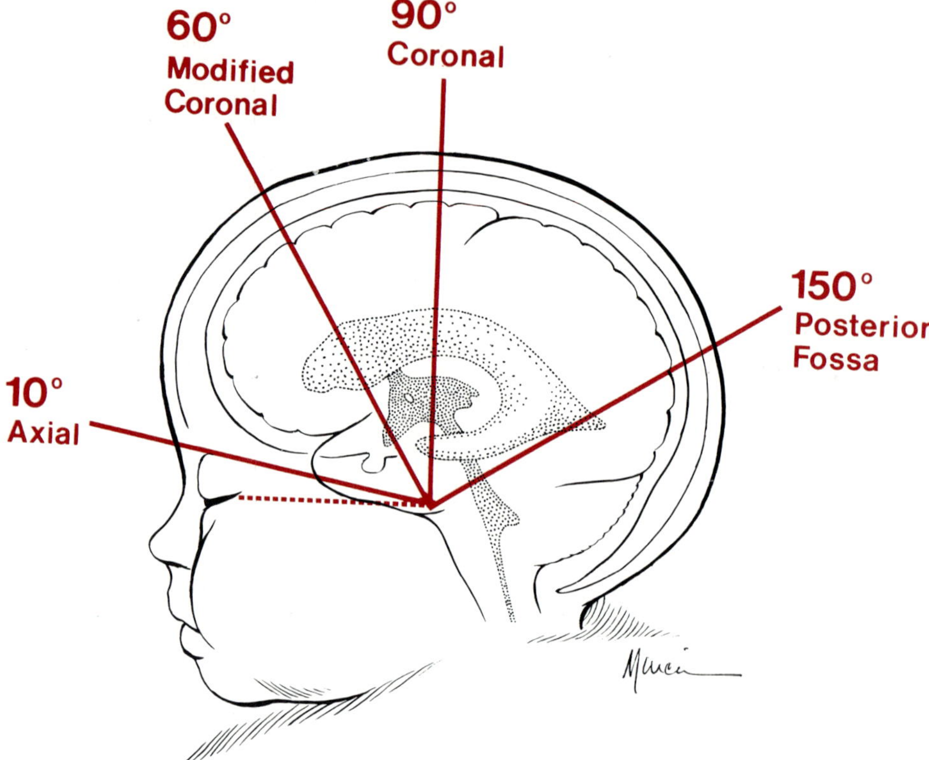

Figure 3.3 Scanning angles. Scanning angle for axial scan—10° from canthomeatal line (*dotted line*). Scanning angles for coronal and modified coronal scans—90° and 60°, respectively, from canthomeatal line. Posterior fossa scanning angle—150° from canthomeatal line and perpendicular to clivus.

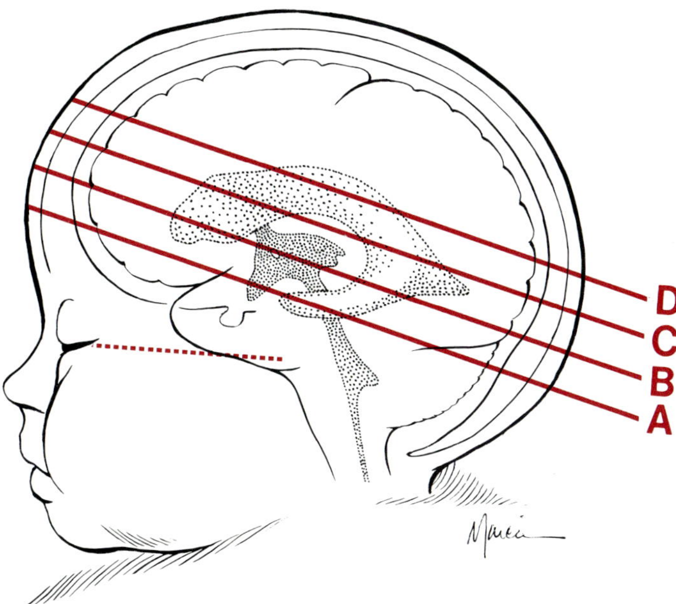

Figure 3.4 Axial scan planes. Axial planes parallel to line 10° from canthomeatal line and comparable to usual CT brain scan images. Scans performed at 5-mm intervals starting at level 1 cm above external auditory meatus and working toward top of head.

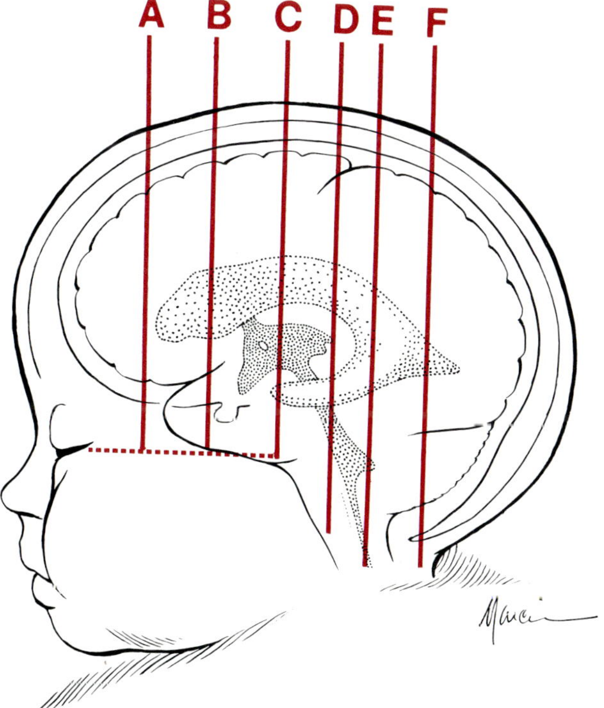

Figure 3.5 Coronal scan planes. Coronal planes at angles 90° from canthomeatal line (*dotted line*). Scans performed at 5-mm intervals starting as far anterior as can make contact in anterior fontanelle and working posteriorly, scanning through anterior fontanelle and sagittal suture.

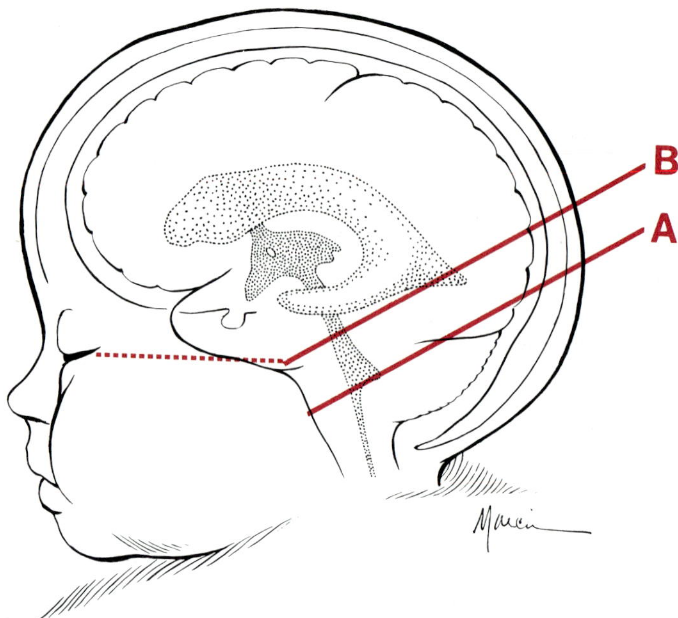

Figure 3.6 Posterior fossa scan planes. Posterior fossa planes at 150° from canthomeatal line (*dotted line*). Scans performed at 5-mm intervals as low as can make contact in posterior fontanelle and working superiorly.

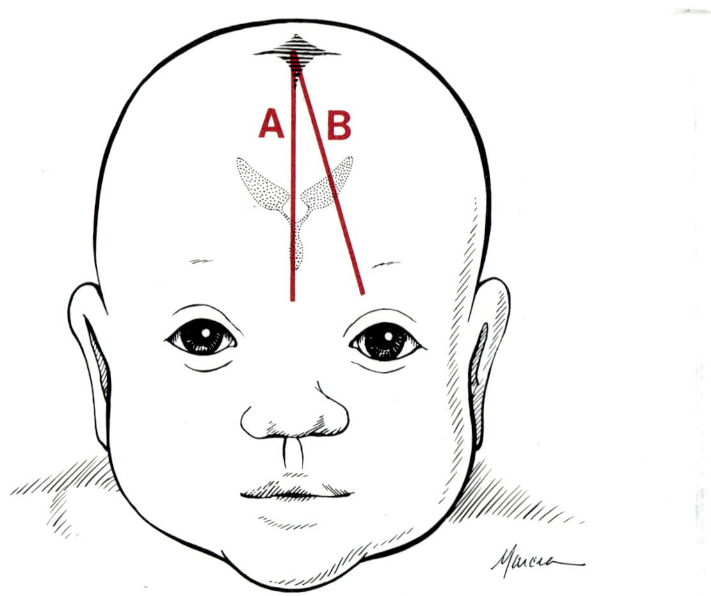

Figure 3.7 Sagittal scan planes through midline (*A*) and through axis of lateral ventricle (*B*) by angling anteromedial to posterolateral.

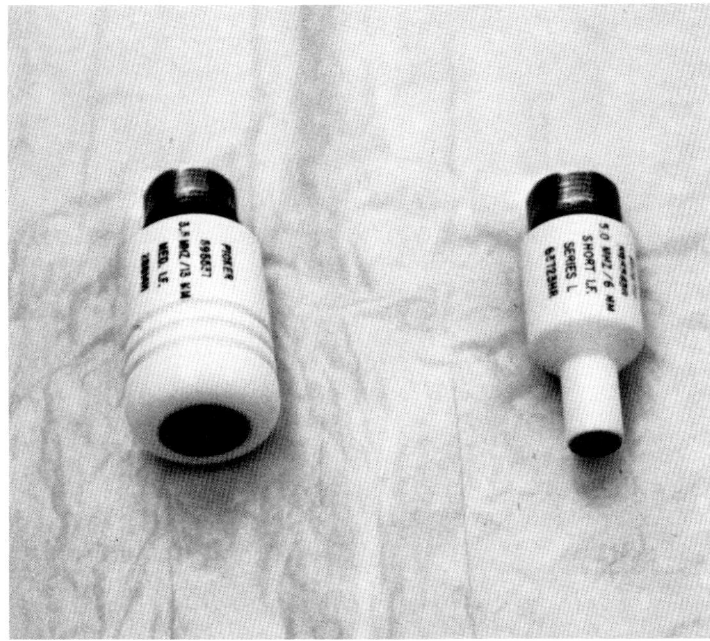

Figure 3.8 Transducers of different frequencies. A 5 MHz, 6 mm, short internal focus transducer (*right*) is used for newborn infants. Small transducer end allows maximum maneuverability for sector sweep in fontanelle. The 3.5 MHz, 13 mm, medium-focus transducer (*left*) used for older infants with larger heads.

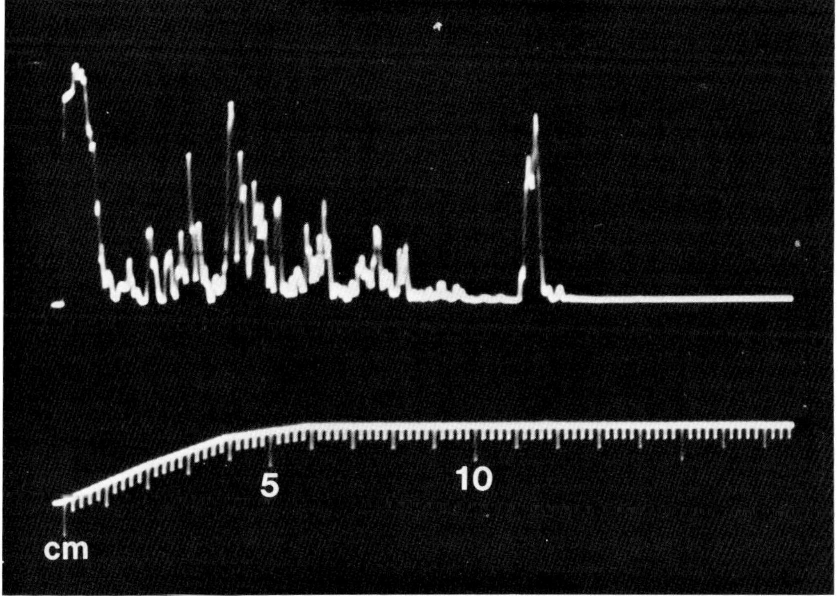

Figure 3.9 A-mode newborn coronal scan. TGC curve set with mild slope (3 dB) from 0 to 6 cm depth. Overall gain varies depending on type of equipment. Overall gain and TGC curve then adjusted until homogeneous echoes throughout brain.

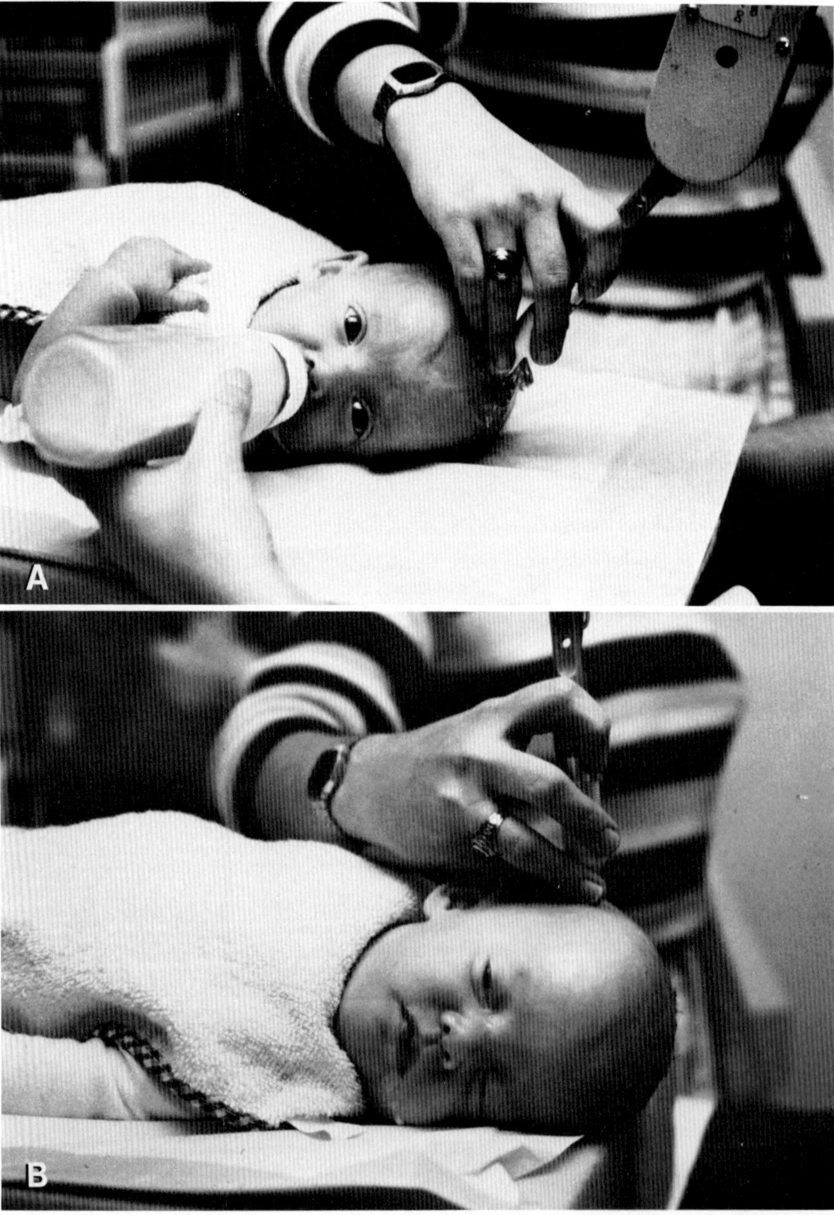

Figure 3.10 Coronal view—scanning technique. Sonographer makes single-sweep, sector scan through anterior fontanelle or sagittal suture (*A*). If necessary, outline of head then filled in by scanning over convexity and side of head (*B*). See diagram (*C*) on facing page.

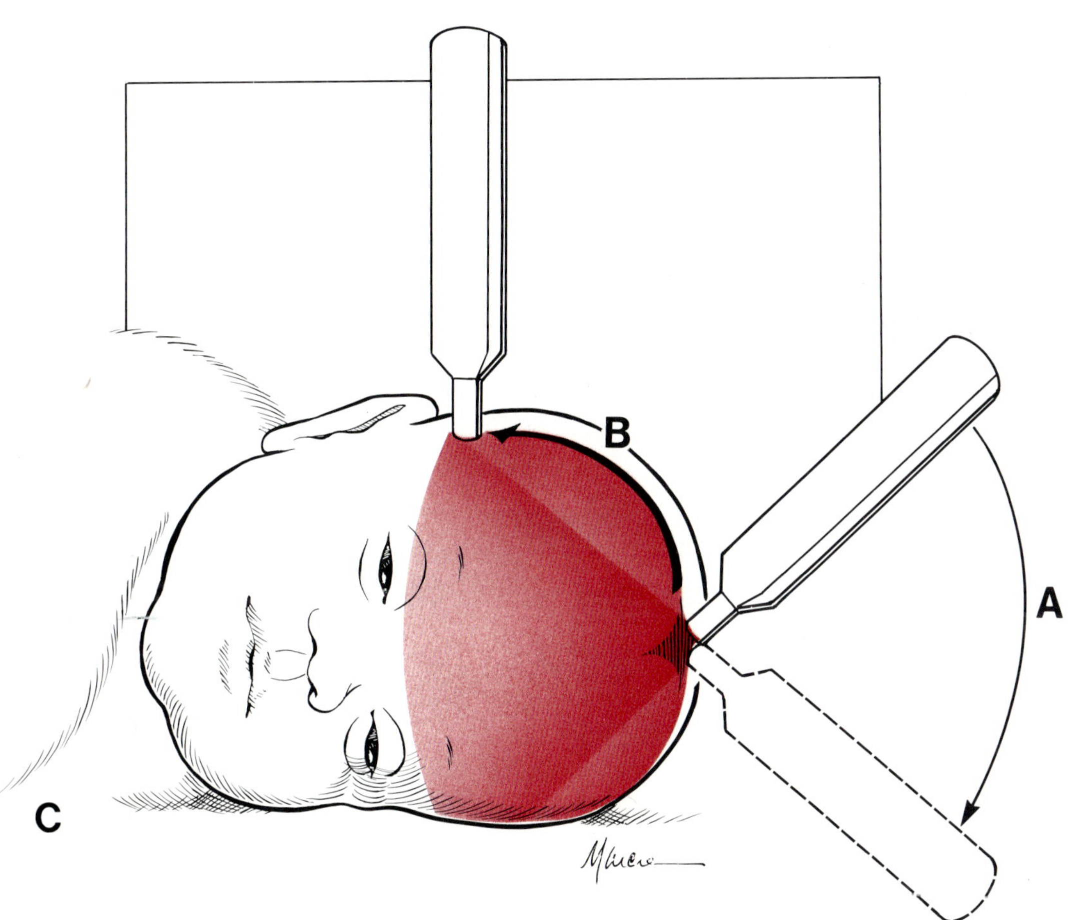
B
A
C

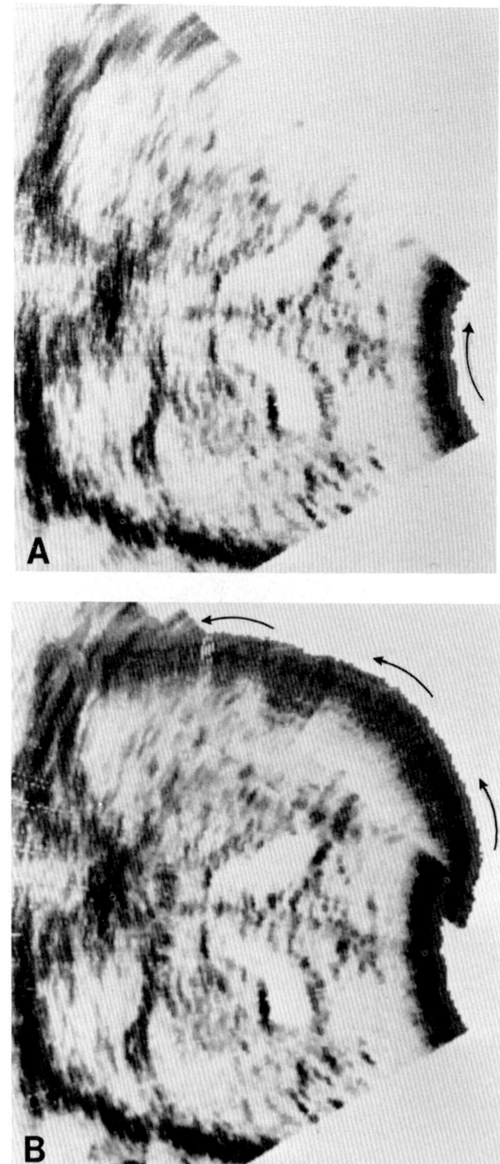

Figure 3.11 Coronal scans produced by these scanning motions. Sector (*A*) and compound (*B*) scans.

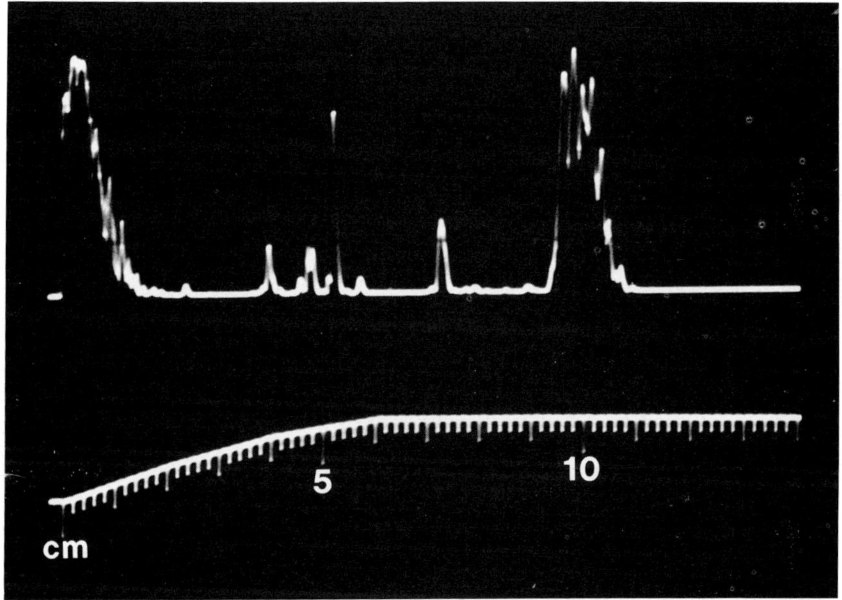

Figure 3.12 A-mode newborn axial scan. TGC curve adjusted with slightly greater slope from 0 to 6 cm depth (3–3.5 dB). Slightly higher overall gain sometimes necessary for axial scan.

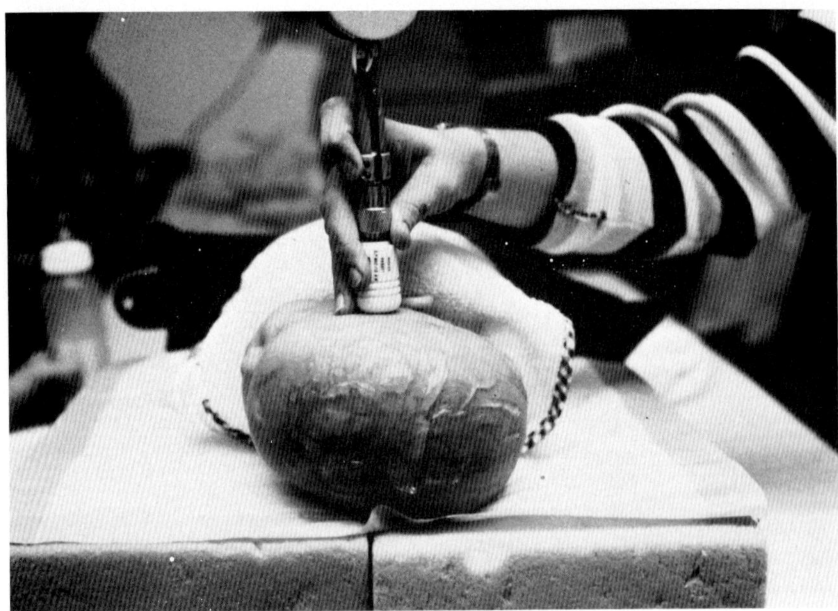

Figure 3.13 Axial view—baby being scanned. Sonographer scans over parietal, frontal, and occipital areas using compounding technique.

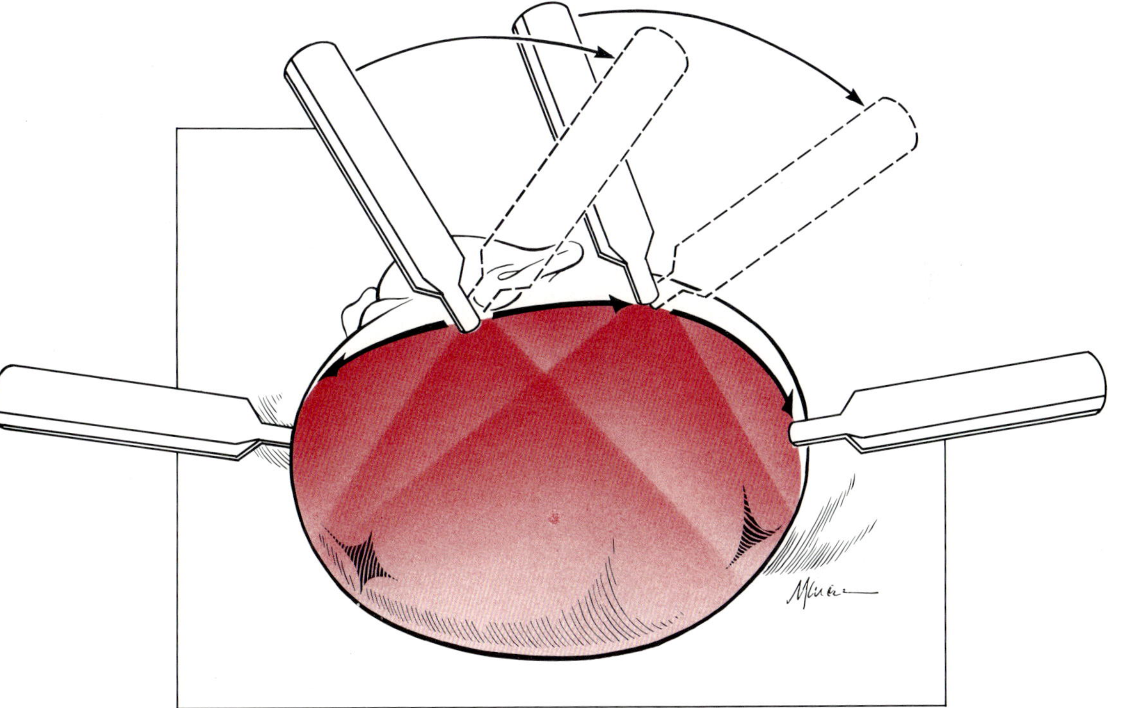

Figure 3.14 Axial scanning technique. Image first obtained by scanning over side of head using compounding technique. As encounter windows such as coronal and lambdoid sutures, sector sweeps made through these areas. If necessary, anterior and posterior portions of outline of head then filled in by continuous scanning over frontal and occipital bones.

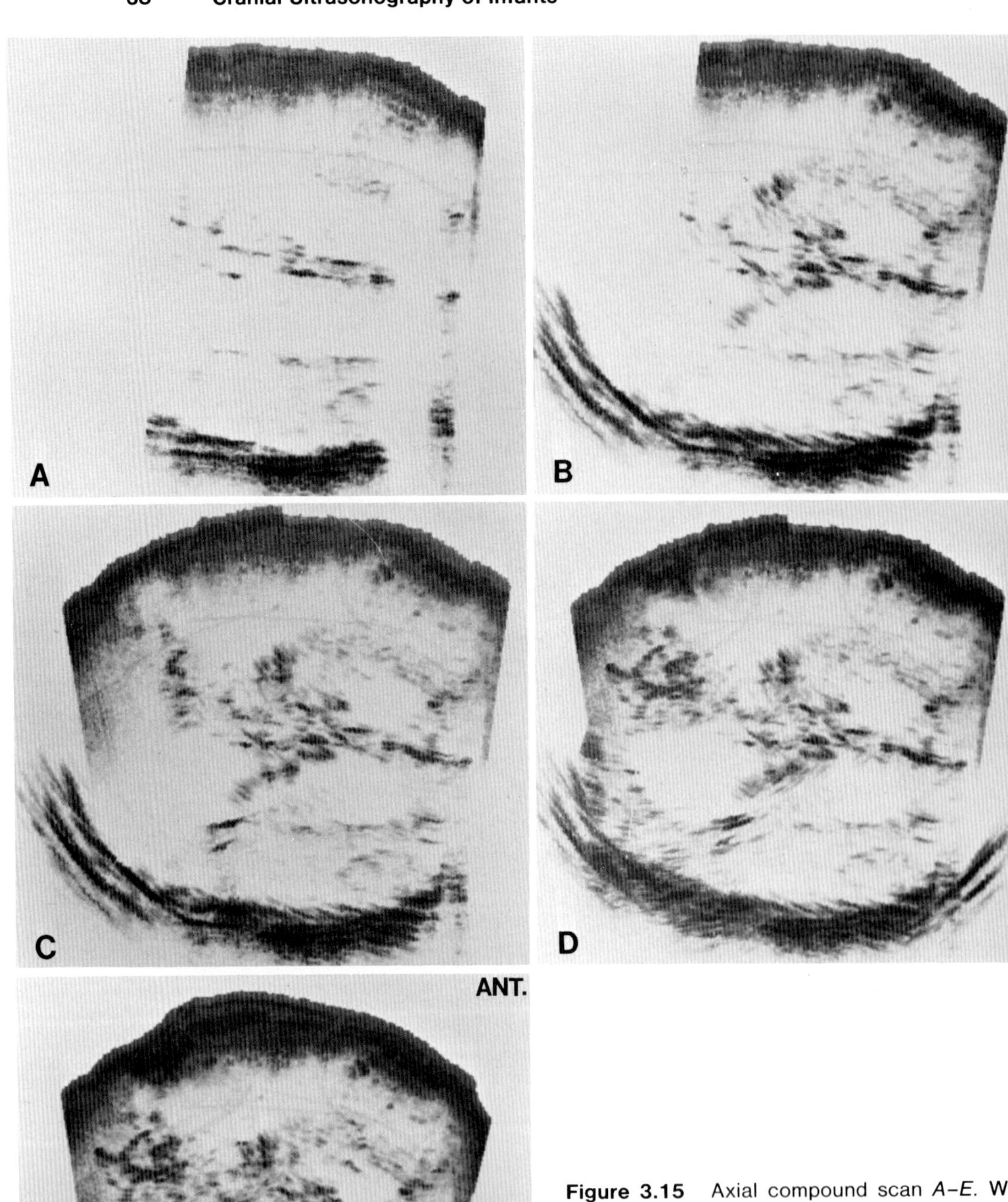

Figure 3.15 Axial compound scan *A–E*. Wit each sweep more information added.

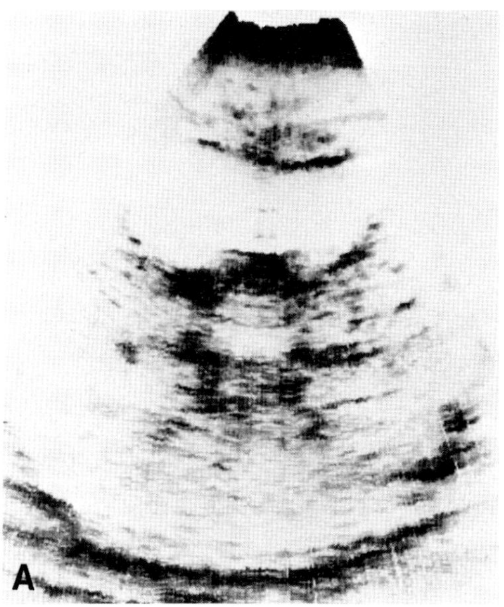

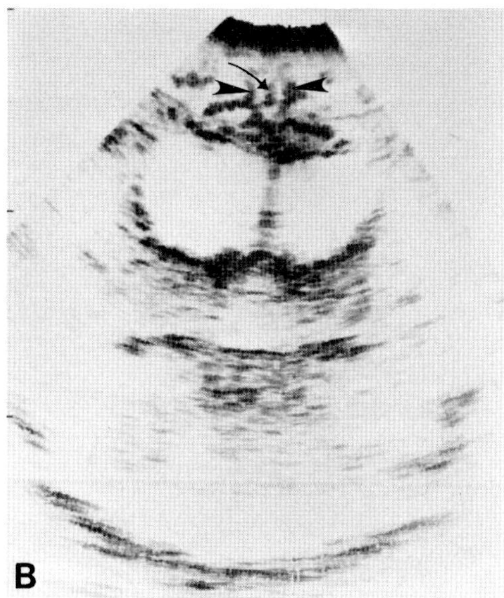

Figure 3.16 Coronal scans with 3.5 and 5.0 MHz transducers showing near and far fields in same patient. (*A*) Scan with 3.5 MHz transducer. Deep structures such as ventricles and posterior fossa well visualized; however, near-field structure such as interhemispheric fissure obscured. (*B*) Scan with 5 MHz transducer. Prominent interhemispheric fissure (*arrowheads*) and falx cerebri (*arrow*) in near-field clearly demonstrated, whereas structures in far-field not well seen.

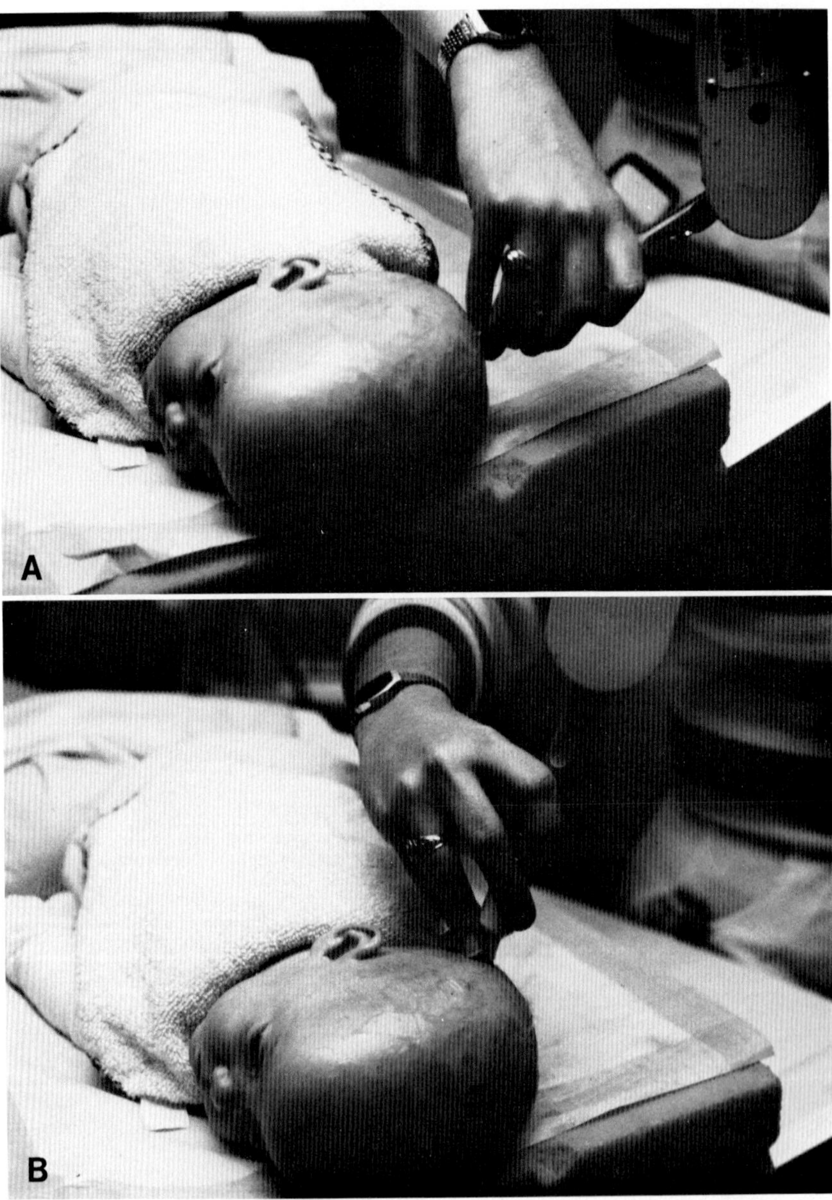

Figure 3.17 Posterior fossa view-scanning technique. Sonographer makes sector sweep through posterior fontanelle (*A*) and then lateral portions of head filled in by continuous scanning toward side of head (*B*). See diagram (*C*) on facing page.

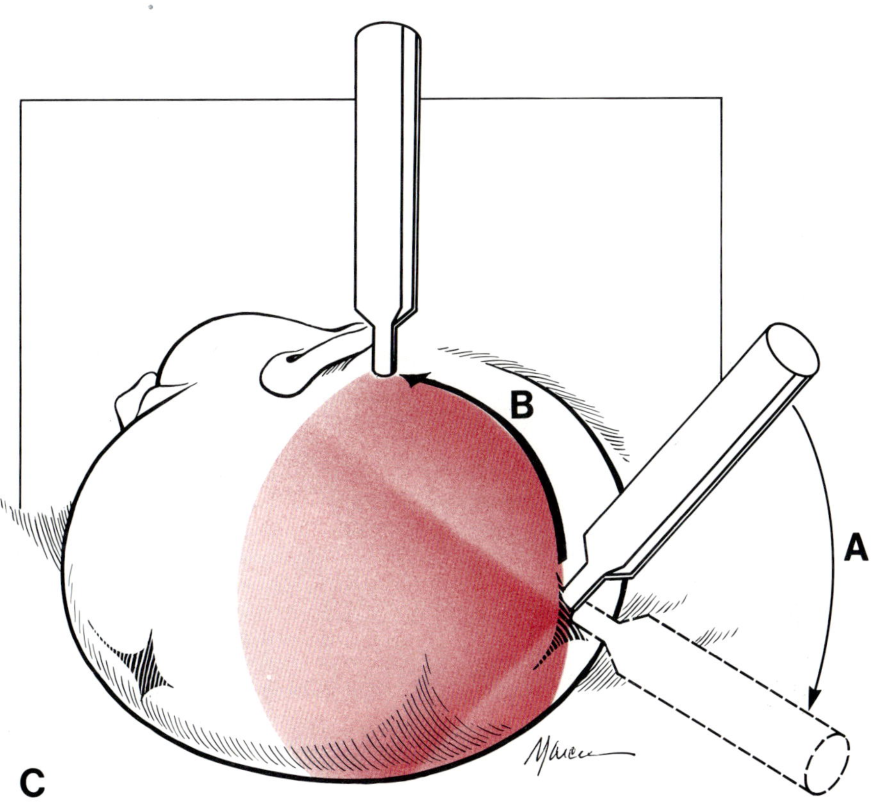
B
A
C

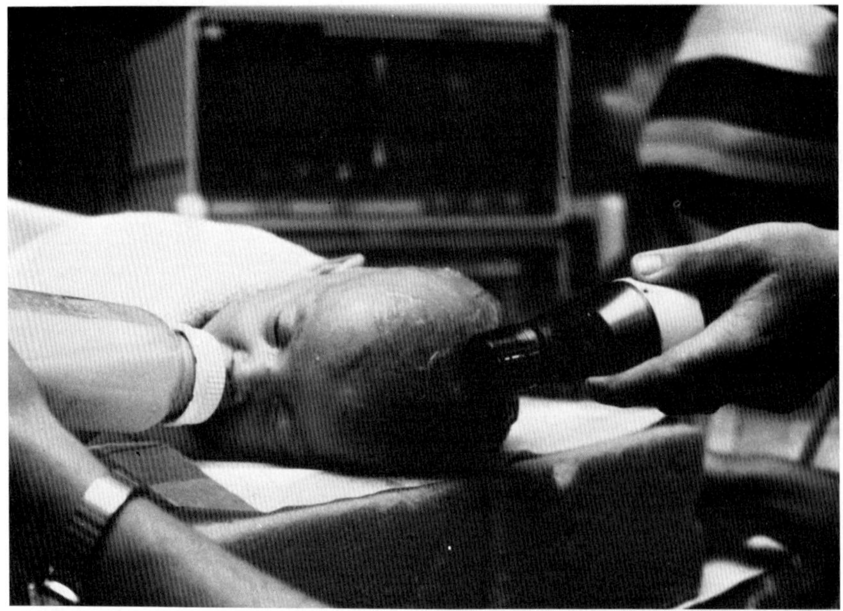

Figure 3.18 Real-time coronal view. Baby being scanned through anterior fontanelle.

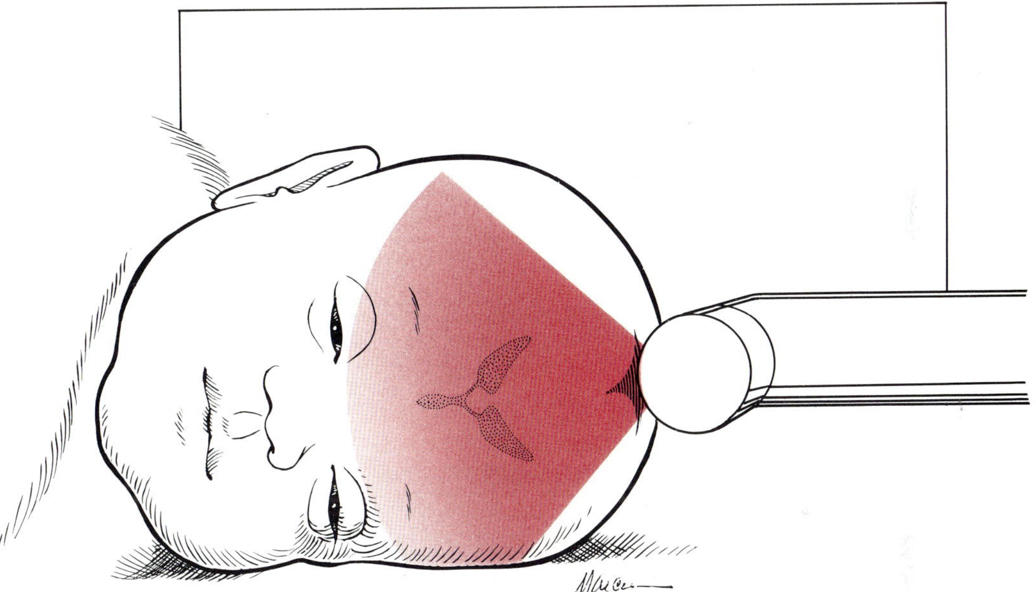

Figure 3.19 Real-time coronal scanning technique. Scans obtained through anterior fontanelle starting anteriorly and working posteriorly. Transducer angled to front and back of head for more anterior and posterior views.

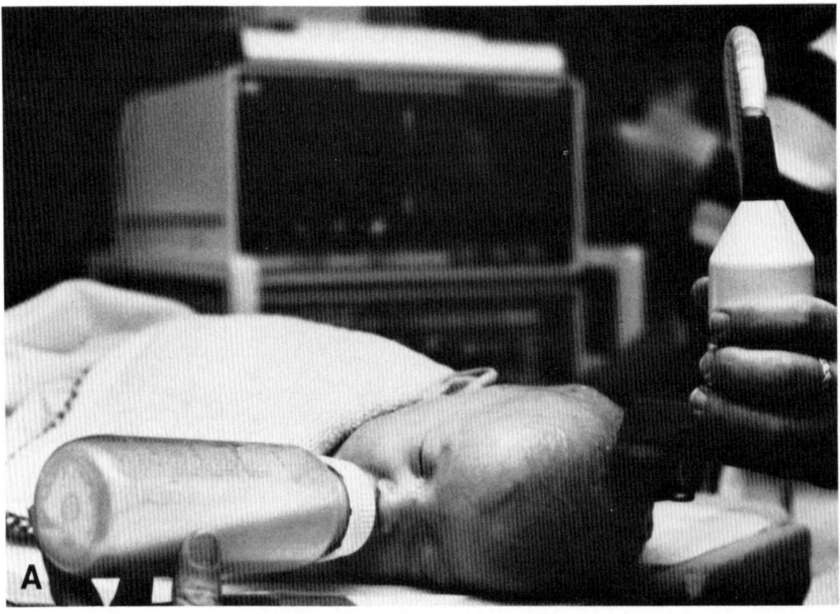

Figure 3.20 Real-time sagittal scanning technique. (*A* and *B*) Midline sagittal scan obtained through anterior fontanelle in midline. (*C*) Parasagittal scans obtained by angling transducer to right and left.

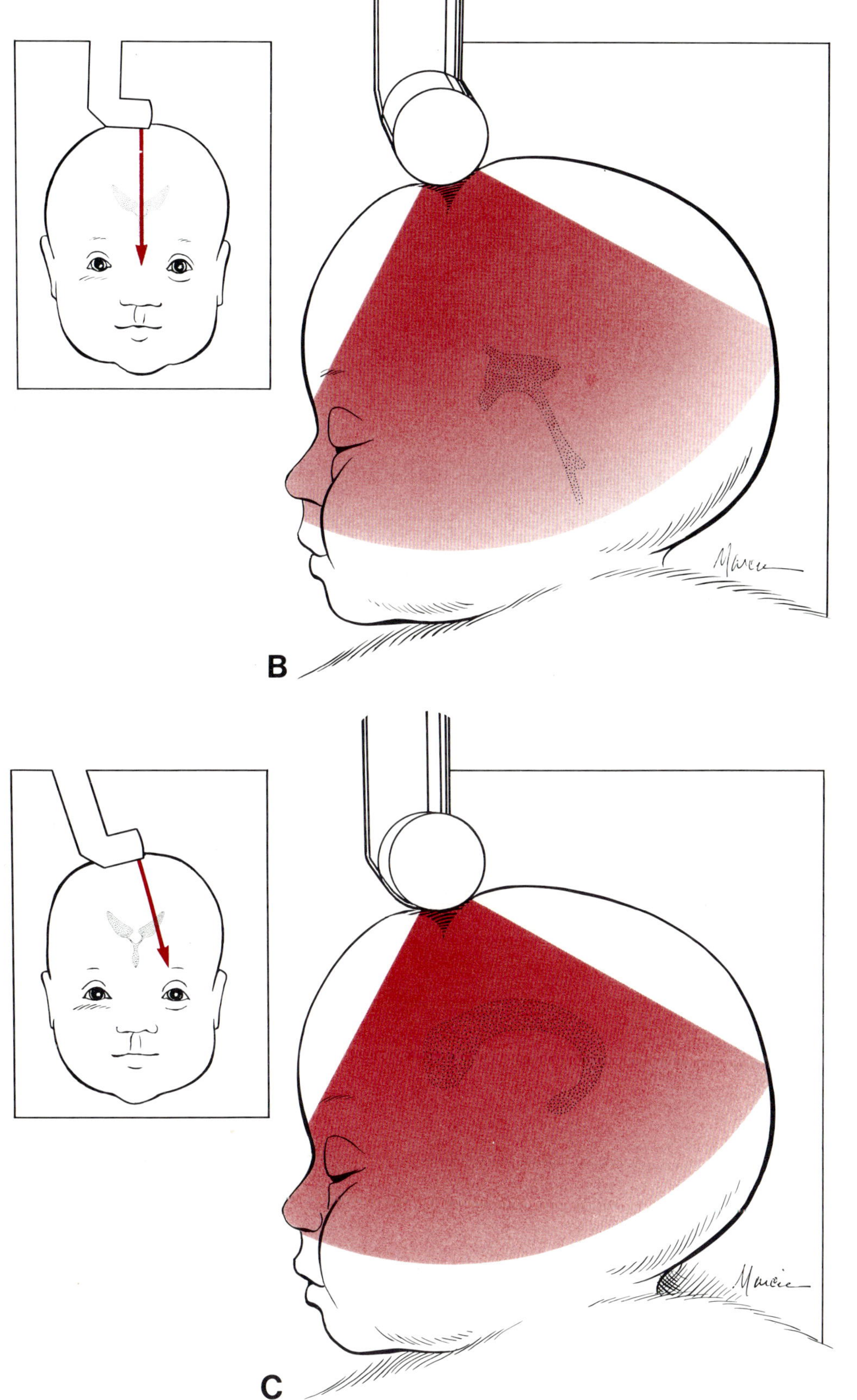
B
C

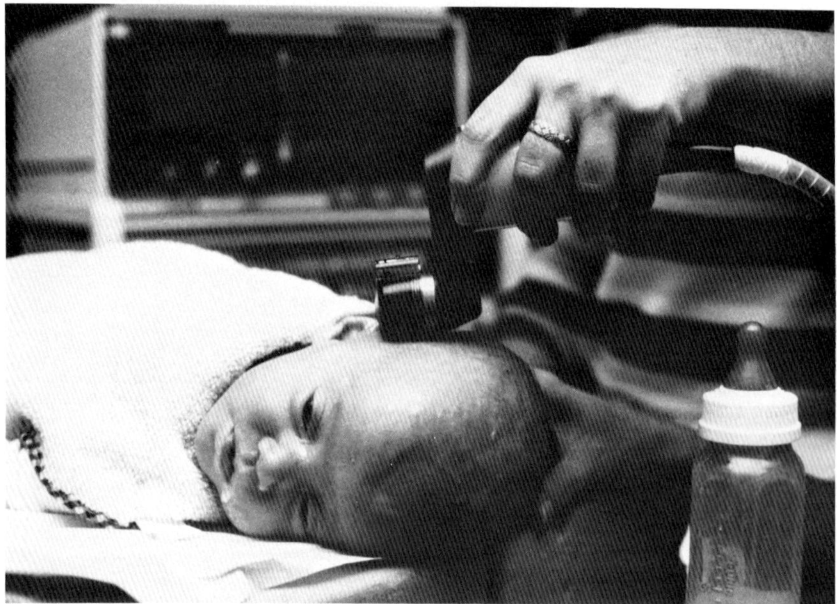

Figure 3.21 Real-time axial view. Baby being scanned through parietal bone.

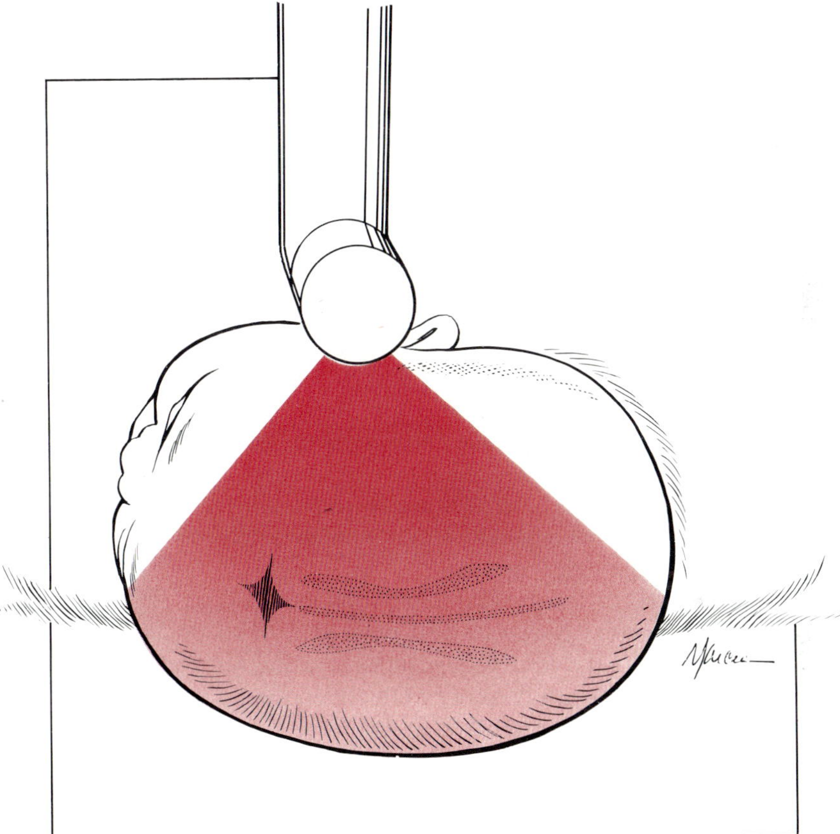

Figure 3.22 Real-time axial scanning technique. Scans obtained through parietal bone at various levels from external auditory meatus towards top of head.

CHAPTER 4

Normal Anatomy

Our patients are routinely scanned in several projections including axial, coronal, and sagittal views (Fig. 4.1). Additional views such as the modified coronal (60°) and posterior fossa views (150°) are used in selected cases particularly when posterior fossa abnormalities or a dilated fourth ventricle are suspected.

Axial Sections

A series of axial scans is performed at a 10° angle from the canthomeatal line at 5-mm intervals, starting at 1 cm above the level of the external auditory meatus (Fig. 4.2). These correspond to the routine computerized tomography (CT) images. Representative axial scans are shown in Figure 4.3. Shown alongside for reference are corresponding sections of an adult human brain.[1] We chose a patient with minimally enlarged ventricles so that the anatomy is more easily seen.

On the most caudad scan (Fig. 4.3*A*) a bilobed midline structure corresponds to the cerebral peduncles and brain stem. This structure is mildly echogenic relative to the more echogenic surrounding structures. The area of increased echogenicity just posterior to the brain stem represents the vermis of the cerebellum. The cerebellum is highly echogenic compared to the cerebrum and other brain tissue.

A scan 1 cm superior to the previous level (Fig. 4.3*B*) shows two relatively homogeneous, faintly echogenic structures lying on either side of the midline that represents the area of the thalamus. The lateral walls of the third ventricle are identified as parallel linear echoes in the midline at this level. The third ventricle is slitlike in the normal patient.

The next higher scan (Fig. 4.3*C*) is at the level of the bodies and atria of the lateral ventricles. A strong linear echo complex from the falx cerebri and septum pellucidum is identified. The lateral ventricles are anechoic areas on either side of the falx and their lateral walls are seen as linear collections of echoes. The choroid plexuses of the lateral ventricles are identified as echogenic structures in their floor.

The highest axial scan (Fig. 4.3*D*) is through the top of the lateral ventricles. The midline strong linear echo collection represents the falx cerebri and extends the whole length of the visualized head. In the normal infant, the ratio of the distance between the midline and the lateral wall of the ventricle, and the distance between the midline and the inner table of the skull, lies in the range of 0.25–0.35 at the level of the body.[2] The fine echogenicity of the cerebral tissue is seen between the lateral ventricle and the inner table of the skull.

Coronal Sections (90°)

A series of coronal scans is performed at 90° from the canthomeatal line starting as far anterior as we can make contact in the anterior fontanelle and working posteriorly at 5-mm intervals (Fig. 4.4). Figure 4.5 shows coronal sections (90°) at intervals from front to back with corresponding sections of the adult brain. The first coronal section (Fig. 4.5*A*) is through the frontal lobes. The fine low-level echoes represent cerebral tissue, while the diffuse medium-level echoes represent sulci and vascular structures. The densely echogenic bony floor of the anterior fossa is inferior to the frontal lobes. The falx cerebri is identified as a linear echogenic structure in the midline between the frontal lobes.

The next more posterior scan (Fig. 4.5*B*) is through the frontal horns of the lateral ventricles which are sonolucent structures on either side of the midline. In the normal patient the ventricles are slitlike. A cystic space between the lateral ventricles is the cavum septi pellucidi, a normal structure which is often seen in infancy. The heads of the caudate nuclei are moderately echogenic areas inferolateral to the lateral ventricles. The Sylvian fissures are seen as Y-shaped echogenic structures.

The next more posterior scan is through the level of the bodies of the lateral ventricles (Fig. 4.5*C*) which are fluid-filled structures on either side of midline. The temporal lobes can be identified separate from the midbrain and pons. The hippocampal gyri are their most medial gyri. The Sylvian fissures are seen as Y-shaped echogenic structures above the temporal lobes. The third ventricle is not well seen, presumably due to the ultrasound beam projecting parallel to its walls rather than perpendicularly.

On the next scan (Fig. 4.5*D*), through the bodies of the lateral ventricles, the echogenic structures in the floor of the lateral ventricles are the choroid plexuses. The septum pellucidum is an echogenic linear structure separating the lateral ventricles in the midline. The body of the corpus callosum lies above, and forms the roof of, the lateral ventricles. Two linear structures on either side of the midline represent the cingulate sulci.

On the next scan more posteriorly (Fig. 4.5*E*) the atria of the lateral ventricles are identified with the temporal horns leading into them. The echogenic choroid plexuses are within the ventricles. The falx cerebri midline linear echo separates into an inverted V-shaped echogenic structure representing the tentorium cerebelli. The cerebellum lies inferior to the tentorium.

On the most posterior scan (Fig. 4.5*F*) the tentorium cerebelli is identified, with moderately echogenic cerebrum of the occipital lobe above it and the densely echogenic cerebellum inferior to it.

Sagittal Sections

Sagittal scans are obtained by scanning through the anterior fontanelle in the midline and to the right and left (Fig. 4.6).

A midline sagittal section is shown (Fig. 4.7*A*) with a corresponding view from a pneumoencephalogram on another patient for comparison. A patient with mildly enlarged ventricles is shown so that the anatomy is easier to see. In the normal patient the third and fourth ventricles are not clearly identified. In midsagittal plane the third ventricle is identified as a sonolucent structure above the echogenic bony sella turcica. The massa intermedia is demonstrated in cross section as an echogenic dot. The foramen of Monro connects the third ventricle to one of the lateral ventricles, which is partially demonstrated. The fourth ventricle is demonstrated inferiorly with the densely echogenic cerebellum forming its roof. The cisterna magna is the fluid space inferior to the cerebellum.

The next scan (Fig. 4.7*B*) is a parasagittal scan angled off midline through one of the lateral ventricles. The lateral ventricle is identified as a J-shaped fluid-filled structure with part of the echogenic choroid plexus demonstrated in its floor. Brain gyri and sulci are also demonstrated on the scan. The temporal lobe is seen with the bony floor of the middle fossa as an echogenic line. The moderately echogenic head of the caudate nucleus is demonstrated inferior to the frontal horn of the lateral ventricle and the thalamus is demonstrated inferior to the body of the lateral ventricle.

Contact scans in the sagittal plane can be obtained but are technically difficult and are not routinely performed.

Modified Coronal Views (60°)

The 60° coronal view is obtained in many patients because the ventricular anatomy is well visualized on this view. All four ventricles can be demonstrated on a single scan through the level of the third and fourth ventricles. This angle is a compromise between the axial and 90° coronal views. Good contact can be made through the anterior fontanelle using this angle, and the posterior brain can be better visualized than on the 90° coronal scans.

Figure 4.9 shows modified coronal sections (60°) at intervals from front to back with corresponding sections of the adult brain. The first modified coronal section (Fig. 4.9*A*) is through the frontal and temporal lobes. The fine, low level echoes represent cerebral tissue and the frontal horns of the lateral ventricles are identified on this section. The falx cerebri is seen as a linear echogenic structure in the midline between the frontal lobes.

The next more posterior scan (Fig. 4.9*B*) is through the bodies of the lateral ventricles. The lobes of the thalami are seen on either side of the slitlike third ventricle. The temporal lobe and cerebellum are identified on this view. The normal fourth ventricle is slitlike and is not demonstrated. The Sylvian fissure is demonstrated as a Y-shaped structure.

On a more posterior scan (Fig. 4.9*C*) the atria of the lateral ventricles are identified with the temporal horns leading into them. The echogenic choroid plexuses are seen within the ventricles. The cerebellum is identified and is more echogenic than the cerebral tissue.

With communicating hydrocephalus or obstruction at the fourth ventricular outlets, all four dilated ventricles can be demonstrated on the modified coronal view (Fig. 4.10).

Posterior Fossa Views

A series of scans is performed at 5-mm intervals through the posterior head at 150° from the canthomeatal line. This is done by scanning over the occipital region angling toward the clivus and base of the skull (Fig. 4.11). The view is performed in selected cases in which posterior fossa abnormalities or a dilated fourth ventricle are suspected.

Figure 4.12 shows posterior fossa views at two different levels with corresponding sections of the adult brain. On the more caudal scan (Fig. 4.12 *A*) the densely echogenic hemispheres of the cerebellum are identified with the moderately echogenic occipital lobes adjacent. The brainstem is seen between the densely echogenic bony clivus and the cerebellum as a mildly echogenic bilobed structure. The fourth ventricle is not shown in normal patients on this view.

A slightly higher posterior fossa view (Fig. 4.12*B*) demonstrates the moderately echogenic occipital lobes of the cerebrum separated from the densely echogenic cerebellum by the V-shaped tentorium cerebelli. The mildly echogenic pons is again identified as a bilobed structure adajcent to the bony clivus.

Cavum Septi Pellucidi and Vergae

The cavum septi pellucidi (CSP) is a fluid-filled space between the leaves of the septum pellucidum and the cavum vergae is its posterior extension behind the columns of the fornix.[3] Pathologic studies have shown that a macroscopically visible CSP is present in 100% of premature infants.[4,5] The incidence decreases sharply at 2 months of age post term and by 6 months of age the incidence is that of an adult population—15–20%.[3]

The CSP is a normal structure commonly visualized on head ultrasonography in newborns (Fig. 4.13). In a recent study[6] we visualized the cavum septi pellucidi in 42% of all newborns and 62% of premature infants. We have noted that the CSP disappears in many infants at approximately 2–4 weeks post term.

It is important to recognize the CSP and to distinguish it from a dilated third ventricle. This is especially true with head ultrasound performed during intrauterine life, because mistaking a normal CSP for dilatation of the ventricular system could cause unnecessary alarm.

Summary

With A-mode and bistable equipment the walls of the ventricles and midline structures could be identified because of their strongly reflective surfaces. With the development of B-mode gray scale equipment we are now able to recognize many more anatomic structures within the brain as shown in this chapter. Future technical improvements in the resolving capabilities of our equipment, along with further experience gained by sonographers interpreting these images, will certainly result in the recognition and identification of even more anatomic structures. The vascular anatomy of the brain as seen by real-time ultrasonography is only beginning to be studied and is difficult to demonstrate on static images. Further interest in this area will lead to identification of normal vessels and changes in their position and pulsations with disease processes.

References

1. Matsui T, Hirano A. *An Atlas of the Human Brain for Computerized Tomography*. Tokyo: Igaku-Shoin, 1978.
2. Kossoff G, Garrett WJ, Radavanovich G: Ultrasonic atlas of normal brain of infant. Ultrasound Med Biol 1974; 1:259–266.
3. Shaw C, Alvord E. Cava septi pellucidi et vergae: their normal and pathological states. Brain 1969; 92:213–233.
4. Larroche JC, Baudey J. Cavum septi lucidi, cavum vergae, cavum veli interpositi: cavites de la ligne mediane. Biol Neonat 1961; 3:193–236.
5. Tenchini L. *Contributo alla storia dei progressi dell'anatomia e della fisiologia del cervello.* Naples, 1880; 174.
6. Farruggia S, Babcock DS. The cavum septi pellucidi: its appearance and incidence with cranial ultrasonography in infancy. Radiology 1981; 139:147–150.
7. Babcock DS, Han BK, LeQuesne GW. B-Mode gray scale ultrasound of the head in the newborn and young infant. AJR 1980; 134:457–468.
8. Babcock DS, Han BK. The accuracy of high resolution real-time ultrasonography of the head in infancy. Radiology 1981; 139:665–676.

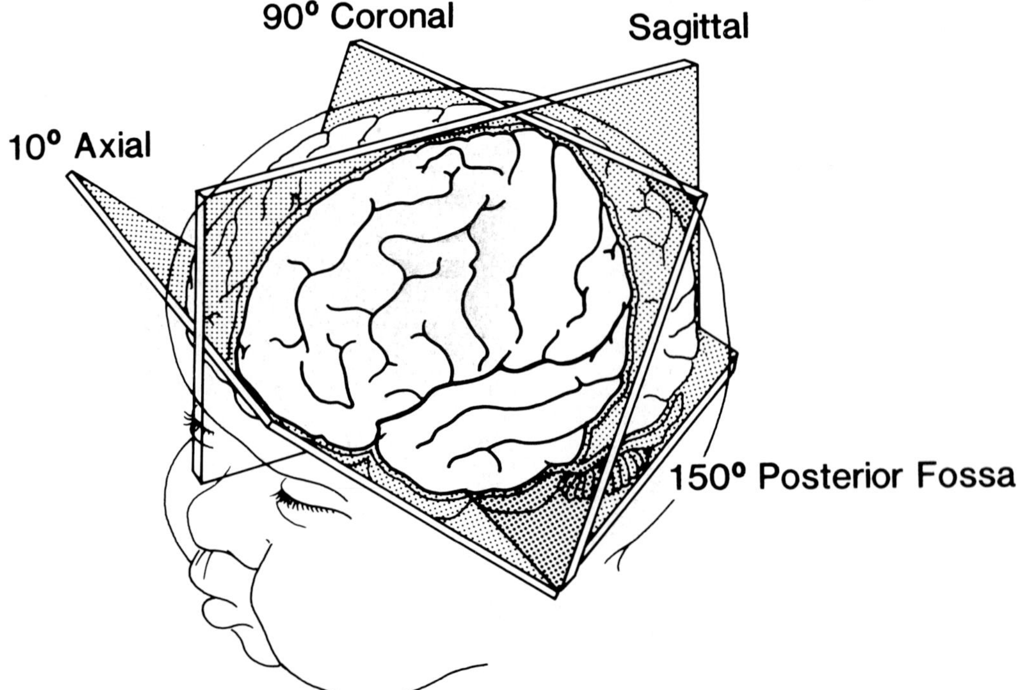

Figure 4.1. Scan angles. Axial, coronal, posterior fossa and sagittal. (Reproduced with permission from D. S. Babcock and B. K. Han: *Radiology*, *139:*665–676, 1981.[8])

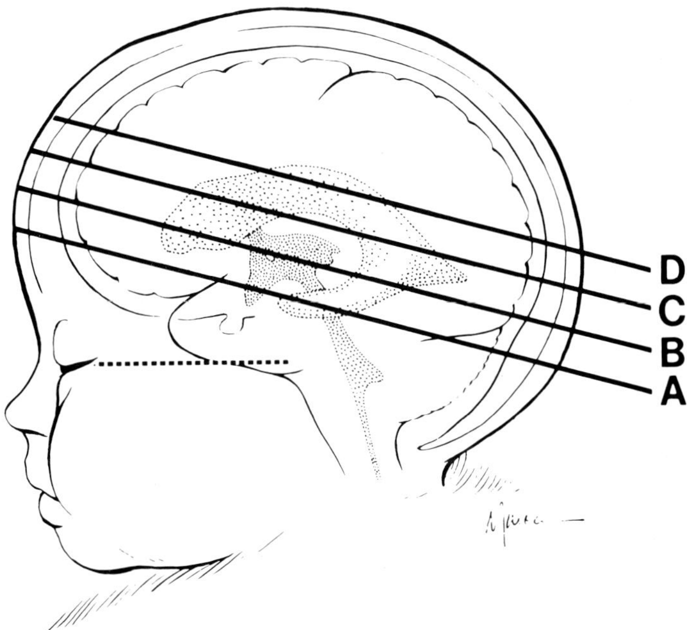

Figure 4.2. Axial scanning planes.

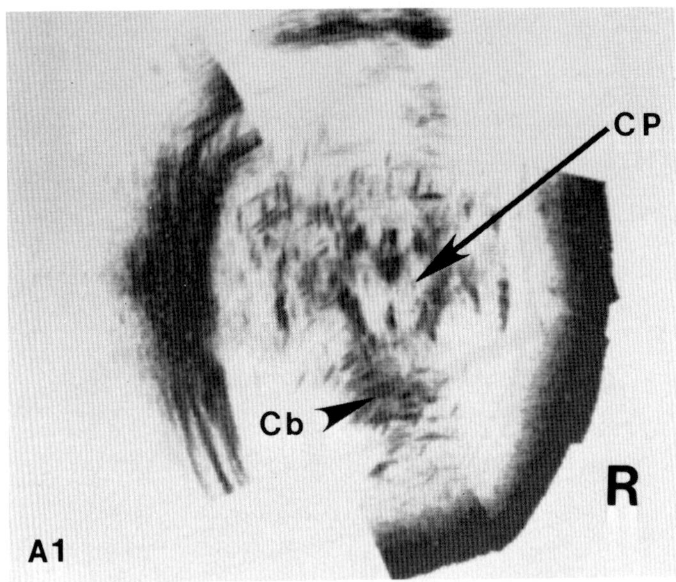
CP
Cb
R
A1

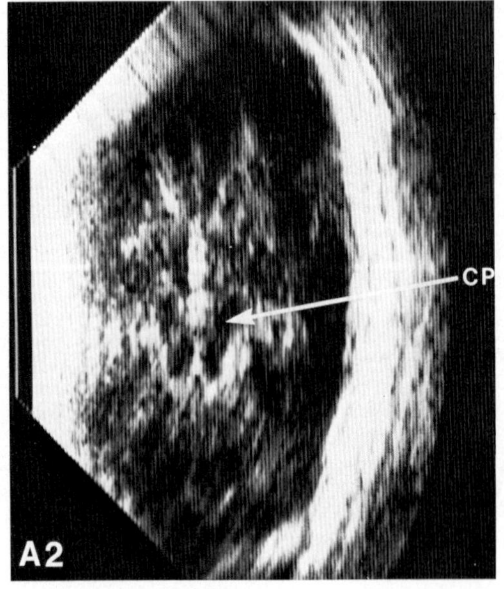
CP
A2

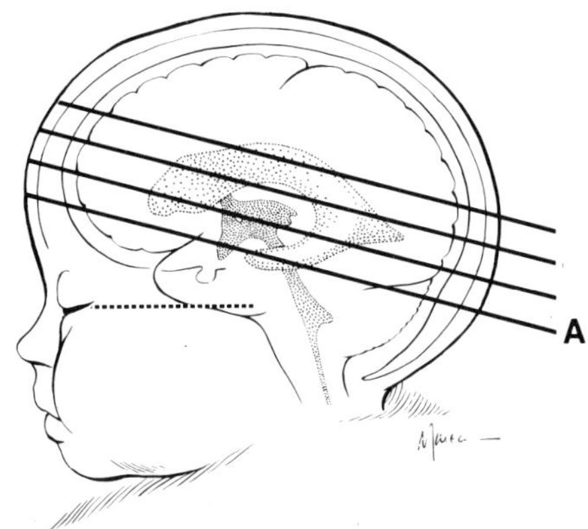

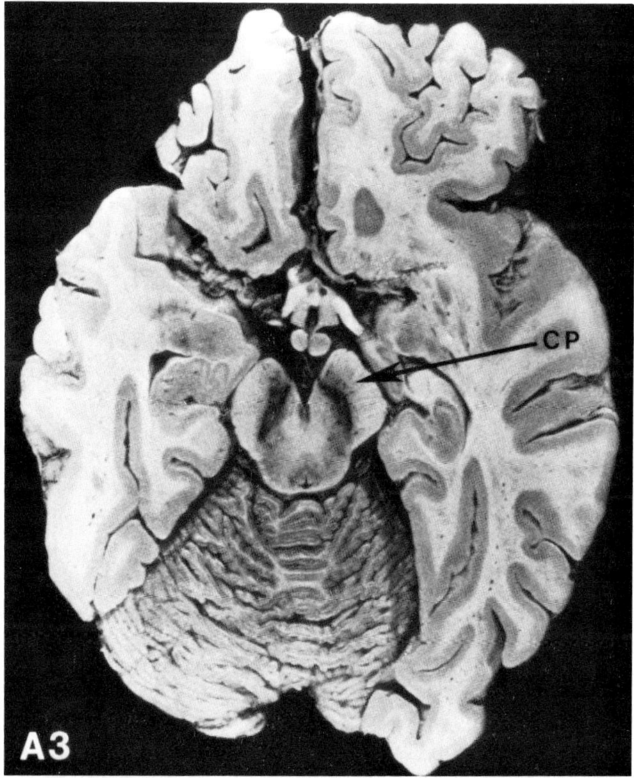

Figure 4.3*A* Normal low axial contact scan (*1*) sector real-time scan (2) and corresponding anatomic section (*3*) show bilobed midline structure representing cerebral peduncles (*CP*). Echogenic vermis of cerebellum (*Cb*). (*1*) Reproduced with permission from D. S. Babcock, B. K. Han, and G. W. Lequesne: *American Journal of Roentgenology*, *134*:457–468, 1980.[7] ((*3*) Reproduced with permission from T. Matsui and A. Hirano: *An Atlas of the Human Brain for Computerized Tomography.* Tokyo: Igaku-Shoin, 1978.[1])

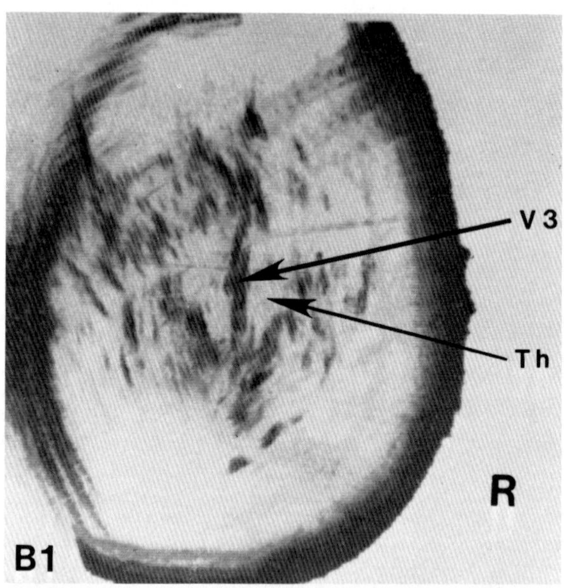
V3
Th
R
B1

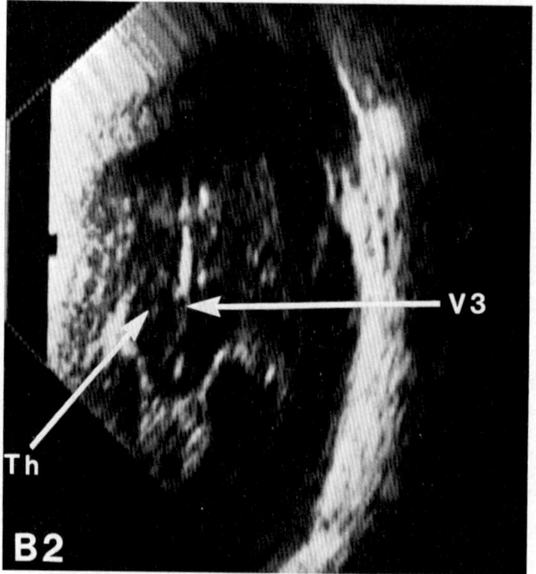
V3
Th
B2

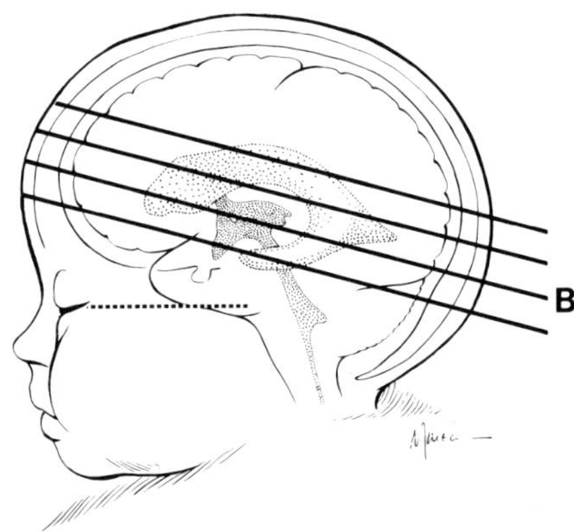

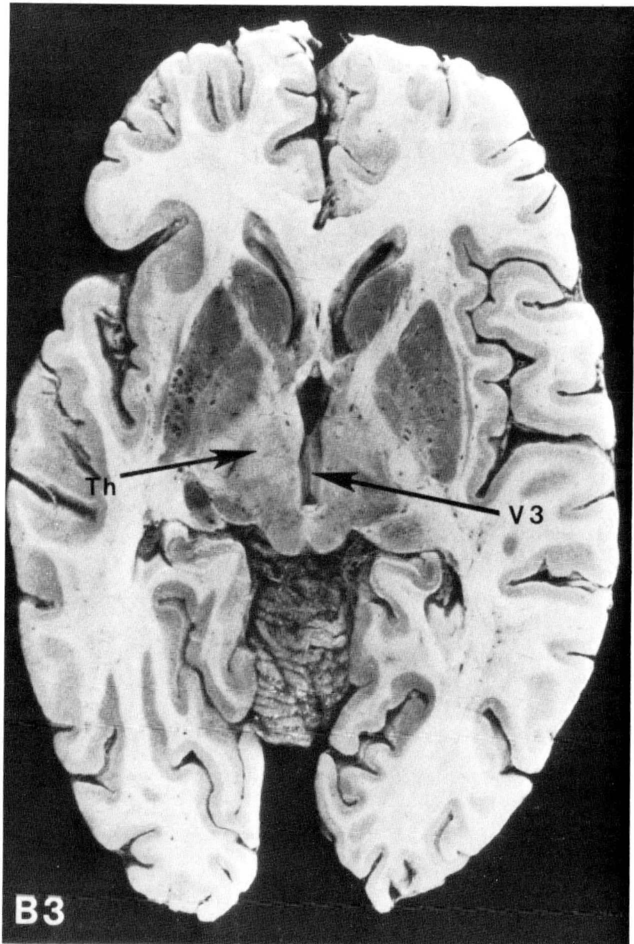

Figure 4.3*B* Normal axial contact scan (*1*), sector real-time scan (*2*), and corresponding anatomic section (*3*) through level of third ventricle (*V3*) and thalamus (*Th*). ((*1*) Reproduced with permission from D. S. Babcock, B. K. Han, and G. W. LeQuesne: *American Journal of Roentgenology*, *134:*457–468, 1980.[7] (*3*) Reproduced with permission from T. Matsui and A. Hirano: *An Atlas of the Human Brain for Computerized Tomography.* Tokyo: Igaku-Shoin, 1978.[1])

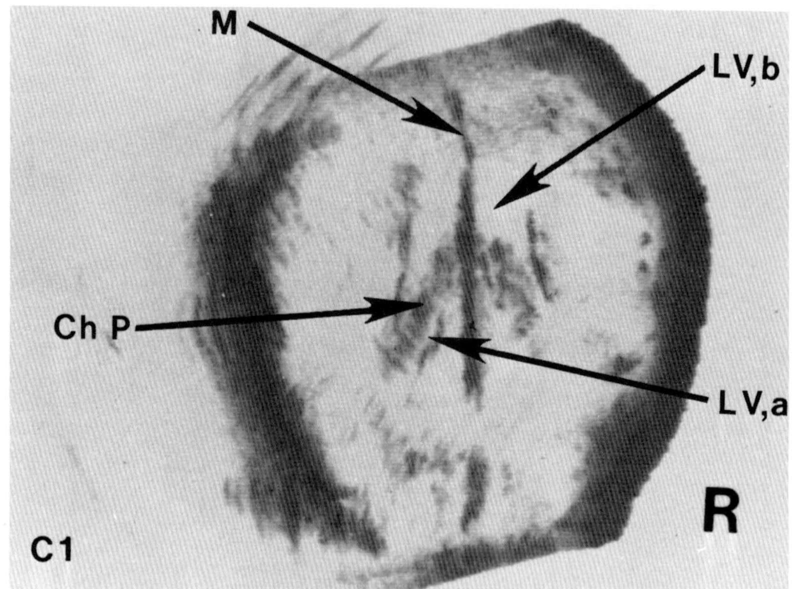
M
LV,b
Ch P
LV,a
R
C1

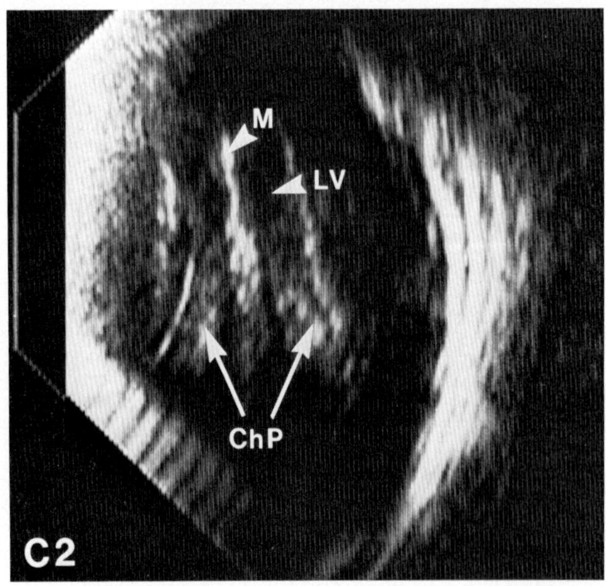
M
LV
ChP
C2

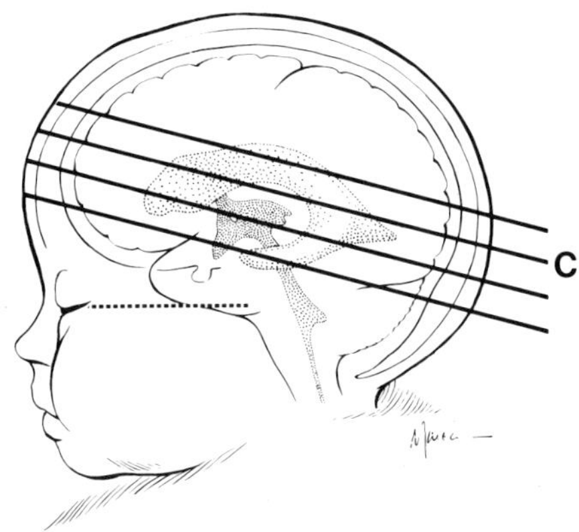

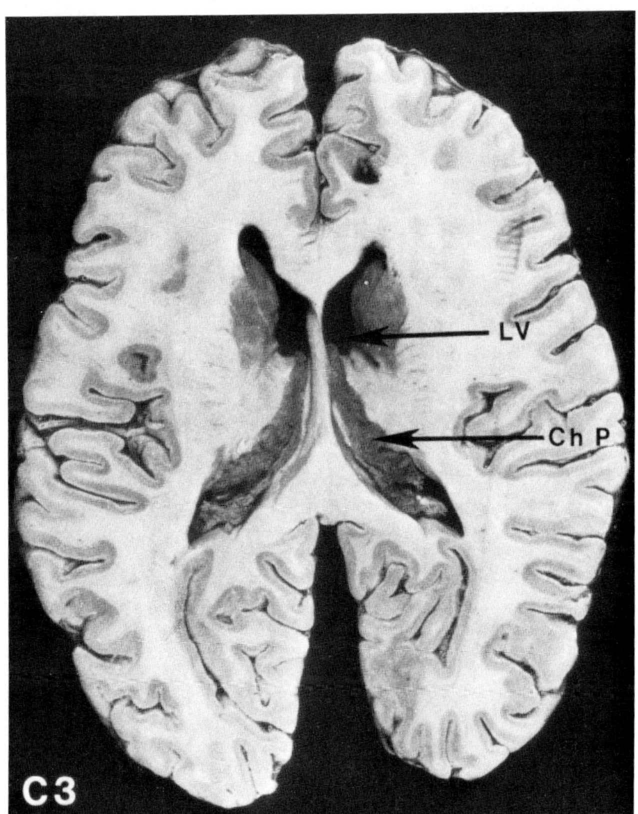

Figure 4.3C Normal axial contact scan (*1*), sector real-time scan (*2*) and corresponding anatomic section (*3*) at level of bodies (*LV*, *b*) and atria (*LV*, *a*) of lateral ventricles. Midline strong linear echoes represent falx cerebri and septum pellucidum (*M*). Choroid plexuses (*ChP*) seen as echogenic structures in floor of lateral ventricles. ((*1*) Reproduced with permission from D. S. Babcock, B. K. Han, and G. W. LeQuesne: *American Journal of Roentgenology*, *134:*457–468, 1980.[7] (*3*) Reproduced with permission from T. Matsui and A. Hirano: *An Atlas of the Human Brain for Computerized Tomography.* Tokyo: Igaku-Shoin, 1978.[1])

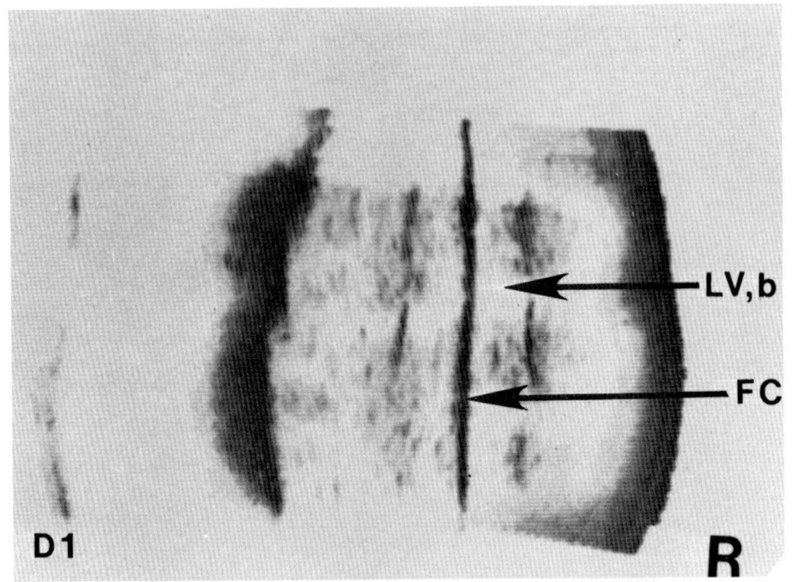
LV,b
FC
D1
R

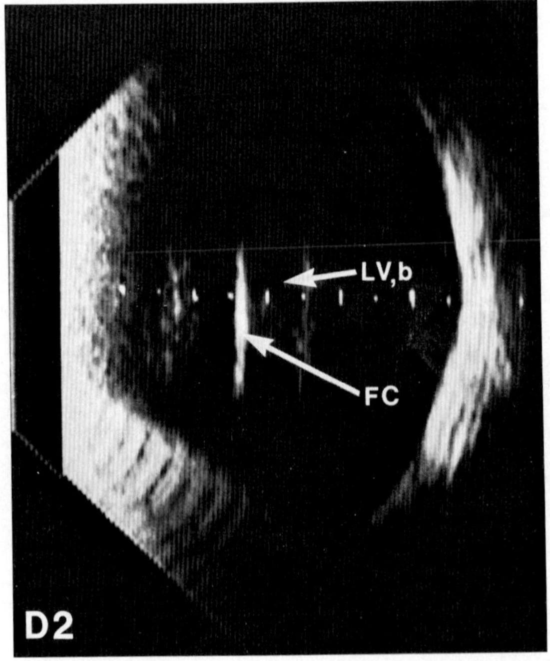
LV,b
FC
D2

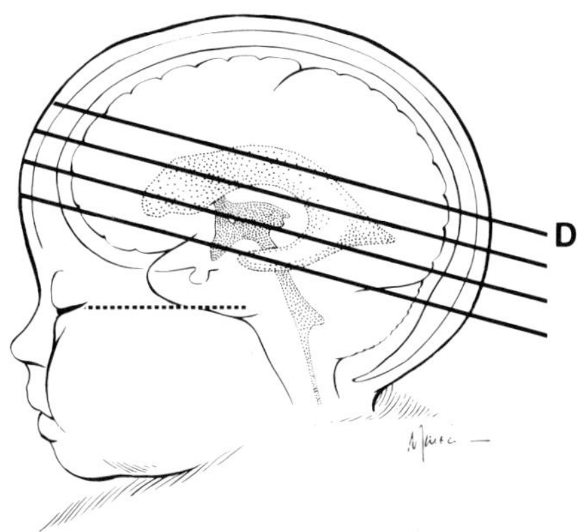

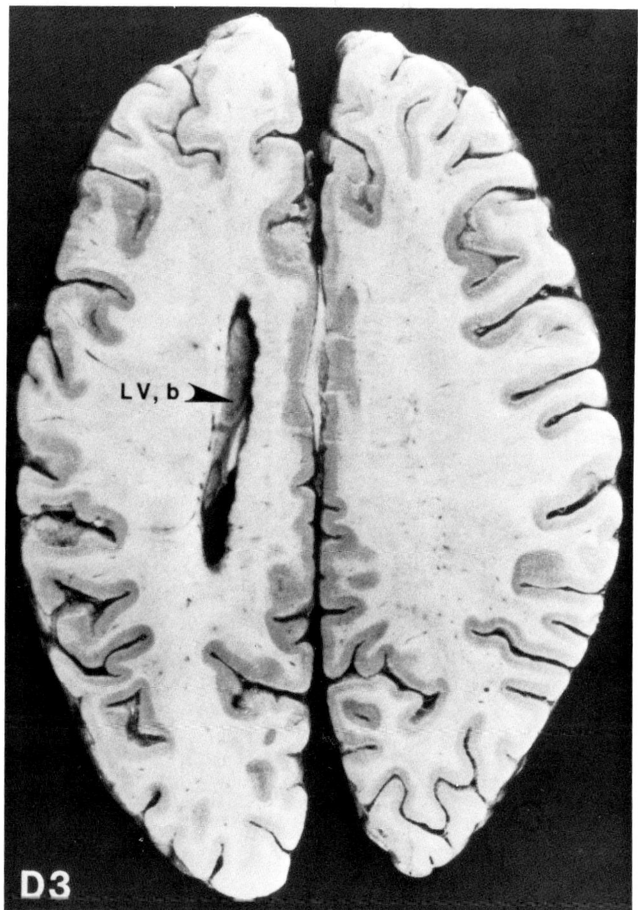

Figure 4.3*D* Normal axial contact scan (*1*), sector real-time scan (*2*), and corresponding anatomic section (*3*) through top of lateral ventricles. Midline falx cerebri (*FC*) with bodies of lateral ventricles (*LV,b*) on either side. ((*1*) Reproduced with permission from D. S. Babcock, B. K. Han, and G. W. LeQuesne: *American Journal of Roentgenology*, *134:*457–468, 1980.[7] (*3*) Reproduced with permission from T. Matsui and A. Hirano: *An Atlas of the Human Brain for Computerized Tomography*. Tokyo: Igaku-Shoin, 1978.[1])

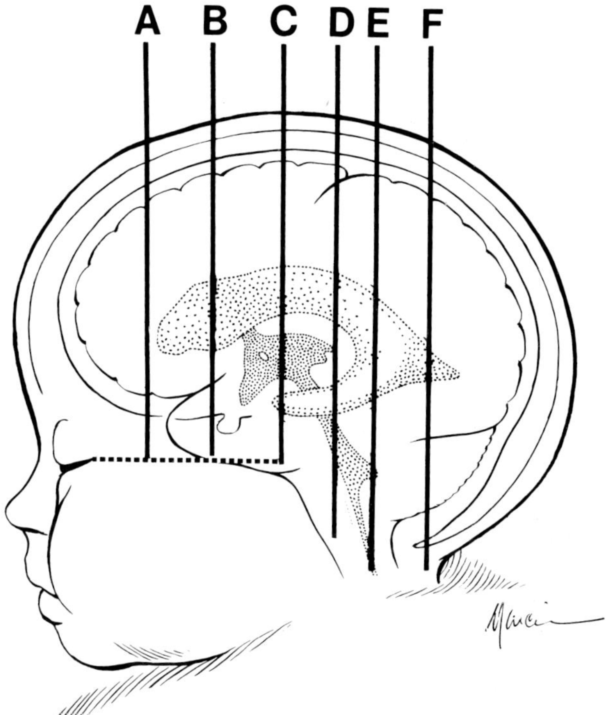

Figure 4.4 Coronal (90°) scanning planes.

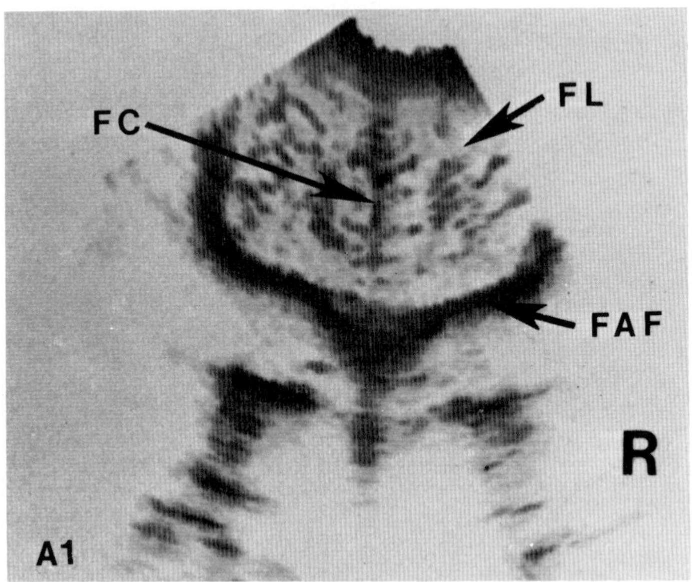
FC
FL
FAF
R
A1

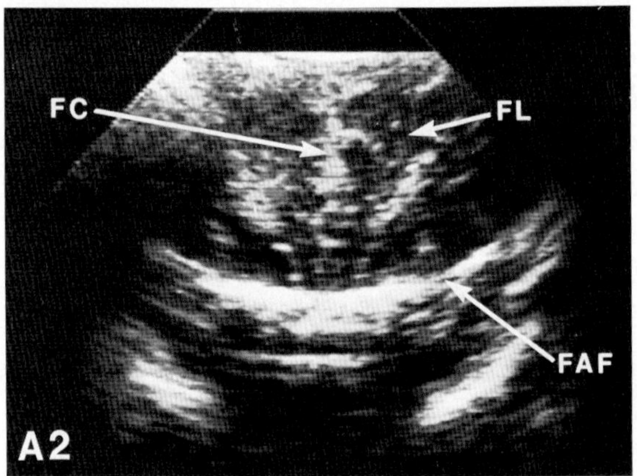
FC
FL
FAF
A2

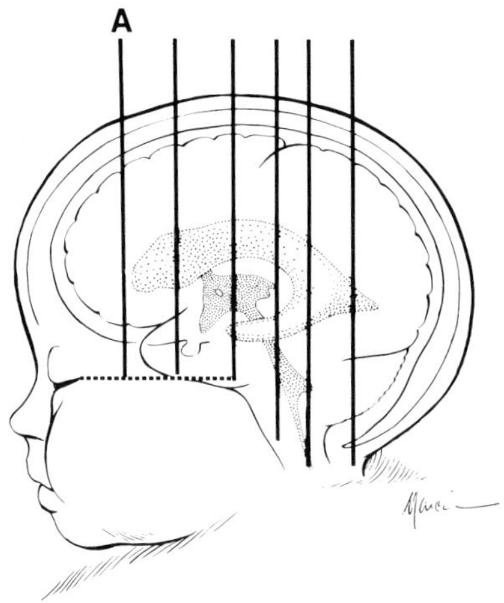

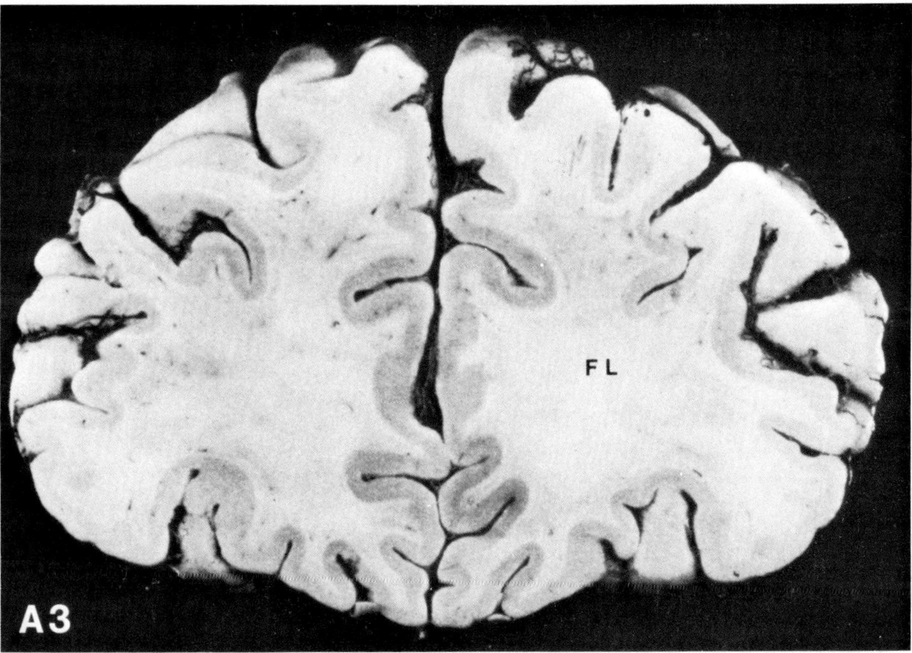

Figure 4.5*A* Normal anterior coronal contact scan (*1*), sector real-time scan (*2*), and corresponding anatomic section (*3*) through frontal lobes (*FL*). Echogenic bony floor of anterior fossa (*FAF*) inferior. Midline linear echoes of falx cerebri (*FC*). ((*1*) Reproduced with permission from D. S. Babcock, B. K. Han, and G. W. LeQuesne: *American Journal of Roentgenology*, *134:*457–468, 1980.[7] (*3*) Reproduced with permission from T. Matsui and A. Hirano: *An Atlas of the Human Brain for Computerized Tomography.* Tokyo: Igaku-Shoin, 1978.[1])

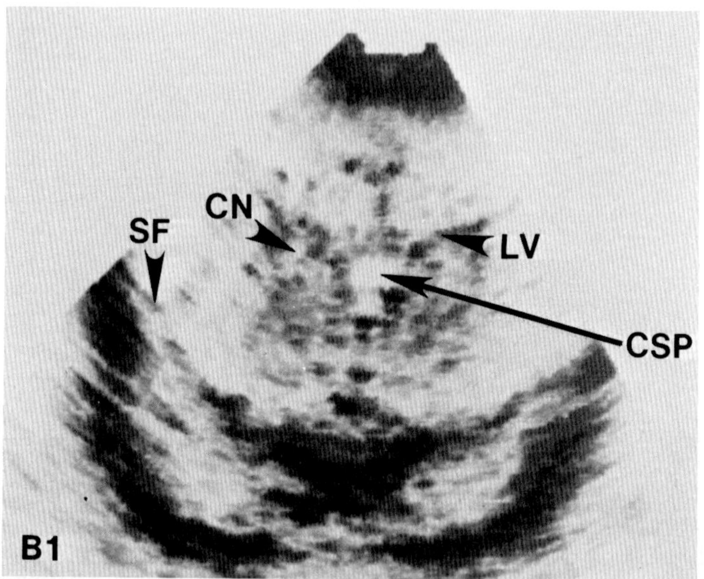
CN
SF
LV
CSP
B1

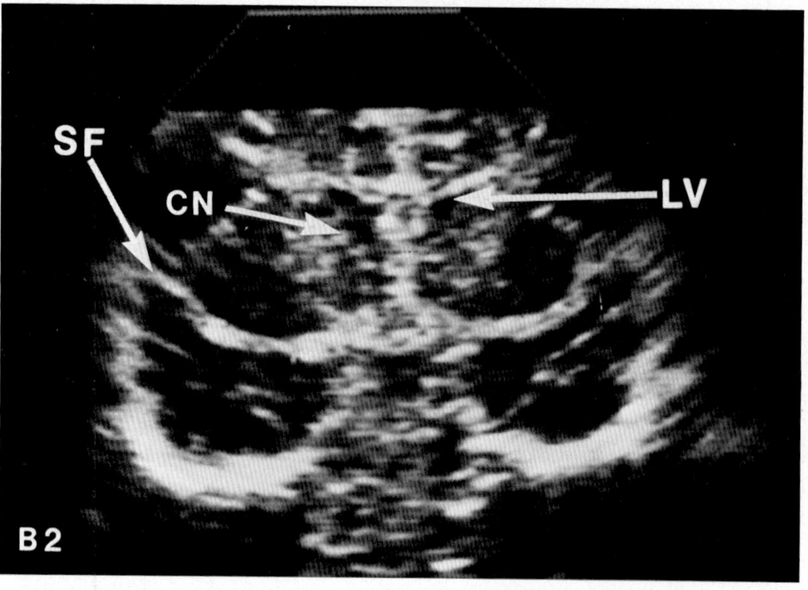
SF
CN
LV
B2

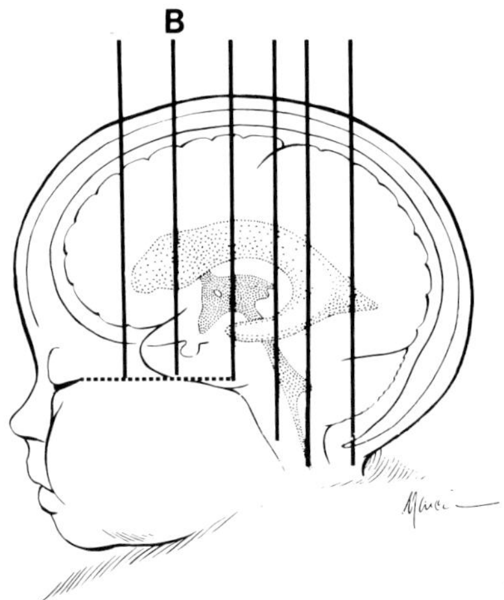

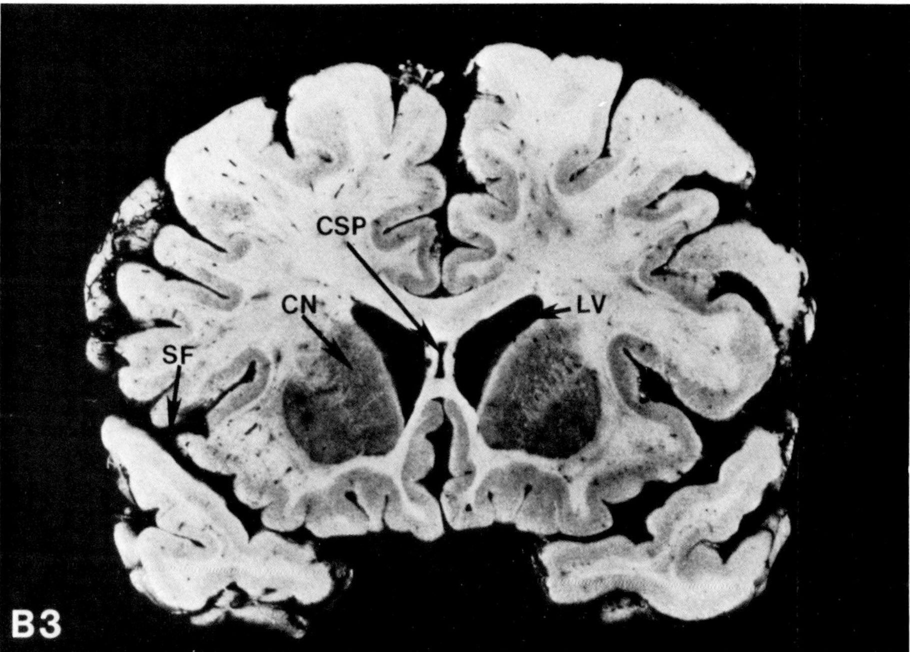

Figure 4.5*B* Normal coronal contact scan (*1*), sector real-time scan (*2*), and corresponding anatomic section (*3*) through frontal horns of lateral ventricles (*LV*). Cavum septi pellucidi (*CSP*) midline cystic structure. Sylvian fissures (*SF*) produce Y-shaped echoes. Moderately echogenic heads of caudate nuclei (*CN*) seen inferolateral to lateral ventricles. ((*3*) Reproduced with permission from T. Matsui and A. Hirano: *An Atlas of the Human Brain for Computerized Tomography.* Tokyo: Igaku-Shoin, 1978.[1])

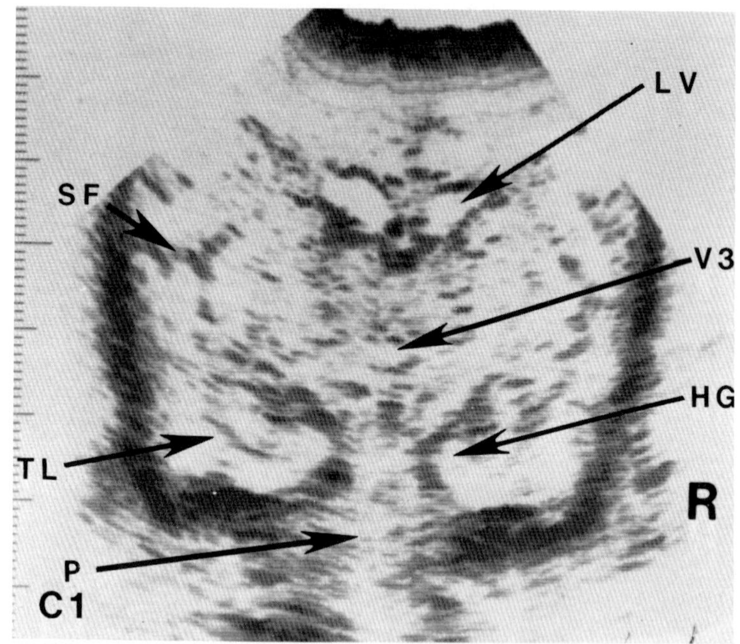
LV
SF
V3
HG
TL
R
P
C1

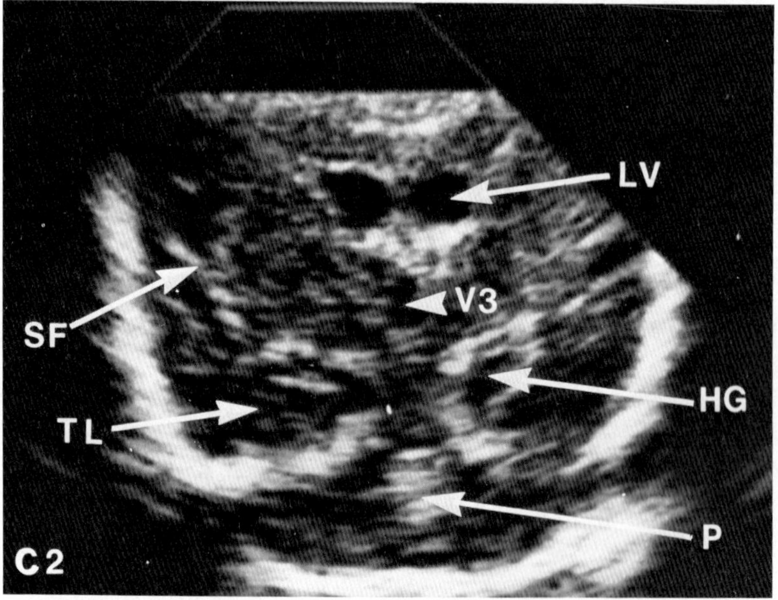
LV
SF
V3
HG
TL
P
C2

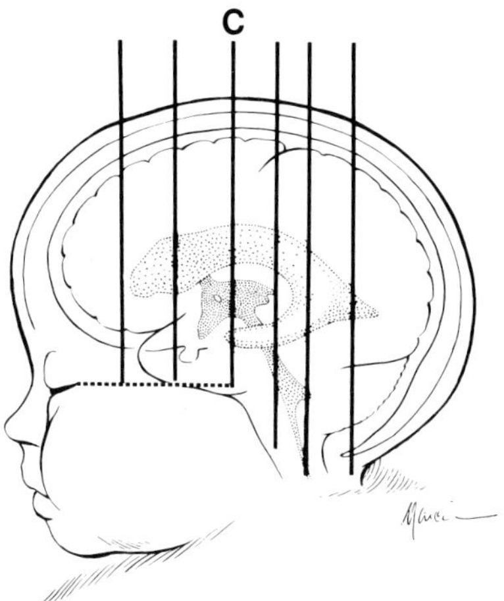

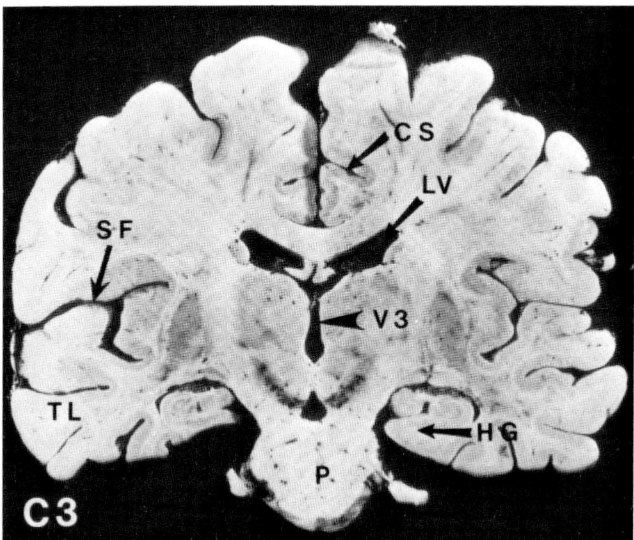

Figure 4.5 *C* Normal coronal contact scan (*1*), sector real-time scan (*2*), and corresponding anatomic section (*3*) through lateral ventricles (*LV*) and third ventricle (*V3*). Temporal lobes (*TL*) with most medial gyrus, hippocampal gyrus (*HG*). Pons and midbrain (*P*) inferior. Sylvian fissure (*SF*). (Case with mild hydrocephalus.) ((*1*) reproduced with permission from D. S. Babcock, B. K. Han and G. W. LeQuesne: *American Journal of Roentgenology*, *134*:457–468, 1980.[7] (*2*) Reproduced with permission from D. S. Babcock and B. K. Han, *Radiology*, *139*:665–676, 1981.[8] (*3*) Reproduced with permission from T. Matsui and A. Hirano: *An Atlas of the Human Brain for Computerized Tomography*. Tokyo: Igaku-Shoin, 1978.[1])

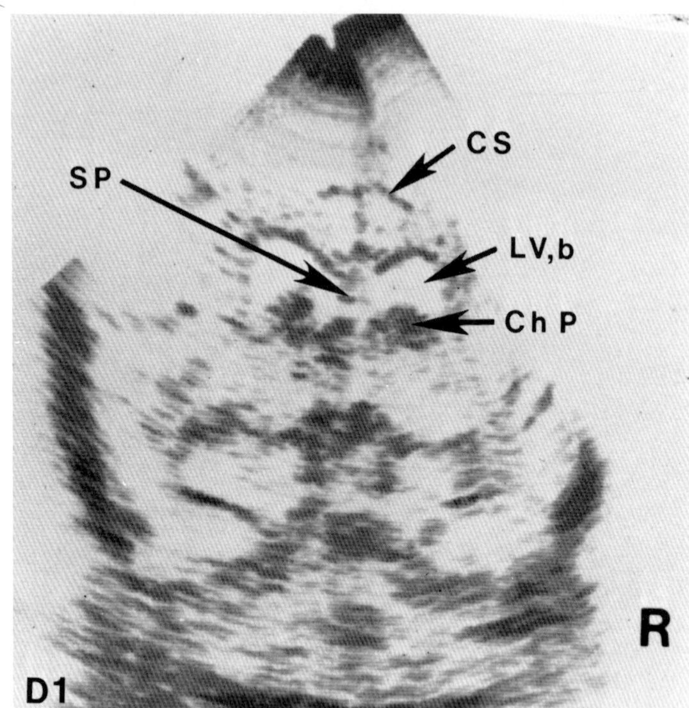
CS
SP
LV,b
Ch P
R
D1

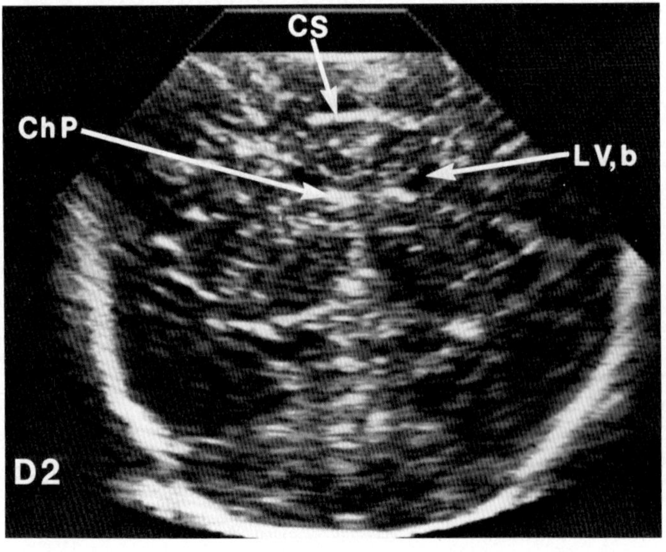
CS
ChP
LV,b
D2

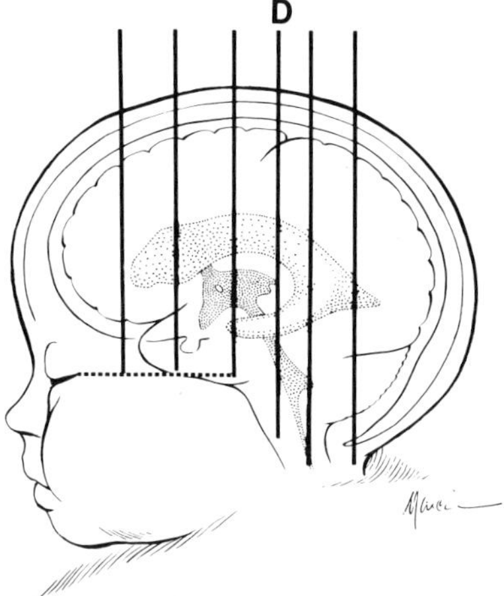

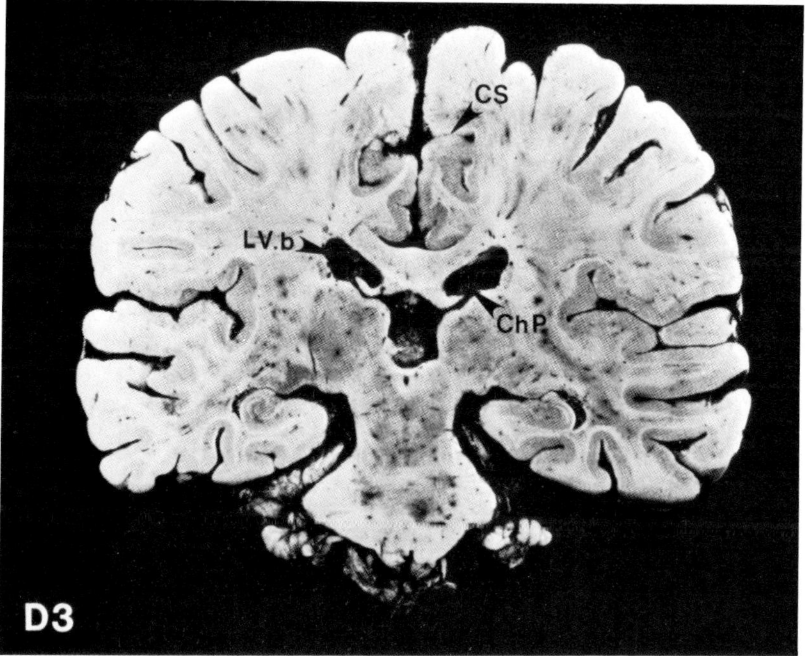

Figure 4.5 *D* Normal coronal contact scan (*1*), sector real-time scan (*2*), and corresponding anatomic section (*3*) through body of lateral ventricles (*LV*, *b*) with echogenic choroid plexus (*ChP*) in floor. Septum pellucidum (*SP*) separates lateral ventricles. Cingulate sulcus (*CS*). ((*1*) Reproduced with permission from D. S. Babcock, B. K. Han, and G. W. LeQuesne: *American Journal of Roentgenology*, *134*:457–468, 1980.[7] (*3*) Reproduced with permission from T. Matsui and A. Hirano: *An Atlas of the Human Brain for Computerized Tomography.* Tokyo: Igaku-Shoin, 1978.[1])

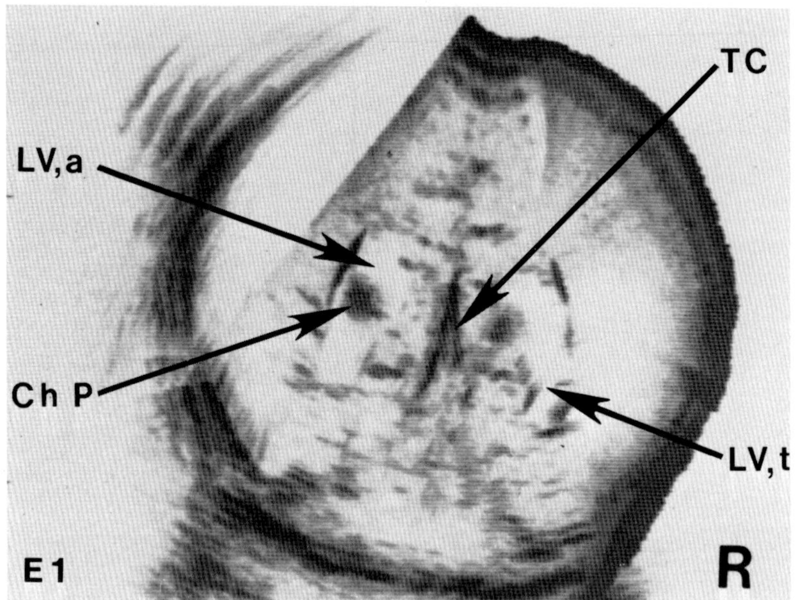
TC
LV,a
Ch P
LV,t
E1
R

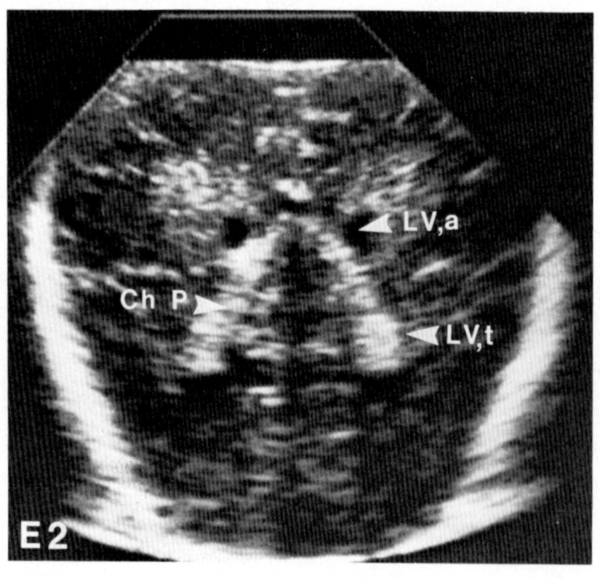
LV,a
Ch P
LV,t
E2

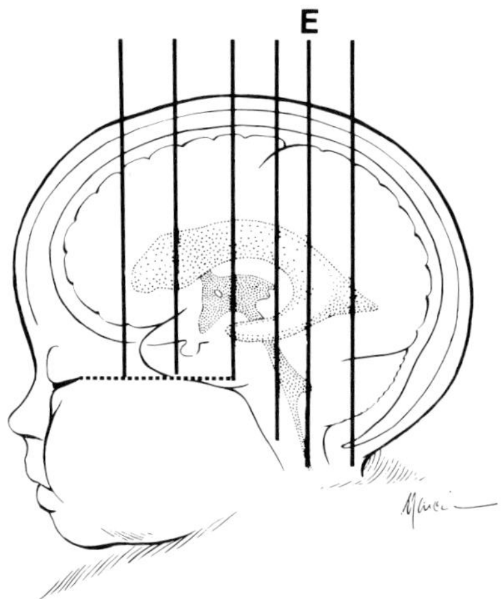

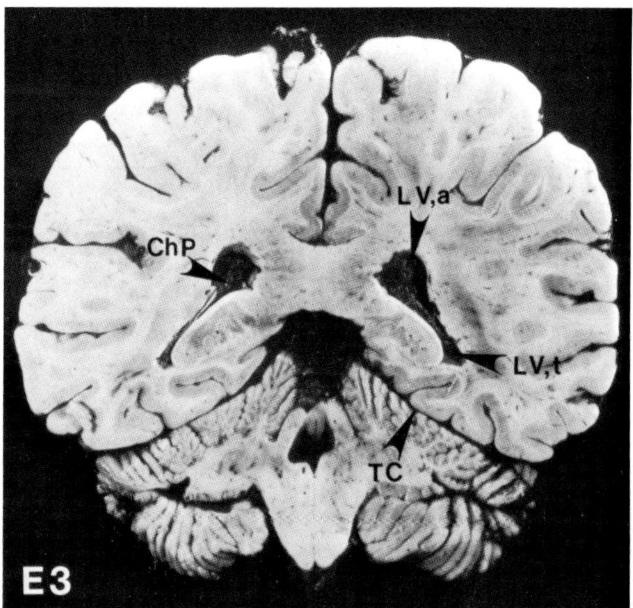

Figure 4.5 *E* Normal coronal contact scan (*1*), sector real-time scan (*2*), and corresponding anatomic section (*3*) through atria of lateral ventricles (*LV, a*) joined by temporal horns (*LV, t*). Choroid plexuses (*Ch P*) and tentorium cerebelli (*TC*). ((*1*) Reproduced with permission from D. S. Babcock, B. K. Han, and G. W. LeQuesne: *American Journal of Roentgenology*, *134*:457–468, 1980.[7] (*2*) Reproduced with permission from D. S. Babcock and B. K. Han: *Radiology*, *139*: 665–676, 1981.[8] (*3*) Reproduced with permission from T. Matsui and A. Hirano: *An Atlas of the Human Brain for Computerized Tomography*. Tokyo: Igaku-Shoin, 1978.[1])

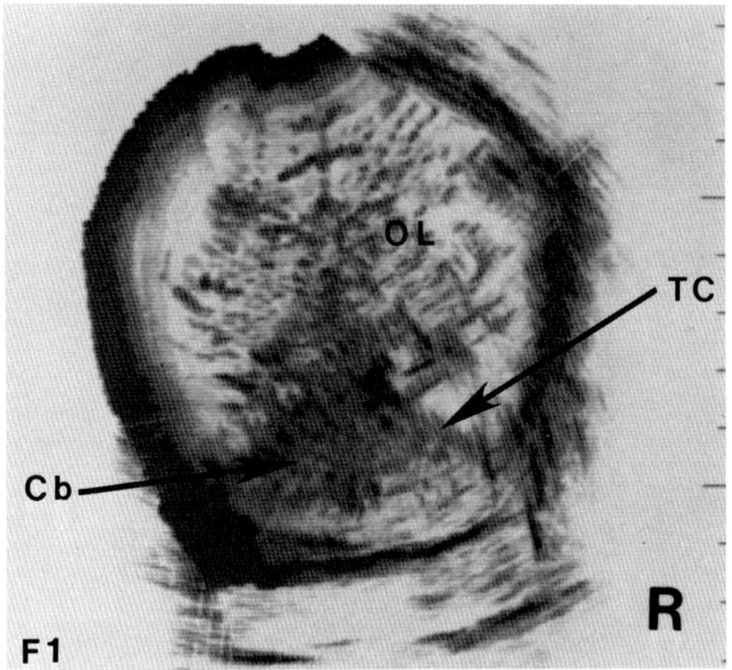
OL
TC
Cb
R
F1

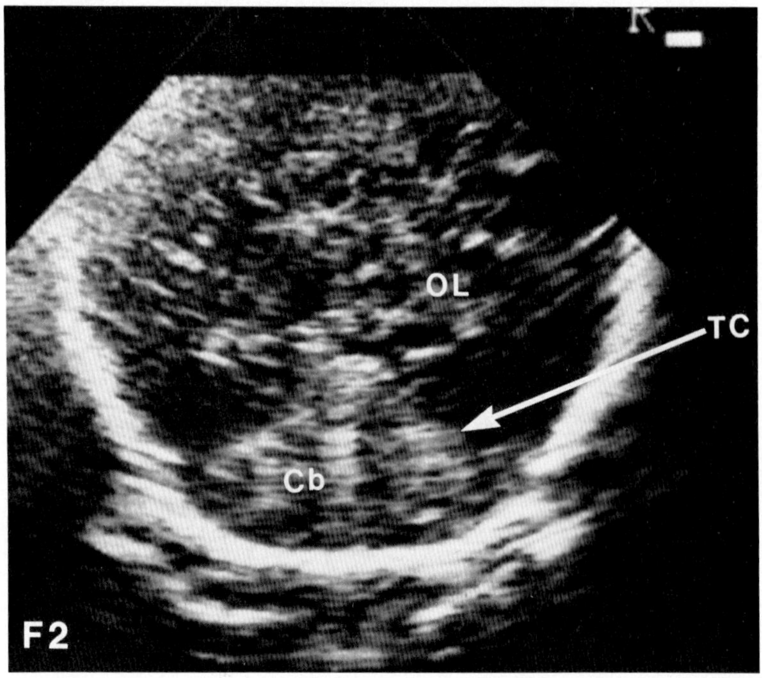
OL
TC
Cb
F2

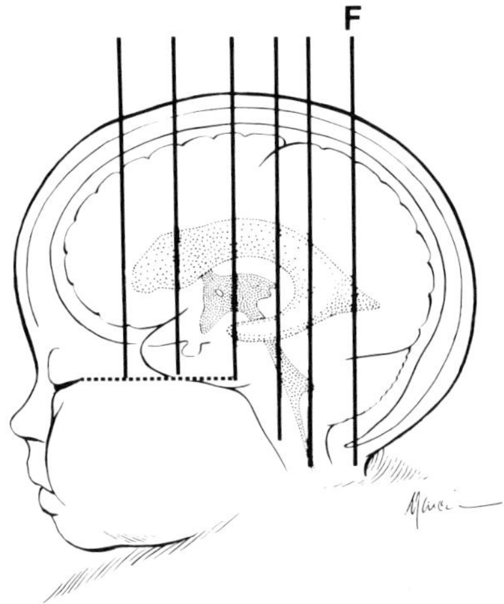

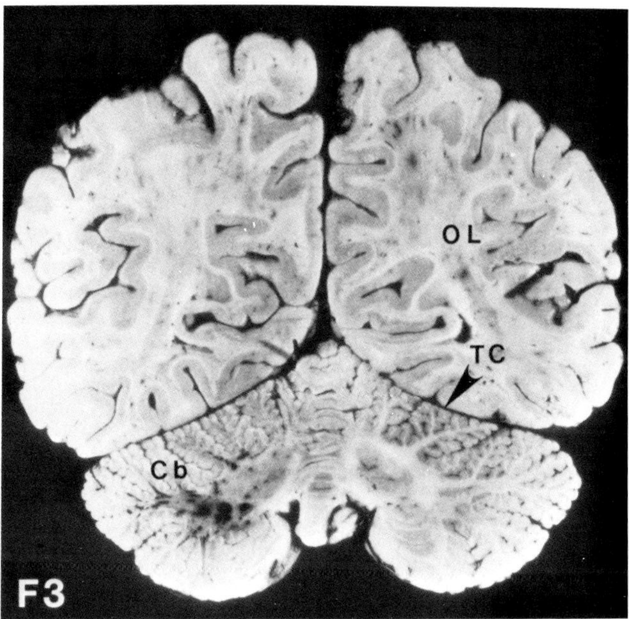

Figure 4.5*F* Normal most posterior coronal contact scan (*1*), sector real-time scan (*2*), and corresponding anatomic section (*3*). Tentorium cerebelli (*TC*) with moderately echogenic occipital lobes (*OL*) above and densely echogenic cerebellum (*Cb*) inferior. ((*1*) Reproduced with permission from D. S. Babcock, B. K. Han, and G. W. LeQuesne: *American Journal of Roentgenology, 134:*457–468, 1980.[7] (*2*) Reproduced with permission from D. S. Babcock and B. K. Han: *Radiology, 139:*665–676, 1981.[8] (*3*) Reproduced with permission from T. Matsui and A. Hirano: *An Atlas of the Human Brain for Computerized Tomography.* Tokyo: Igaku-Shoin, 1980.[1])

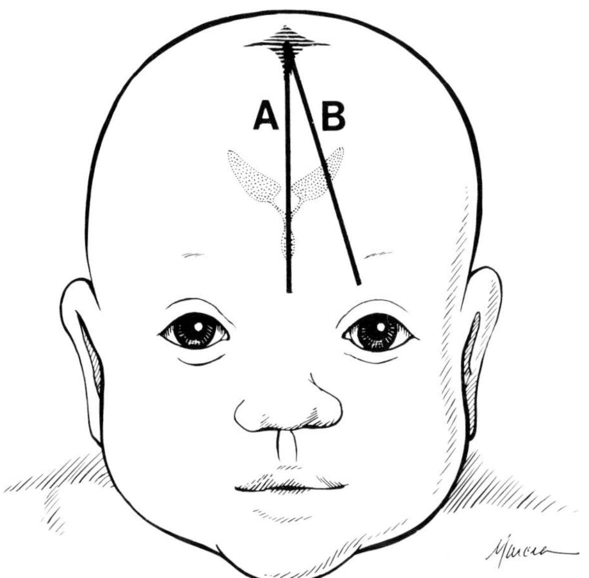

Figure 4.6 Sagittal scanning planes.

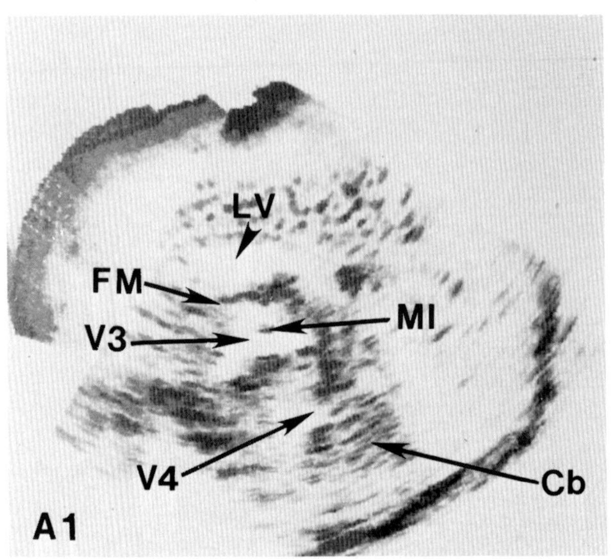
LV
FM
MI
V3
V4
Cb
A1

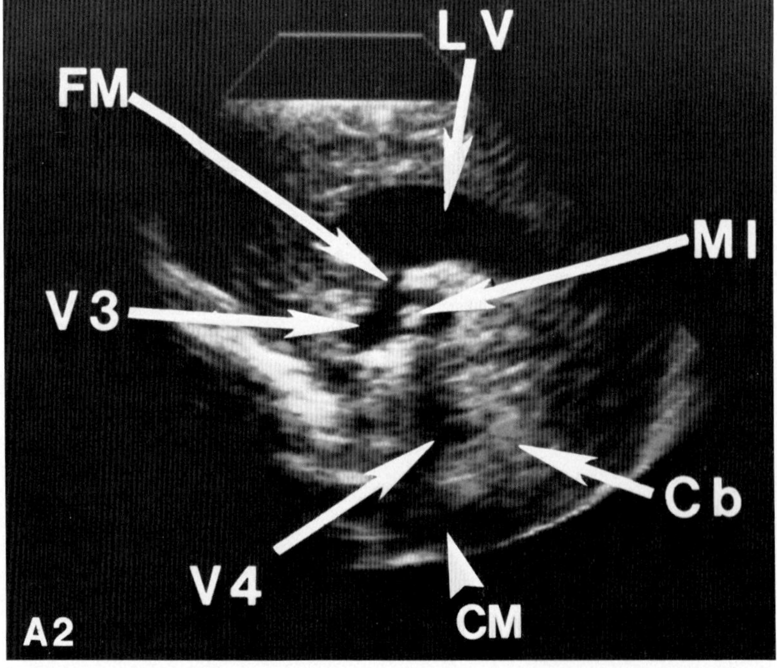
LV
FM
MI
V3
Cb
V4
CM
A2

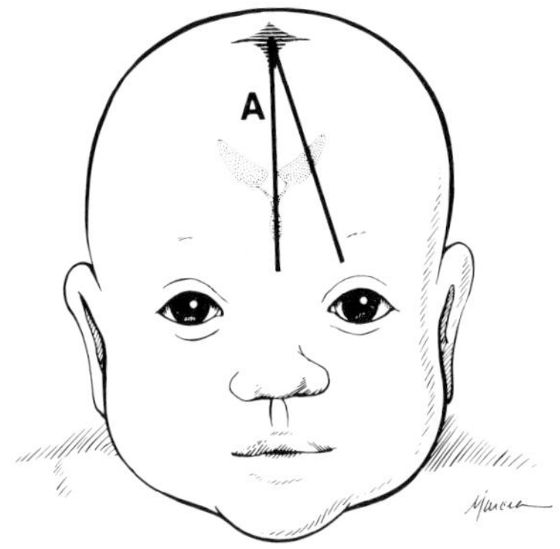

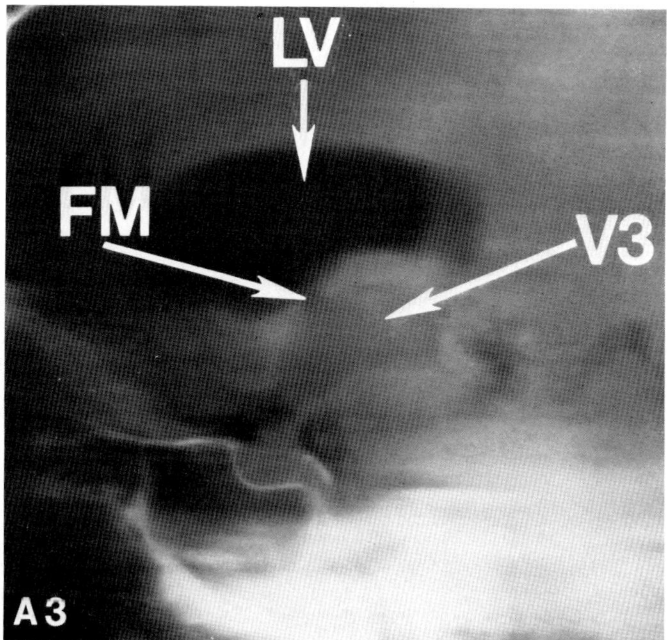

Figure 4.7 *A* Normal midline sagittal contact scan (*1*), sector real-time scan (*2*), and corresponding pneumoencephalogram (*3*). Third ventricle (*V3*). Portion of slightly dilated lateral ventricle (*LV*). Massa intermedia (*MI*) seen as dot in third ventricle. Foramen of Monro (*FM*) connects third ventricle to lateral ventricle. Fourth ventricle (*V4*) demonstrated inferiorly with echogenic cerebellum (*Cb*) forming roof. Cisterna magna (*CM*) seen as sonolucent space inferior to cerebellum. ((*2 and 3*) Reproduced with permission from D. S. Babcock and B. K. Han: *Radiology*, *139:*665–676, 1981.[8])

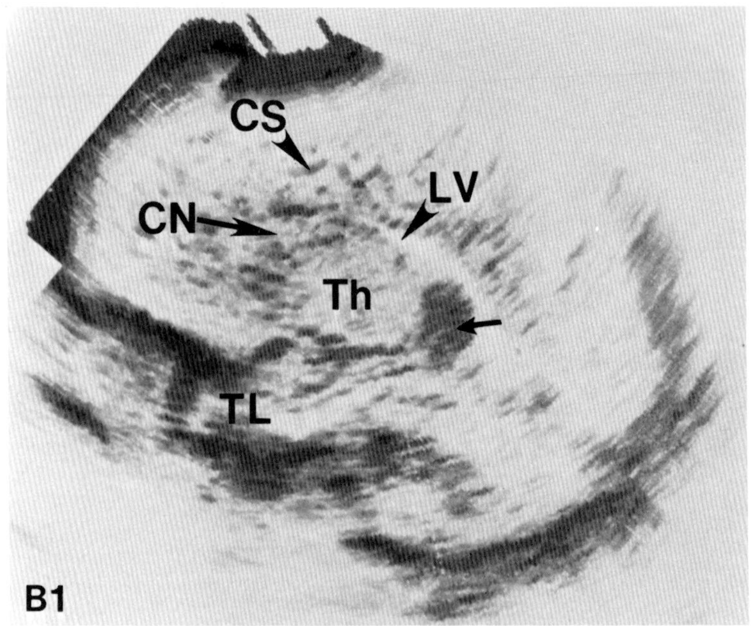
CS
CN
LV
Th
TL
B1

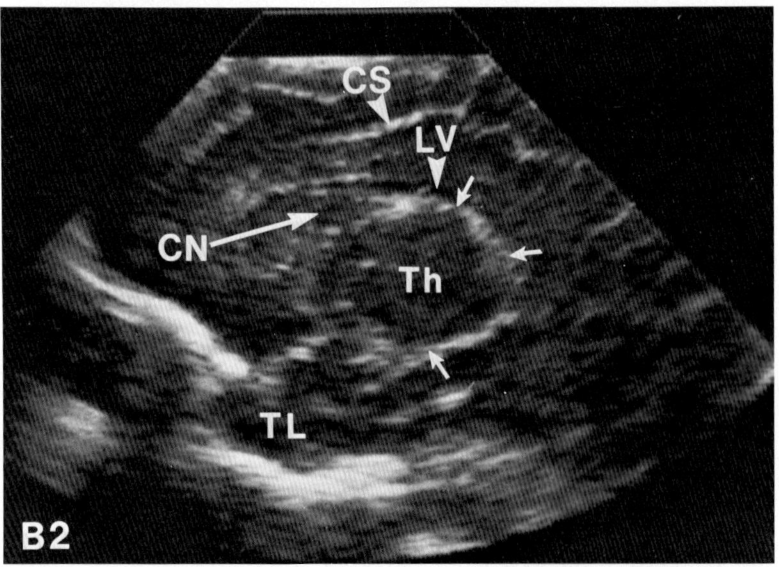
CS
LV
CN
Th
TL
B2

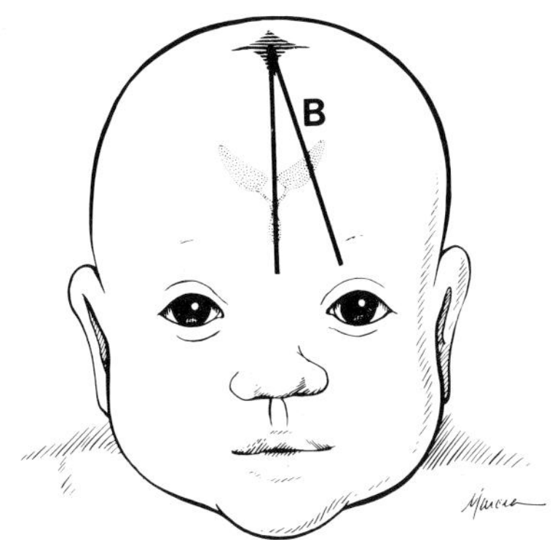

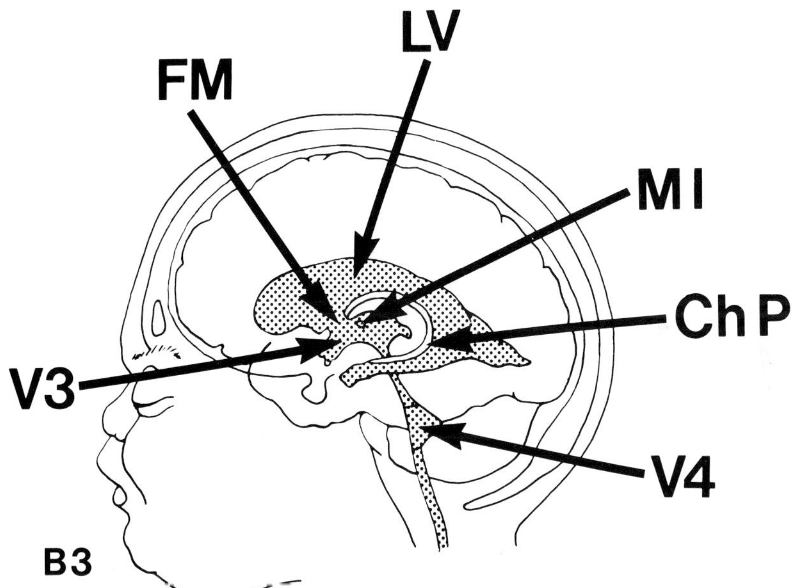

Figure 4.7 *B* Normal parasagittal contact scan (*1*), sector real-time scan (*2*), and corresponding diagram (*3*) through lateral ventricle with choroid plexus (*arrows*) beginning at foramen of Monro and coursing along floor of lateral ventricle into atrium and temporal horn. Moderately echogenic head of caudate nucleus (*CN*) lies inferior to frontal horn of lateral ventricle and anterosuperior to thalamus (*Th*). Thalamus (*Th*) lies inferior to body of lateral ventricle (*LV*). Temporal lobe (*TL*). Cingulate sulci (*CS*). ((*2* + *3*) Reproduced with permission from D. S. Babcock and B. K. Han: *Radiology*, *139*:665–676, 1981.[8])

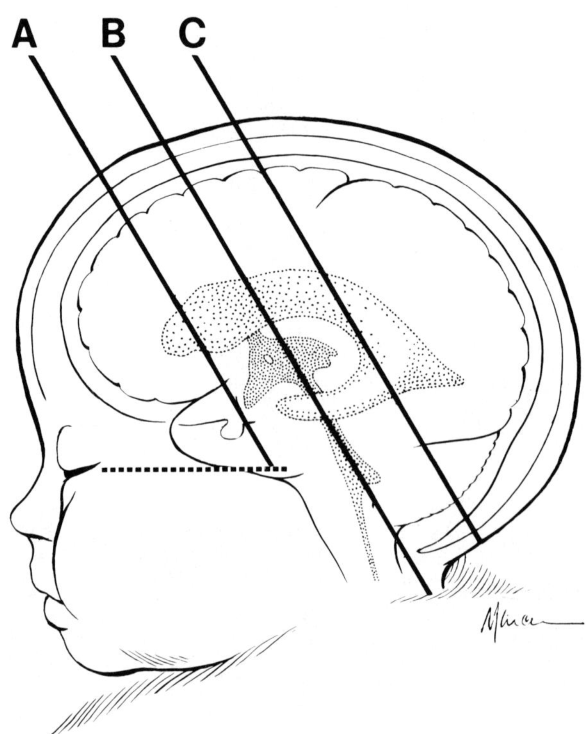

Figure 4.8 Modified coronal (60°) scanning planes.

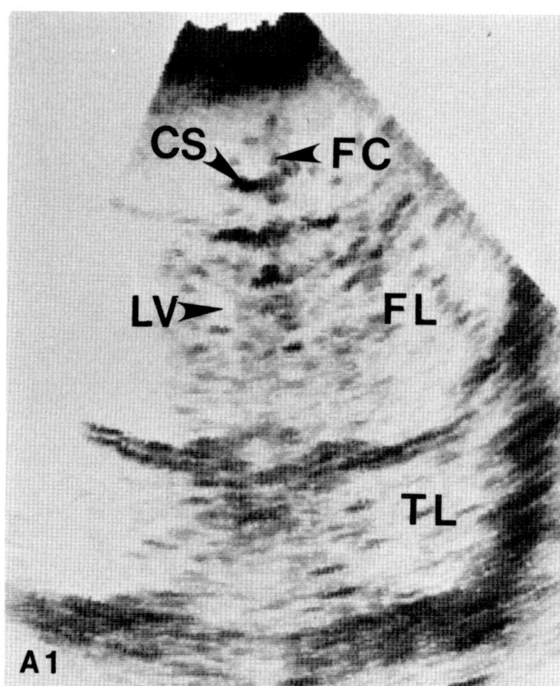

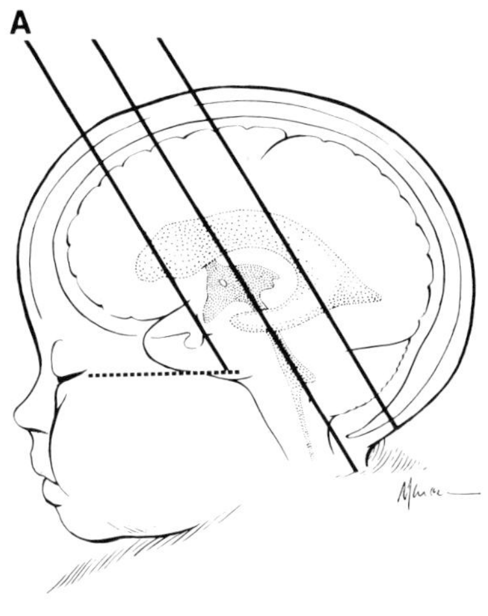

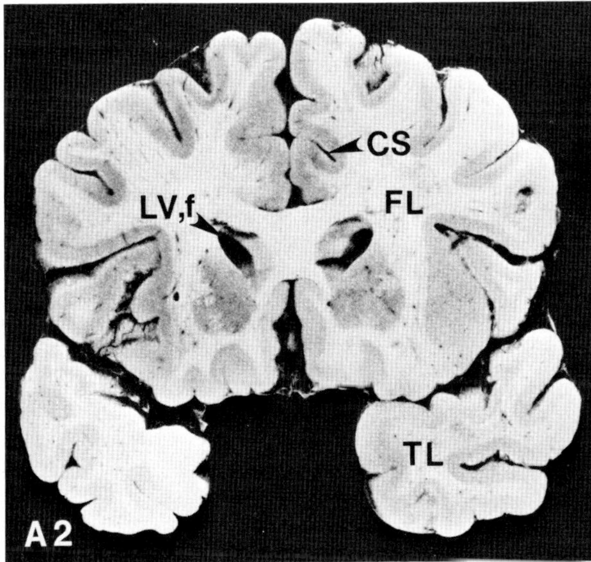

Figure 4.9 *A* Normal anterior modified coronal contact scan (*1*) and corresponding anatomic section (2) through frontal (*FL*) and temporal (*TL*) lobes. Midline linear echoes of falx cerebri (*FC*). Frontal horns of slit-like lateral ventricles (*LV*, *f*). Cingulate sulci (*CS*). ((2) Reproduced with permission from T. Matsui and A. Hirano: *An Atlas of the Human Brain for Computerized Tomography.* Tokyo: Igaku-Shoin, 1978.[1])

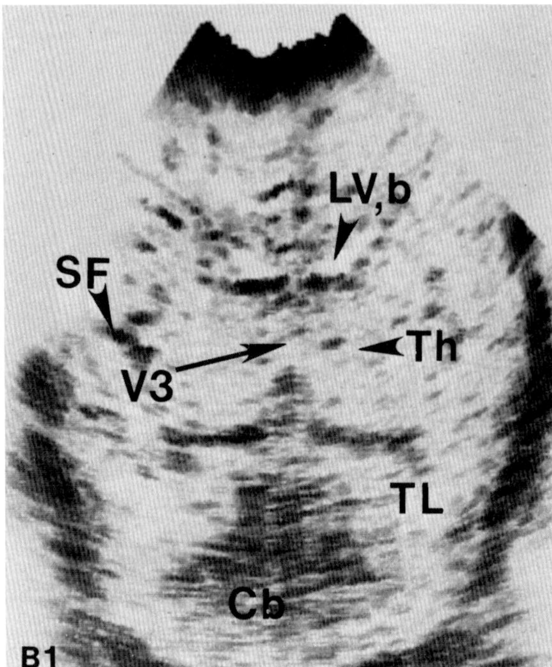

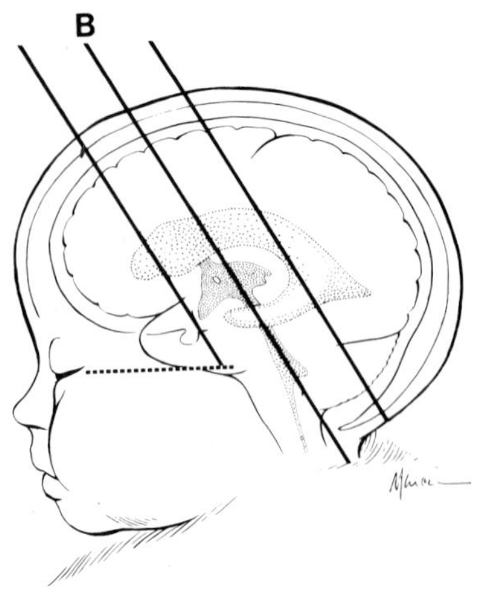

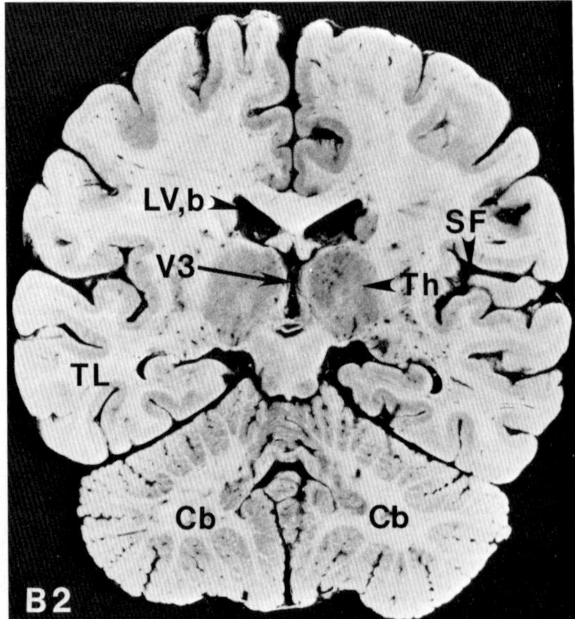

Figure 4.9*B* Normal modified coronal contact scan (*1*) and corresponding anatomic section (*2*) through bodies of lateral ventricles (*LV, b*). Thalamus (*Th*) demonstrated on either side of slit-like third ventricle (*V3*). Temporal lobe (*TL*) and more echogenic cerebellum (*Cb*). Sylvian fissure (*SF*), Y-shaped structure. ((2) Reproduced with permission from T. Matsui and A. Hirano: *An Atlas of the Human Brain for Computerized Tomography*. Tokyo: Igaku-Shoin, 1978.[1])

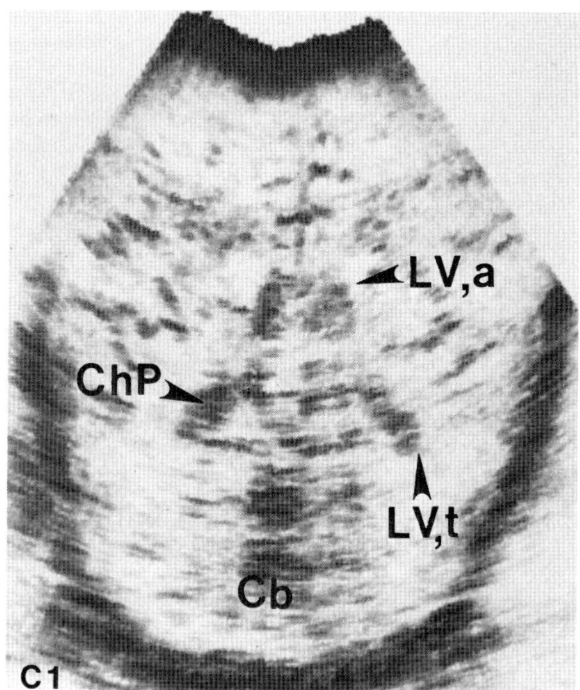

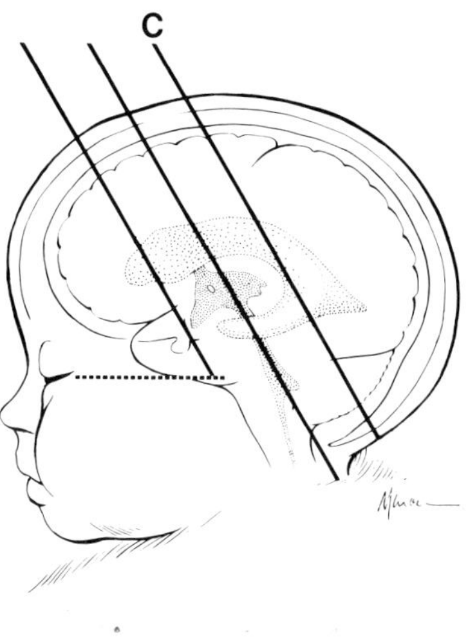

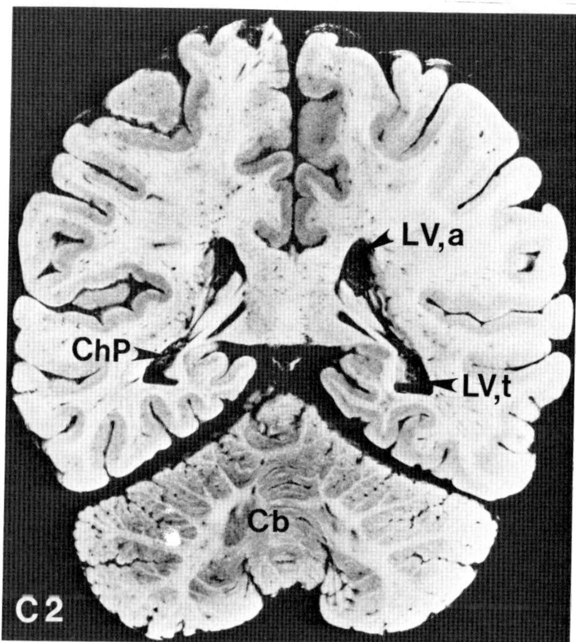

Figure 4.9*C* Normal modified coronal contact scan (*1*) and corresponding anatomic section (*2*) through atria of lateral ventricles (*LV, a*) joined by temporal horns (*LV, t*). Echogenic choroid plexuses (*ChP*) within lateral ventricles. Cerebellum (*Cb*) more echogenic than cerebrum. ((*2*) Reproduced with permission from T. Matsui and A. Hirano: *An Atlas of the Human Brain for Computerized Tomography.* Tokyo: Igaku-Shoin, 1978.[1])

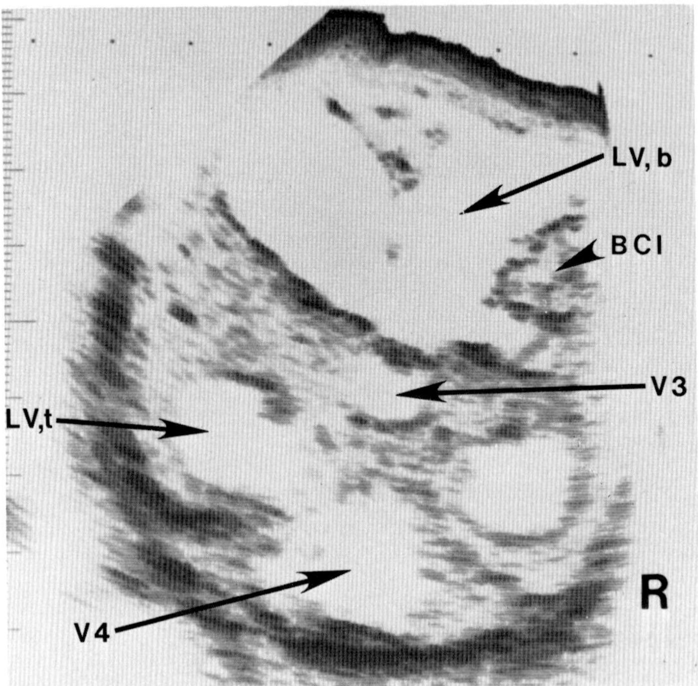

Figure 4.10 Modified coronal scan with moderate hydrocephalus showing all dilated ventricles in one plane. Body (*LV,b*), and temporal horn (*LV,t*) of lateral ventricle. Third ventricle (*V3*). Fourth ventricle (*V4*). Blood clot from previous intraventricular hemorrhage (*BCl*). (Reproduced with permission from D. S. Babcock, B. K. Han, and G. W. LeQuesne: *American Journal of Roentgenology, 134*:457–468, 1980.[7])

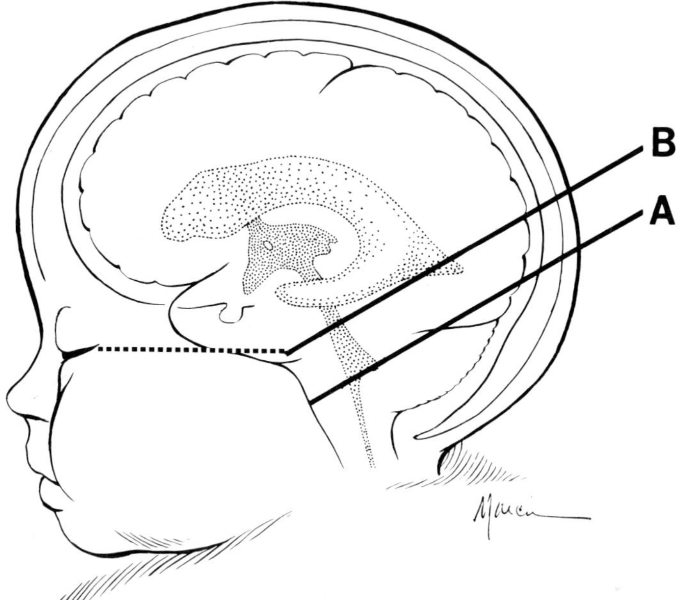

Figure 4.11 Posterior fossa scanning planes.

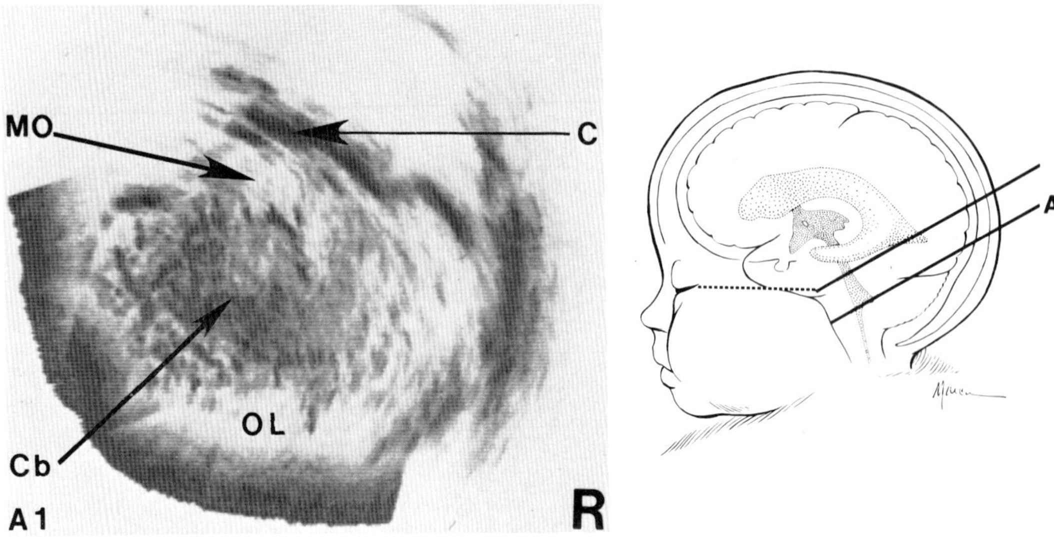

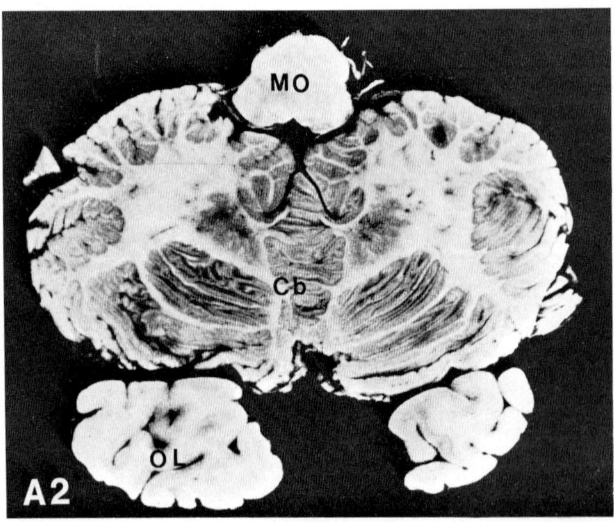

Figure 4.12 *A* Normal low posterior fossa contact scan (*1*) and corresponding anatomic section (*2*). Densely echogenic cerebellum (*Cb*) and moderately echogenic occipital lobes (*OL*). Slightly echogenic medulla oblongata (*MO*) anteriorly. Clivus (*C*). ((*1*) Reproduced with permission from D. S. Babcock, B. K. Han, and G. W. LeQuesne: *American Journal of Roentgenology*, *134:*457–468, 1980.[7] (*2*) Reproduced with permission from T. Matsui and A. Hirano: *An Atlas of the Human Brain for Computerized Tomography.* Tokyo: Igaku-Shoin, 1978.[1])

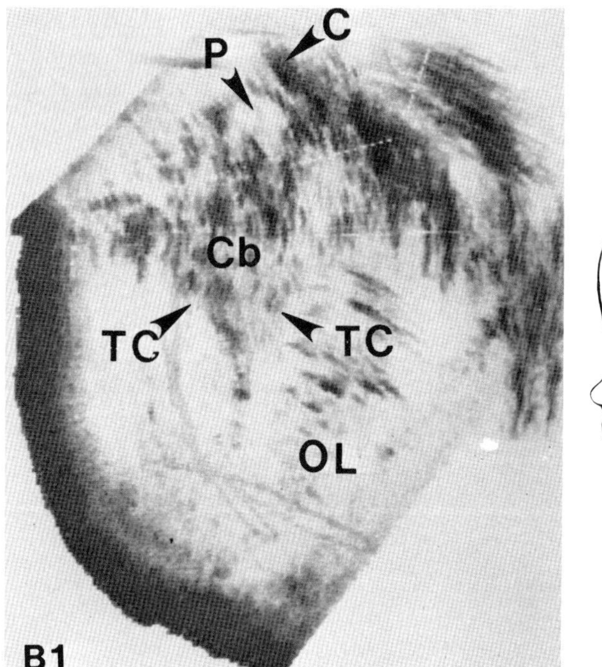

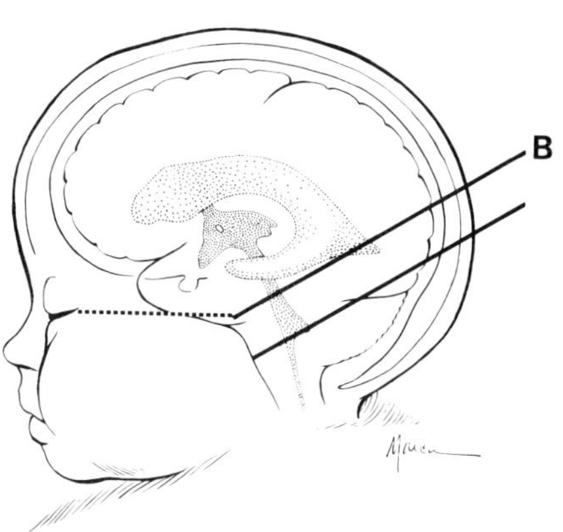

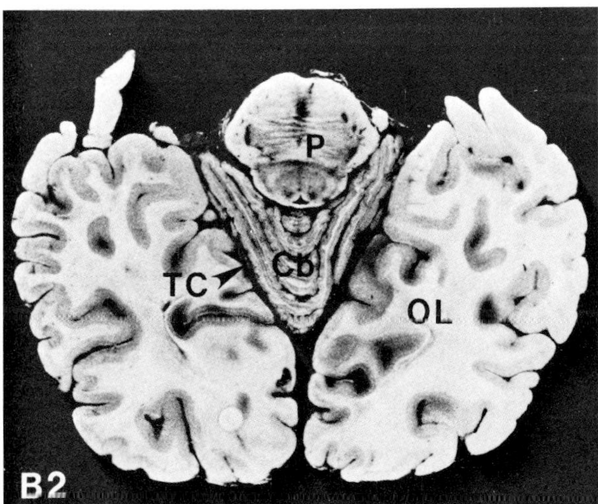

Figure 4.12 ***B*** Normal higher posterior fossa contact scan (*1*) and corresponding anatomic section (*2*) Occipital lobes (*OL*) separated from echogenic cerebellum (*Cb*) by V-shaped tentorium cerebelli (*TC*). Slightly echogenic bilobed pons (*P*) posterior to bony clivus (*C*). ((*2*) Reproduced with permission from T. Matsui and A. Hirano: *An Atlas of the Human Brain for Computerized Tomography.* Tokyo: Igaku-Shoin, 1978.[1])

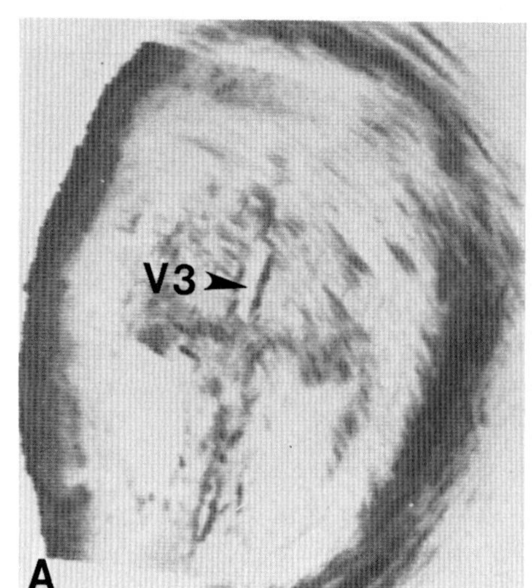
V3
A

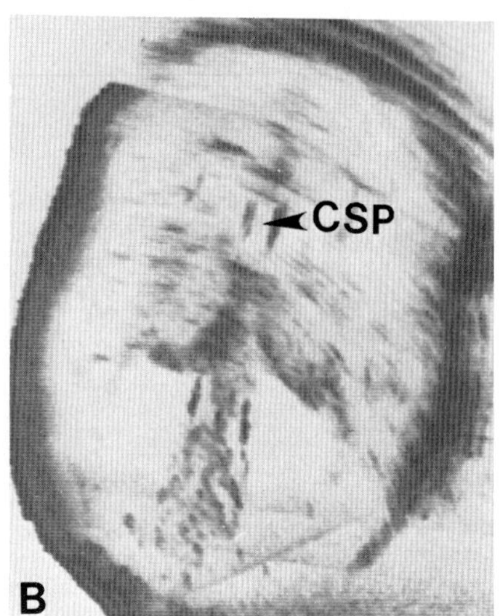
CSP
B

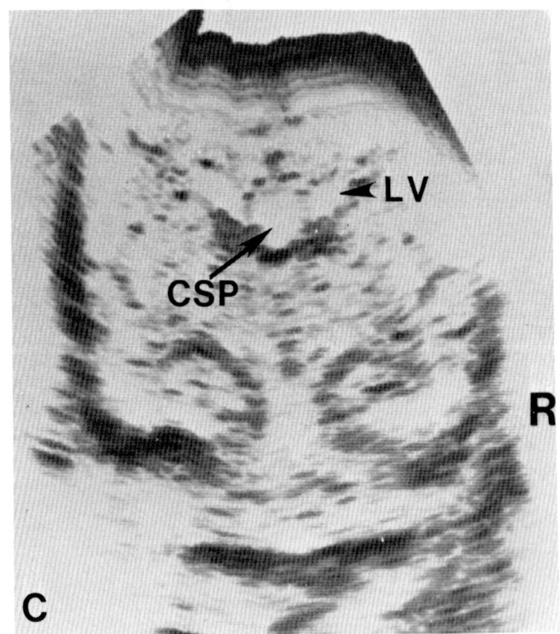
LV
CSP
R
C

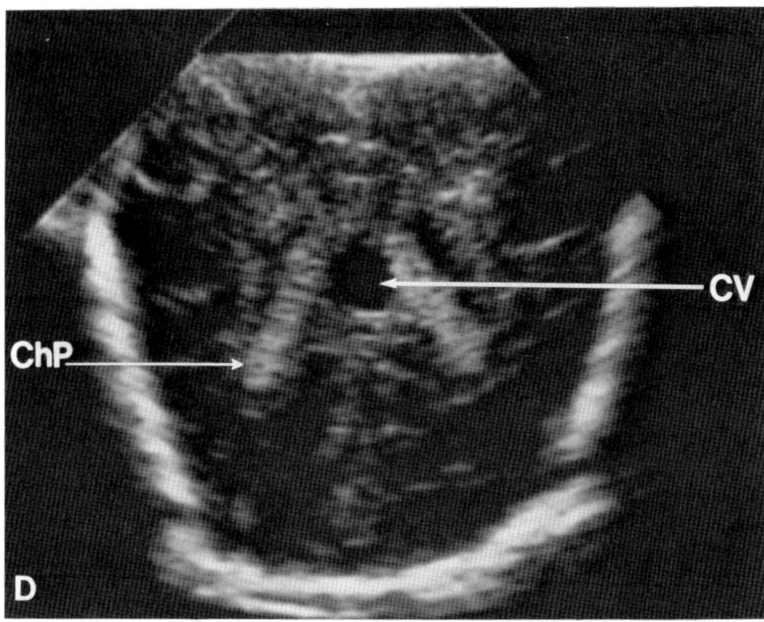

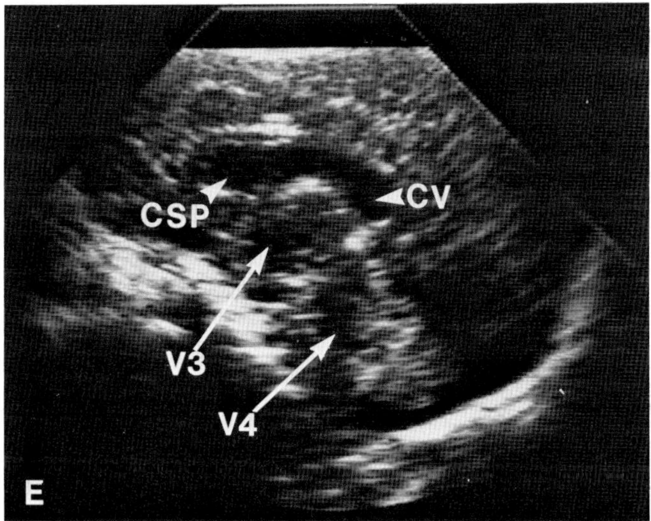

Figure 4.13 Cavum septi pellucidi and vergae. (*A*) Axial scan through lower thalamus. (*B*) Higher axial scan. Cavum septi pellucidi (*CSP*), and dilated third ventricle (*V3*) on different levels and CSP located more anterior and higher than third ventricle. (*C*) Coronal scan through frontal horns of lateral ventricles. (*D*) Posterior coronal scan and (*E*) midline sagittal scan. Cavum septi pellucidi (*CSP*) between frontal horns of lateral ventricles (*LV*). More posteriorly located cavum vergae (*CV*). Choroid plexus (*ChP*) within lateral ventricles. ((*A* and *B*) Reproduced with permission from S. Farruggia and D. S. Babcock: *Radiology*, *139:* 147–150, 1981.[6] (*C*) Reproduced with permission from D. S. Babcock, B. K. Han, and G. W. LeQuesne: *American Journal of Roentgenology*, *134:*457–468, 1980.[7])

CHAPTER 5

Fetal Intracranial Anatomy

Michael L. Johnson, M.D.

In considering imaging of the neonatal brain it should be realized that the brain can be visualized by ultrasound while the fetus is still in utero. With commercially available real-time and static gray scale ultrasound equipment it is possible to visualize intracranial anatomy in the fetus beginning in the second trimester.[1-3] It is also possible to follow the growth and development of the fetal brain throughout gestation. Analysis of vascular anatomy, as visualized by real-time ultrasound, has permitted proper identification of many neural structures. The fetal brain is a rapidly growing organ and there are marked changes apparent in the size of the cerebral ventricles from the 12th week of gestation (menstrual age) until term. Knowledge of fetal intracranial anatomy is important for accurate in utero diagnosis of intracranial pathology and for a better understanding of neonatal anatomy.

Normal Anatomy

The scanning plane must be directed to obtain a true axial section through the fetal skull. This is the same plane used for biparietal diameter measurements. In order to visualize brain parenchyma it is necessary to increase the system gain and utilize a single pass technique or real-time scanner. Serial sections are then obtained from the base of the skull up through the vertex.

The base of the fetal skull is quite easy to demonstrate. The sphenoid wings are seen anteriorly and the petrous ridges posteriorly (Fig. 5.1). With slight caudad angulation the orbits are visualized anteriorly. By scanning slightly rostrally the base of the brain is imaged. The cerebral peduncles are identified as heart-shaped, paired structures of low echogenicity with dense surrounding echoes (Fig. 5.2). The notch of the "heart" is directed anteriorly and contains the basilar artery in the interpeduncular cistern. The pulsation of this vessel can be appreciated by real-time examination and in fact it is possible to follow the pulsations of the basilar artery up into the region of the suprasellar cistern and demonstrate pulsations from the vessels in the circle of Willis. The origins of the middle and anterior cerebral arteries are routinely seen (Fig. 5.2) and the course of these vessels into the Sylvian fissure and anterior interhemispheric fissure can be visualized, respectively. In the posterior aspect of the skull the strongly reflective echoes from the tentorium diverge posteriorly from the cerebral peduncles and outline the region of the cerebellum (Fig. 5.3). The tightly packed fibers of the midbrain result in very few acoustic interfaces and thus a relatively sonolucent appearance. The cisterns, fissures and tentorium on the other hand are very echogenic; possibly due to the multiple interfaces from fat, collagen or connective tissue. Real-time demonstration of vessel pulsation is essential in delineating parenchymal brain anatomy.

By moving the scanning plane 5–10 mm toward the vertex, the region of the thalami can be seen as paired central areas of low to medium echogenicity on either side of the midline (Fig. 5.4). These should not be mistaken for the lateral ventricles which has been previously reported.[4] Between lobes of the thalami lies the third ventricle which is not normally seen in the fetus as it is only a narrow slit when not dilated. Anterior to the thalami are paired sonolucent structures representing the frontal horns. These are the most anterior inferior projections of the lateral ventricular system. A cystic structure is often seen anterior to the thalami and between the frontal horns. This represents the cavum septi pellucidi, which is a normal anatomic structure and present in all babies. It is also seen in neonates and should not be mistaken for the third ventricle.[2] In the lateral aspect of the brain at this level and slightly anterior to the thalami is a dense linear echo representing the Sylvian fissure (Fig. 5.4). Real-time examination will demonstrate pulsation of the middle cerebral artery in this fissure.

A more rostral scan, 5–10 mm above the thalami, will demonstrate the bodies of the lateral ventricles (Fig. 5.5). This portion of the brain is not easy to scan and effort on the part of the examiner is necessary to reliably visualize the lateral ventricles. In most cases the lateral walls of the ventricles are seen as linear echoes paralleling the central midline echo. The central midline echo is thought to be generated by the interhemispheric fissure and septum pellucidum.[1] The medial walls of the lateral ventricles are much more difficult to demonstrate and require increased gain and slight angulation of the scanning plane. It is important to realize that the distance from the midline echo to the lateral wall of the ventricle is not the width of the lateral ventricle as the medial wall is not imaged. Nevertheless, it is possible to measure an index of ventricular size and determine whether fetal ventricles are normal or enlarged.[1]

By measuring from the middle of the midline echo to the first echo of the lateral wall of the lateral ventricle, an index of the lateral ventricular width (LVW) is obtained. As ventricular size should always be compared with the amount of brain parenchyma present, the cerebral hemispheric width (HW) should be measured at the same level. This is represented by the distance from the middle of the midline echo to the bright echo from the inner table of the calvarium. These measurements should be made on the hemisphere away from the transducer, at the point where the hemispheric dimension is greatest (Fig. 5.5). A ratio of lateral ventricular width to hemispheric width (LVW/HW) can then be calculated. In the term gestation the average LVW measured 1.2 cm with a HW of 4.3 cm and a ratio of 28%.[1] At term the LVW/HW ratio ranged between 23 and 35% and ventricular dilatation is considered present if the LVW/HW ratio exceeds 35% in the term fetus. It is interesting that this ventricular ratio is not constant throughout gestation.

In fact, prior to 20 weeks gestation the ventricles occupy more than 50% of the hemisphere. This is terribly important to recognize in the patient being evaluated for possible fetal hydrocephalus with a history of previous neurologic defects. Figure 5.6*A* is a scan through the lateral ventricles in a 17-week fetus. The mother had a previous child with congenital hydrocephalus and was considering termination of the pregnancy if this fetus was similarly affected. The lateral ventricular width measured 0.8 cm with a hemispheric width of 1.7 cm. The LVW/HW ratio was 47% which was above the limits established for term infants and appeared dilated. We felt it was important to establish normal values for this gestational age prior to any decision and found that all babies between 15 and 18 weeks gestation had large ventricles and large ratios (Table 5.1). In fact, at 15 weeks the LVW/HW ratio can be as high as 71% with a mean of 56%.[1] The fetus in Figure 5.6*A* was followed and 5 weeks later (gestational age of 22 weeks) the LVW still measured 0.8 cm, but the HW had increased to 2.5 cm and the LVW/HW ratio had decreased to 32%, which is well within normal limits (Fig. 5.6*B*). This fetus was normal at the time of delivery. This growth pattern has been previously noted by neuroanatomists,[5, 6] but not appreciated by ultrasonologists. In the young fetus the diencephalon, including the ventricles, occupies most of the calvarium. As the fetus matures, the cerebral hemispheres (telencephalon) grow more rapidly resulting in a decrease in the LVW/HW ratio with increasing gestational age (Table 5.1). The size of the lateral ventricle increases only slowly until term, but the hemispheric width nearly triples

Table 5.1
Normal Values for Lateral Ventricular Width (LVW) and Hemispheric Width (HW)[a]

Menstrual Age (wk)	Lateral Ventricular Width (cm)	Hemispheric Width (cm)	Ratio (LVW/HW) (% ± 2 SD)
15	0.75	1.4	56(40–71)
16	0.86	1.5	57(45–69)
17	0.85	1.5	52(42–62)
18	0.83	1.8	46(40–52)
19	—	—	—
20	0.82	1.9	43(29–57)
21	0.76	2.2	35(27–43)
22	0.82	2.6	32(26–38)
23	0.83	2.5	33(24–42)
24	0.83	2.7	31(23–39)
25	1.1	3.0	34(26–42)
26	0.9	3.0	30(24–36)
27	0.9	3.0	28(23–34)
28	1.1	3.3	31(18–45)
29	1.0	3.4	29(22–37)
30	1.0	3.4	30(26–34)
31	1.0	3.4	29(23–36)
32	1.1	3.6	31(26–36)
33	1.1	3.4	31(25–37)
34	1.1	3.8	28(23–33)
35	1.1	3.8	29(26–31)
36	1.1	3.9	28(23–34)
37	1.2	4.1	29(24–34)
Term	1.2	4.3	28(22–33)

[a] From M. L. Johnson et al.[1]

from the 15th week until term. Great care must be exercised in evaluating a fetus for hydrocephalus prior to 20 weeks gestation. The patient should be examined as early as possible (15–16 weeks) and then reexamined at 20–22 weeks to determine the direction the ventricles and hemisphere are growing. In a normal fetus the LVW/HW ratio should decrease significantly in 4–5 weeks and should be less than 50% by 21 weeks. The ratio should not increase during this time.

Another important anatomic feature to recognize in the young fetus is the prominent size and echodensity of the choroid plexus (Fig. 5.7). From 12 to 18 weeks the choroid plexus may completely fill the lateral ventricles and the choroid should not be mistaken for a tumor or brain parenchyma as has been previously reported.[4]

Fetal Intracranial Pathology

Many of the intracranial abnormalities detected in the neonate and discussed in detail in other chapters of this textbook have been diagnosed in utero.[7–11] Certainly it is now possible to detect most cystic masses within the fetal cranium and we have correctly diagnosed hydrocephalus, encephalocele, Dandy-Walker cyst, arachnoid cysts and posterior fossa cysts.[1, 7, 8] Other lesions, such as hydranencephaly,[8, 9] microcephaly,[10, 11] and anencephaly[7, 10] have also been diagnosed in utero. We have not, as of yet, detected a solid brain tumor in utero, nor have we detected intracranial hemorrhage prior to delivery.

The in utero diagnosis of intracranial pathology can be very difficult due to the multiple artifacts which can be produced within the fetal skull and careful attention to technique and normal anatomy is essential. Reverberation echoes can be mistakenly interpreted as lateral ventricles or mass lesions and increased gain near the transducer can produce noise within a cystic lesion which will mask it or give the appearance of unilateral hydrocephalus. An example of reverberation artifact is shown in Figure 5.8. The curved echo within the skull is due to the sound pulse traveling back and forth twice from the transducer to the outer skull table of the fetus. As the distance of the skull from the maternal skin surface increases, the artifact bends. This artifact is quite obvious, but many are much more subtle and will lead to misdiagnosis if the examiner is not extremely careful. We will often repeat an examination in hopes of finding the fetus in a better position and use different transducers and different equipment.

Hydrocephalus can be diagnosed reliably even in the fetus with a normal biparietal diameter and no enlargement of the skull (Fig. 5.9). We have accurately diagnosed hydrocephalus before 20 weeks gestation in at least six pregnancies and this has significantly affected the obstetrical management of these patients. We have had no false negative or false positive diagnoses for hydrocephalus. With careful scanning, it is possible to determine if the third and fourth ventricles are enlarged and it is always important to examine the entire length of the fetal spine searching for a neural tube defect. With isolated hydrocephalus, the amniotic fluid α-fetoprotein will not be elevated and management decisions will rest solely on the ultrasound diagnosis. Body computed tomography is not necessary in the evaluation of fetal hydrocephalus if good real-time ultrasound equipment is available.

The evaluation of fetal intracranial anatomy is possible in all pregnancies and ultrasound is sufficiently reliable and accurate to make a major impact on management decisions in the obstetrical patient. Any fetus with a questionable ultrasound examination in utero should be examined with ultrasound in the neonatal period.

References

1. Johnson ML, Dunne MG, Mack LA, Rashbaum CM. Evaluation of fetal intracranial anatomy by static and real-time ultrasound. J Clin Ultrasound 1980; 8:311–318.
2. Denkhaus H, Winsberg F. Ultrasonic measurements of the fetal ventricular system. Radiology 1979; 131:781–786.
3. Hadlock FP, Deter RL, Park SK. Real-time sonography: ventricular and vascular anatomy of the fetal brain in utero. AJR 1981; 136:133–137.
4. Hobbins JC, Venus I. Congenital anomalies. Clin Diagn Ultrasound 1979; 3:95.
5. Lemire RJ, Loeser JD, Leech RW, et al. *Normal and Abnormal Development of the Human Nervous System.* New York: Harper & Row, 1975; 95.
6. Moore KL. *The Developing Human. Clinically Oriented Embryology* (Ed. 2). Philadelphia: W. B. Saunders, 1977.
7. Dunne MG, Johnson ML. The ultrasonic development of fetal abnormalities in utero. J Reprod Med 1979; 23:195–206.
8. Rumack CM, Johnson ML. Antenatal diagnosis of neonatal diseases. Clinics in Ultrasound (1981) in press.
9. Lee TG, Warren BH. Antenatal diagnosis of hydranencephaly by ultrasound: Correlation with ventriculography and computed tomography. J Clin Ultrasound 1977; 5:271.
10. Garrett WJ, Fisher CC, Kossoff G. Hydrocephaly, microcephaly and anencephaly diagnosed in pregnancy by ultrasound echography. Med J Aust 1975; 2:587.
11. Kurtz AB, Wapner RJ, Rubin CS, et al: Ultrasound criteria for in utero diagnosis of microcephally. J Clin Ultrasound 1980; 8:11–16.

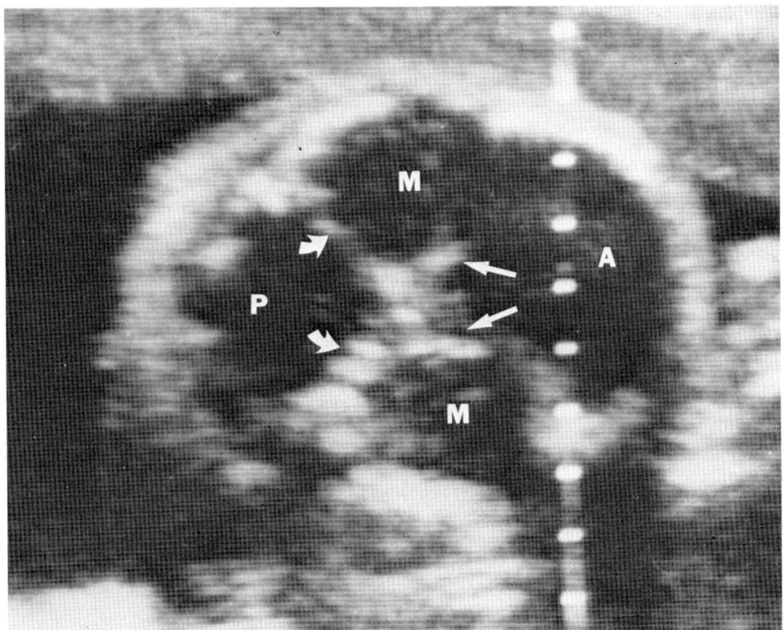

Figure 5.1 Axial scan through base of skull in 28-week fetus with occiput to the left of image. The anterior (*A*), middle (*M*), and posterior (*P*), cranial fossae are visualized. The petrous ridges are seen posteriorly (*curved arrows*) and the sphenoid wings (*straight arrows*) are imaged anteriorly.(Reproduced with permission from M. L. Johnson et al.: *Journal of Clinical Ultrasound*, *8*:311–318, 1980.[1])

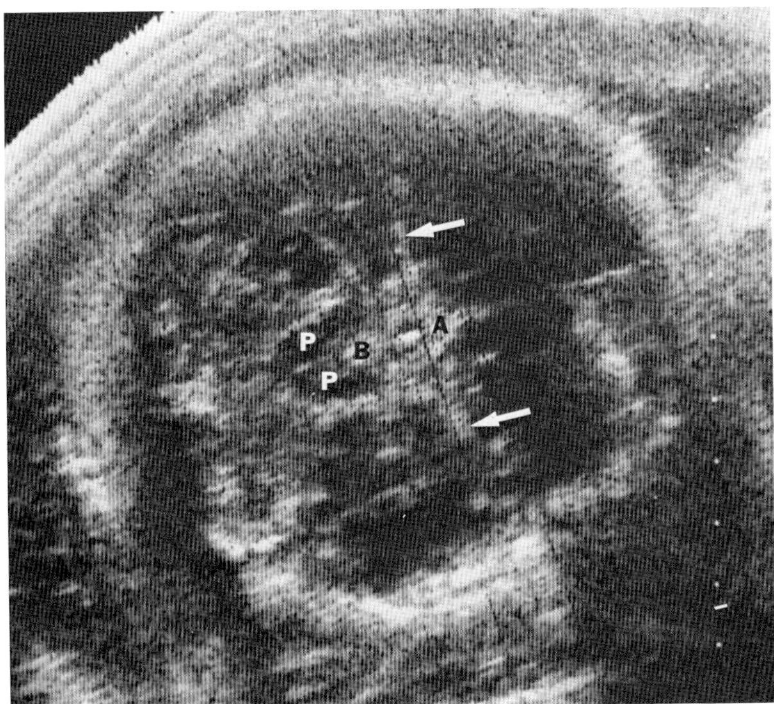

Figure 5.2 Axial scan through the base of the brain in a 35-week fetus demonstrating the area of the supracellar cistern. The basilar artery (*B*) is anterior to the cerebral peduncles (*P*). The communicating vessels of the circle of Willis form an echogenic circle connecting the basilar artery to the region of the anterior cerebral artery (*A*). The middle cerebral arteries (*arrows*) are traversing out laterally. (Reproduced with permission from M. L. Johnson et al.: *Journal of Clinical Ultrasound*, *8*:311–318, 1980.[1])

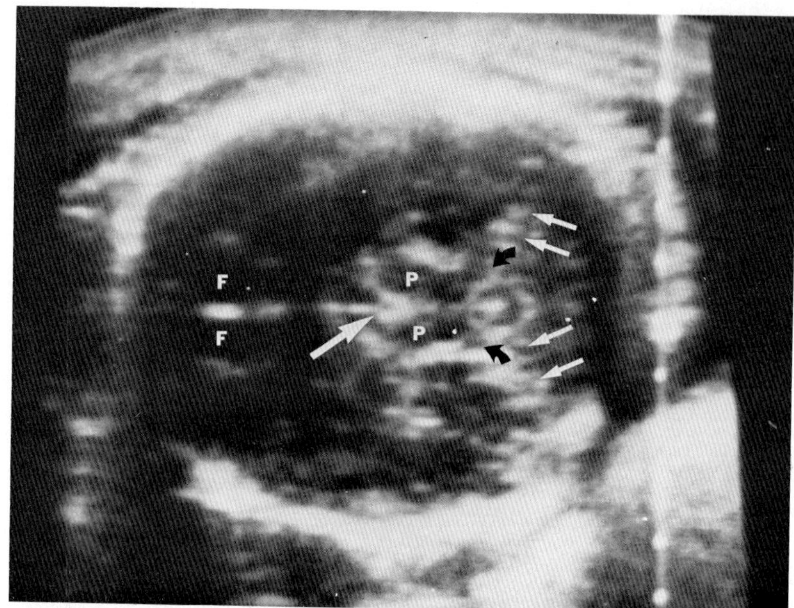

Figure 5.3 Axial scan at the level of the cerebral peduncles (*P*) in 32-week fetus with occiput to the right of image. The tentorium produces strongly reflective echoes (*small white arrows*) which diverge posteriorly. The basilar artery is located in the interpeduncular cistern (*large white arrow*) and the cerebellar peduncles (*black arrows*) are seen projecting posteriorly from the cerebral peduncles into the posterior fossa. The frontal horns (*F*) of the lateral ventricles are seen anteriorly. (Reproduced with permission from M. L. Johnson et al.: *Journal of Clinical Ultrasound*, *8:*311–318, 1980.[1])

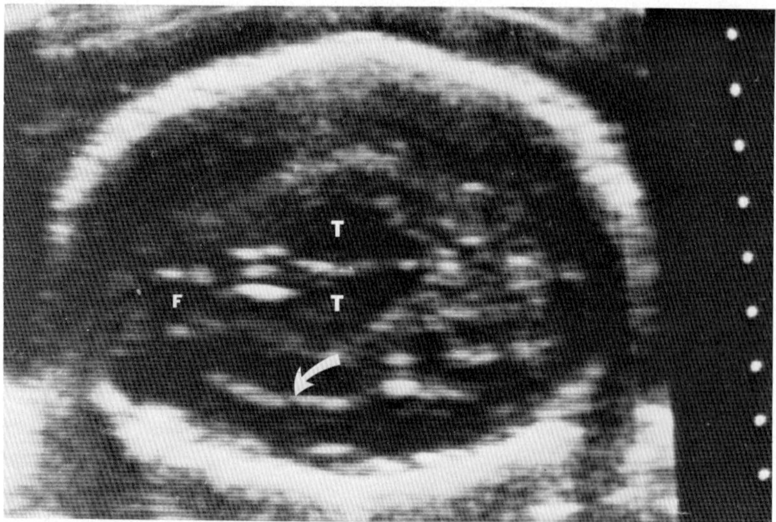

Figure 5.4 Single pass scan through the level of the thalami (*T*) in 31-week fetus. Occiput is to right of scan. Anterior to the thalami is the region of the columns of the fornix. The frontal horns (*F*) are poorly seen. The Sylvian fissure appears as a dense echogenic line (*arrow*) in the hemisphere contralateral to the transducer. (Reproduced with permission from M. L. Johnson et al.: *Journal of Clinical Ultrasound*, *8:*311–318, 1980.[1])

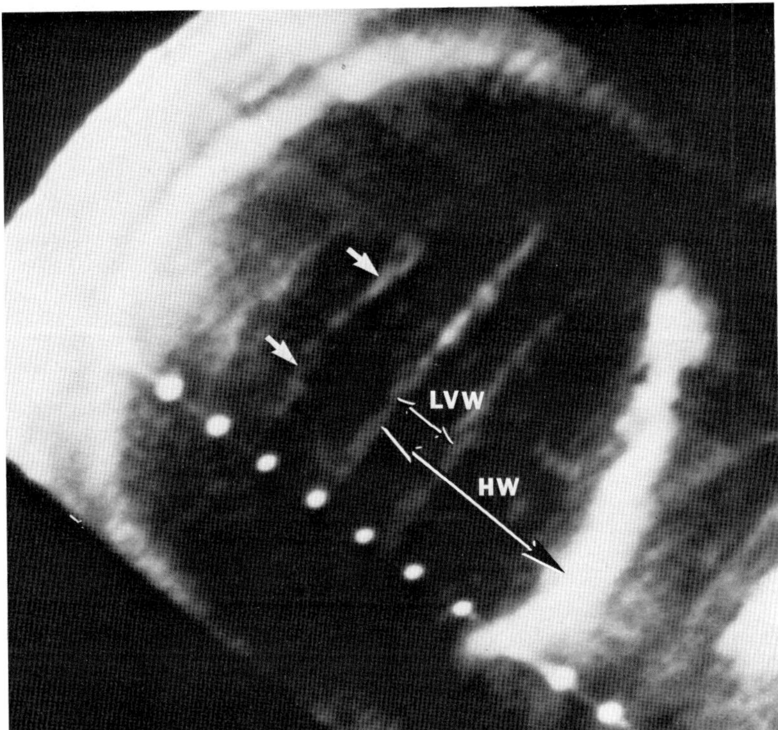

Figure 5.5 Scan through lateral ventricles of term fetus. The lateral walls of the ventricles (*white arrows*) parallel the central midline echo. Occiput is to the left and posterior. Lateral ventricular width (*LVW*) is measured from the midline echo to first strong echo from lateral wall of lateral ventricle. Hemispheric width (*HW*) is measured from the midline echo to the first echo from the inner table of the skull. The lateral ventricular ratio is LVW/HW. The measurements are made at the point of maximal hemispheric dimension.

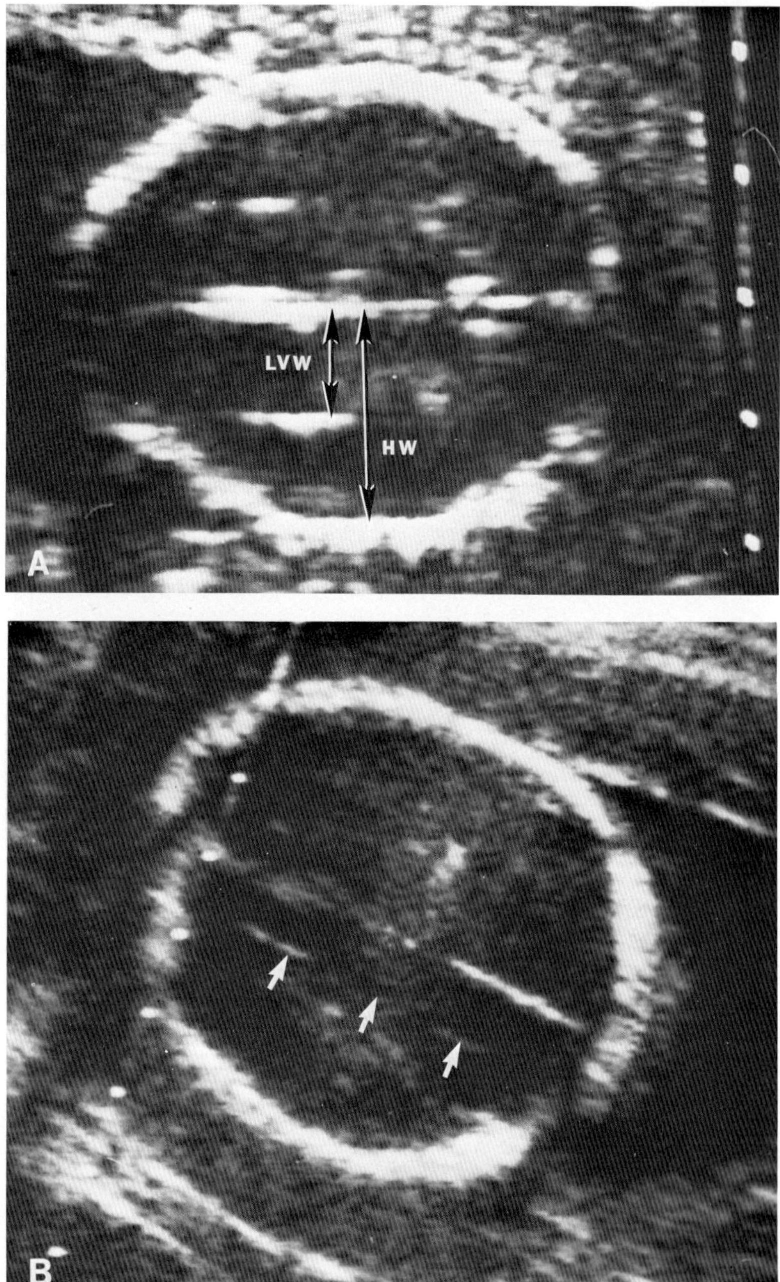

Figure 5.6 (*A*) Single pass scan through the lateral ventricles in a 17-week fetus. The lateral ventricular ratio measured 47%. (*B*) Scan of same infant 5 weeks later at 22 weeks gestational age. The lateral ventricular ratio now measures 32%. The lateral wall of contralateral ventricle is visualized (*arrows*). Ipsilateral lateral ventricle is obliterated by noise.

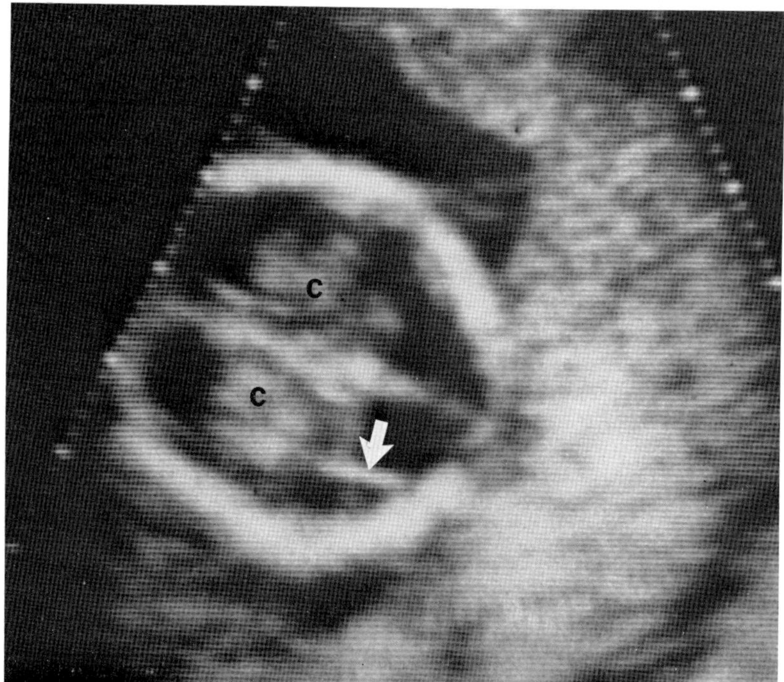

Figure 5.7 Real-time scan through level of lateral ventricles in a 16-week fetus. The lateral wall of the lateral ventricle is a dense straight line (*arrow*). Within the lateral ventricle is the densely echogenic choroid plexus (*C*) which is very prominent at this gestational age. (Reproduced with permission from M. L. Johnson et al.: *Journal of Clinical Ultrasound*, *8*:311–318, 1980.[1])

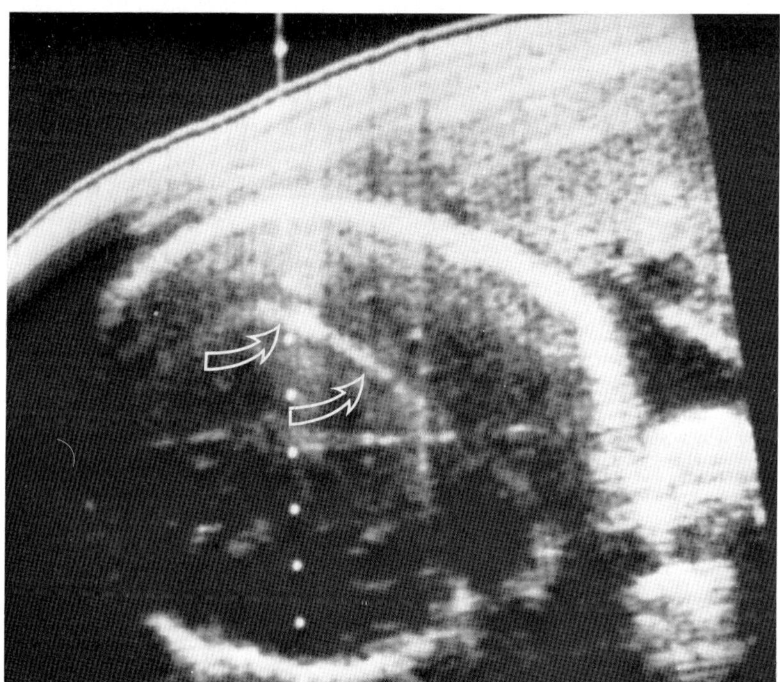

Figure 5.8 Single pass scan through fetal head at term demonstrating reverberation artifact (*arrows*). As the distance from the maternal skin surface to the fetal skull echo increases, the artifact bends posteriorly. Occiput is to the left of scan. (Reproduced with permission from M. L. Johnson et al.: *Journal of Clinical Ultrasound*, *8*:311–318, 1980.[1])

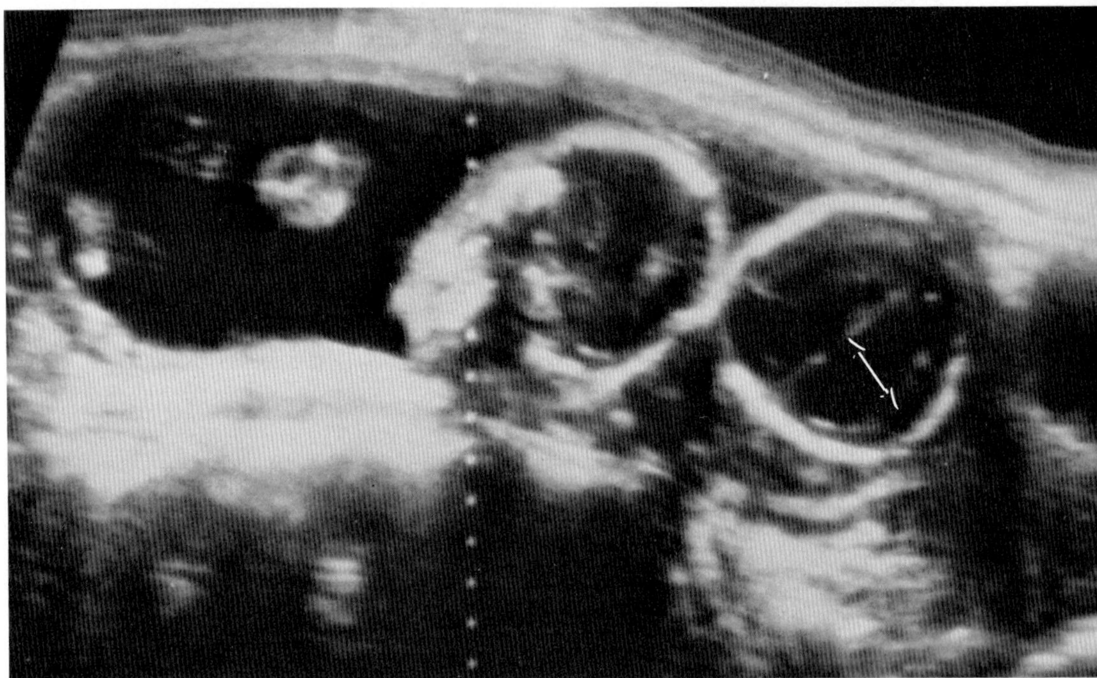

Figure 5.9 Longitudinal scan through gravid uterus at 22 weeks gestation. The lower twin had dilatation of the lateral ventricles noted at 18 weeks gestation and confirmed at 22 weeks. The lateral ventricle (*arrow*) measures 1.9 cm and the hemispheric width is 2.8 cm for a ventricular ratio of 68%. The infant had gross hydrocephalus at the time of delivery. (Reproduced with permission from M. L. Johnson et al.: *Journal of Clinical Ultrasound*, *8*:311–318, 1980.[1])

CHAPTER 6

Automated Water Delay Head Scanning

Kai Haber, M.D.

Various methods of generating cross-sectional anatomic images by pulsed-echo ultrasound have been developed. The vast majority of diagnostic ultrasound instruments in clinical use today employ direct contact of the ultrasonic transducer to the patient's skin with only a thin intervening layer of mineral oil or other suitable coupling agent. An alternative to contact scanning involves interposition of a long water path between the transducer and the patient. This chapter will describe such a system which is commercially available and detail its applicability to intracranial imaging in neonates and young children.

Historical Perspective

Among the first instruments developed for B-mode cross-sectional ultrasonic imaging were systems which utilized water path technology. The pioneers in medical ultrasonics, Howry, Bliss, and Holmes, developed the so-called "Somascope" in 1950.[1, 2] Although excellent images were obtained, this system was quite cumbersome and clinically impractical, requiring total submersion of the anatomical area of interest in a large circular water tank (Fig. 6.1). A single ultrasonic transducer was mechanically moved back and forth on a horizontal track. The horizontal track assembly in turn was transported on a circular track around the 360° circumference of the water tank. Thus, the first compound two-dimensional ultrasonic images for medical diagnosis were produced. Because this "wet" system appealed mainly to mermaids and these were in short supply in Denver hospitals in the early 1950s, the water tank was modified into a semicircular pan. The patient was examined in the upright position with the area to be imaged applied to a flexible plastic membrane acting as a dam and indenting the straight side of the semicircular water pan (Fig. 6.2). Coupling was achieved by application of KY jelly. Because the system was still cumbersome and precluded examination of sick patients unable to sit upright, the University of Colorado group channeled its main efforts into development of contact scanners.

In 1961, Dr. George Kossoff of the Australian Government National

Acoustics Laboratories began development of advanced water-delay pulsed-echo technology. In his early systems, the patient was also either sitting or standing coupled to a membrane stretched over an opening in the side of a tub. Compound scans were achieved by a single transducer which was mechanically sectored through an arc while riding back and forth on a horizontal rail[3]. Dr. Kossoff, who in 1969 developed gray scale ultrasonic imaging, continued work on water-offset technology and in 1975 built an automated general purpose echoscope utilizing eight transducers and called the Octoson.[4, 5]

Instrumentation Description and Examination Technique

The Octoson utilizes eight large diameter transducers submerged in a large water tank covered by a plastic membrane, on which the patient lies (Fig. 6.3). The movement of the array of transducers and the scanning functions are carried out remotely from the control console. The array of transducers has 5° of motion freedom so that it can be placed anywhere in the tank for the examination of various body areas at multiple angles.

A water-offset system allows the use of large diameter crystals, dramatically increasing returning echo-collecting efficiency. Crystal diameter is 55 mm, as compared to standard static scan crystal dimensions of 13 or 19 mm. The large aperature of the transducers together with the water offset permits focusing in the transition zone at the junction of the near and far fields, thus avoiding the acoustically complex near field and taking advantage of the long focal zone available in this region. Using a large transducer in direct contact with the patient would result in poor coupling and a short focal zone (Fig. 6.4). In comparing the large aperture transducer in a water delay system with a smaller standard sized contact transducer, there is a larger usable focal zone in the water-delay system (Fig. 6.5). This obviates the need for transducers with varying depths of focus. The transducers operate at 2.9 MHz.

The eight transducers are linked together so that they are mechanically sectored in unison. They are pulsed in sequence. Each transducer sectors through an arc of 55° and one line of sight is generated for each 0.1° of sector (Fig. 6.6). Thus, there are 4400 lines of sight for each image.

Images can be generated utilizing all eight transducers or any combination thereof. The scan is obtained in from 0.5 to 2.0 sec, depending on the number of transducers being fired.

There is a microprocessor which can be programmed so that serial echograms can be obtained automatically in any desired plane. Routinely, we obtain semi-axial and coronal scans at 5-mm intervals. The semi-axial scans are made in the same plane as those used for conventional computerized tomography (CT) studies. Slice thickness is between 2 and 4 mm, depending upon the amount of gain used. An entire head study can be generated in less than 5 minutes. The axial scans are viewed "from the patient's feet." Coronal scans are "face to face" with the patient. The orientation of the image is similar to that used in CT. The limiting factor is not the time necessary for the generation of the scans but the exposure time of the image formater. Because of the mechanical nature of this system and because this system is not dependent upon the manual skill of the operator, images are highly reproducible during one study and also from one examination to another.

Unlike the somewhat limited fields of view generated by real-time sector scanners, Octoson images of the head are panoramic, CT-like presentations. There are major advantages in anatomical orientation, particularly for the referring clinicians. Hard copies are of very high image quality.

The water temperature is between 35° and 37.5° C. This, together with the fact that there is no direct physical contact between the transducer and the neonate, induces sleep or rest. Generally, little or no sedation is required. A small gauze pad or edge of a blanket is placed underneath the eyes on the dependent side (Fig. 6.7). This is done to prevent the mineral oil, which is used as an acoustic couplant, from entering the eye. Generally the examination is performed with the left side down, though frequently right-side-down and occasionally occiput-down, examinations are performed, particularly if intraventricular blood clots or blood casts are suspected.

The advantage of this type of water-delay system is the rapid generation of panoramic echographic views which in many ways are comparable to those obtained with CT. Imaging is not limited by skull contours or the ear, nor is it dependent upon acoustic "windows" such as the fontanelles or sutures. The two disadvantages of this type of instrumentation are the relatively high initial costs and the obvious lack of portability.

Clinical Applications

Diagnostic studies are routinely obtained in children up to the age of 24 months. Even though we have been successful in imaging the intracranial contents in 6-year-olds, this is the exception, rather than the rule. In older children calvarial ossification and increased convolutions of the inner table of the skull produce formidable barriers to penetration and straight line propagation of the ultrasonic pulses.

At the University of Arizona, we have performed over 300 examinations on some 108 patients in the past 2 ½ years. In order to ascertain the accuracy of the ultrasonic images, measurements of normal ventricles, dilated ventricles and certain pathologic fluid collections (Dandy-Walker cyst, subdural hygroma, etc.) were made from both CT and sonographic images.[6] Figure 6.8 is a linear regression analysis demonstrating the excellent correlation between CT and ultrasonic measurements in the first 19 patients.

A great many normal structures are routinely identifiable in both axial (Fig. 6.9) and coronal planes (Fig. 6.10). Because the entire circumference of the head in any given slice is visualized, orientation is simplified, aiding in recognition of both normal and pathologic anatomy.

Ultrasound examination is highly sensitive for detection of even mild degrees of hydrocephalus[7] and is the procedure of choice when clinicians wish to determine the presence or absence of a dilated ventricular system. Figure 6.11 shows a normal infant and three other infants with varying degrees of hydrocephalus.

A communicating form of hydrocephalus is one of the sequelae of intraventricular hemorrhage in neonates, particularly those who are premature. The ventricular dilatation, felt to be secondary to an arachnoiditis as a response to the presence of blood, may be self-limiting and spontaneously regress, may remain stable or may be progressive, sometimes quite rapidly. Serial ultrasound examinations will readily distinguish between these three courses.

In cases of progressive ventricular dilatation and in cases of hydrocephalus persisting despite frequent ventricular taps, placement of a ventriculoperitoneal shunt is frequently indicated. Octoson examinations offer an ideal way to both ascertain the immediate postoperative success of the shunt and to monitor the patient on a long term basis. Frequent serial postoperative ultrasound examinations have revealed some interesting findings about the time course of ventricular decompression following surgical placement of a shunt. We examined patients frequently (often daily) during the first postoperative week. In a series of 11 patients, 81% of the decrease in ventricular size during the first postoperative week occured within the first 24 hours following shunting. We then undertook a study to determine the response on an even shorter time scale. A series of 12 other patients were examined with ultrasound within 90 min after shunt placement and then re-examined 24 hours postoperatively. Fifty-three percent of the decrease in ventricular size noted at 24 hours had already occurred 1 1/2 hours after shunt placement.

Although we do not yet have the necessary number of cases or long enough follow-up to show a statistically significant relationship between initial response to shunting and prognosis for neurological development, initial results are promising at the extremes of response. Figure 6.12 shows a dramatic, rapid, and steady decrease in ventricular size in a child who at 2 years of age appears neurologically normal. Figure 6.13 shows a very poor response to ventriculoperitoneal shunting. At age 20 months, the child appears moderately retarded. Duration of hydrocephalus before shunting, initial degree of ventriculomegaly, and other variables may be important in prognosis as well. Because subtle neurologic changes, particularly reduced intellectual capacities, are difficult to measure in young children, a long term investigation is being undertaken to determine if there is any prognostic value to knowing how the ventricles respond to shunting in the immediate postoperative period.

The full-term infant with severe congenital hydrocephalus in Figure 6.11 had very little demonstrable cortex on the initial ultrasound examination shortly after birth (Fig. 6.14*A*). After surgical shunt placement there were dramatic increases in cortical thickness and decreases in ventricular size on the 2nd (Fig. 6.14*B*) and 4th (Fig. 6.14*C*) postoperative days. Some 6 months later ventricular size was normal (Fig. 6.14*D*) and at 1½ years the child had reached developmental milestones on a timely basis and was neurologically normal.

Increasing head circumference and bulging fontanelles are gross changes reflecting increasing ventricular size over time. They are not nearly as sensitive as serial ultrasonic studies, which are particularly valuable in evaluating the patency and function of permanent ventriculoperitoneal shunts. Figure 6.15 illustrates initial excellent response to shunting (Fig.

6.15, *A* and *B*) and the effects of mechanical shunt failure 2 months after surgery (Fig. 6.15 *C*).

Once a ventriculoperitoneal shunt has been placed, the neurosurgeon is obligated to keep it functional. These children are also, of course, susceptible to the same childhood diseases as any normal infants are. When a shunted infant presents with nonspecific symptoms, such as irritability, the pediatrician must always be concerned about shunt patency. An ultrasound study can quickly assess ventricular size and aid in making the proper diagnosis.

Serial ultrasound examinations after shunting for hydrocephalus are also helpful in detecting complications which may arise postoperatively. Ventricular decompression may cause localized areas of mantle collapse resulting in formation of subdural hygromas (Fig. 6.16). On occasion the degree of collapse of the cerebral mantle can be quite significant (Fig. 6.17). Subgaleal fluid collections can occur if cerebrospinal fluid is under particularly high pressure or if the shunt tube holes become plugged (Fig. 6.18).

The incidence of subependymal and intraventricular hemorrhage in premature infants, particularly those under 1000 g birth weight, is very high.[8] Ultrasound affords a convenient noninvasive method of detecting the results of these hemorrhages.[9, 10] The premature infant in Figure 6.19 shows the typical appearance of subependymal hemorrhage in the region of the germinal matrix.

Intraventricular blood casts are particularly well imaged by ultrasound. The neonate in Figure 6.20 demonstrates moderate hydrocephalus with a blood cast in each lateral ventricle. Note that the cast shifts to the dependent side in each position. Imaging the patient in these different positions, especially with the occiput down, helps to differentiate free floating casts or clots from the equally echogenic choroid plexus.

Sagittal views may be obtained by placing the infant in the upside-down position by holding the feet up and placing the top of the head in contact with the membrane. This does not endear the ultrasonographer to the patient; however, it appears that serial sections in the sagittal plane aid in anatomical display, especially in the middle and posterior cranial fossae.[11]

Changing patient position is also quite helpful in detecting small accumulations of fluid in the subdural space. The strong echoes of the calvarium and the dependent position of the brain makes identification of a subdural hematoma or hygroma on the side against the membrane difficult. In Figure 6.21 the subdural fluid collections are bilateral; but only one can be imaged at a time, that one being on the nondependent side away from the transducers.

Ultrasound may on occasion give information not available from CT. The ultrasound and CT examinations in figure 6.22 both readily demonstrate a left frontal hematoma. Note, however, that the Octoson examination clearly shows a central fluid area representing early liquefaction. This was not discernible on the CT examination. The newborn patient in Figure 6.23 was delivered by Caesarean section because of massive intrauterine hydrocephalus. Initial response to ventriculoperitoneal shunting was good (no images shown). When the patient returned some 4 weeks later with shunt failure, gross hydrocephalus was identified by both CT and echography. Note that an arachnoid cyst was readily demonstrated on the sonogram (Fig. 6.23, *A* and *B*). However, even on the enhanced CT examination (Fig. 6.23*C*), this finding was not as clear. Metrizamide was percutaneously instilled into the cyst (Fig. 6.23*D*) to determine presence or absence of communication with the ventricular system.

Another area in which the Octoson has proven to be clinically very useful is in the detection and diagnosis of congenital intracranial abnormalities. A 2-week-old infant with the Dandy-Walker malformation shows the expected dysplastic cerebellar hemispheres and the cystic replacement of the posterior fossa cyst (Fig. 6.24). The cerebellum has increased echogenicity, particularly in comparison with the brainstem which is, as usual, relatively echo free. A case of agenesis of the corpus callosum shows the typical findings on the axial ultrasound and CT images (Fig. 6.25, *A* and *B*). The third ventricle is interposed between the laterally displaced lateral ventricles. A prenatal ultrasound study in another case demonstrated a large cystic structure which appeared to extend from the fetal head (Fig. 6.26*A*). The infant was delivered by Caesarean section and an encephalocele with a thin stalk was immediately surgically removed without intracranial exploration. Shortly after the operation, the patient's head was examined on the Octoson. The axial CT and Octoson views show hydrocephalus (Fig. 6.26, *B* and *C*). Note the pointed shape of the frontal horns consistent with dysgenesis of the corpus callosum. Compare this with the case of agenesis of the corpus callosum in Figure 6.25. The coronal view (Fig. 6.26*D*) shows the extension from the left lateral ventricle that communicated with the encephalocele. This was not apparent on the axial sonograms or on CT.

Ultrasound is best suited for displaying fluid lesions which are by far the most common type of intracranial pathology in the first 2 years of life. However, solid lesions do occur and these can be successfully imaged by water-delay ultrasound technique. A 4-year-old boy had Wiskott-Aldrich syndrome and primary central nervous system lymphoma which had been previously treated with radiotherapy. Shortly before the ultrasound and CT image in Figure 6.27 were made, a burr hole had been placed to evacuate a subdural fluid collection. The CT and Octoson slices were made at comparable levels. Because of differences in positioning for the two studies, the air-fluid level in the subdural space is in the coronal plane on CT and in the sagittal plane on ultrasound. Note the acoustic shadow "behind" the air. The midline is shifted to the left by the subdural collection and there is a left hemispheric mass. The density of this mass did not change with contrast enhancement and its CT numbers were well below that of calcium. No definitive abnormality is demonstrated. The increased density may be due to hemosiderin deposition (occasionally seen in treated lymphoma) or other high density tissue in the tumor.

A different patient who presented with brain stem symptoms was initially examined by CT (Fig. 6.28*A*). This study showed marked hydrocephalus and a soft tissue mass (glioma) in the region of the brain stem and tentorial notch. A ventricular shunt was placed and a follow-up sonogram was performed (Fig. 6.28*B*). The soft tissue tumor in the region of the tentorial notch is again well seen (Fig. 6.28*C*). Note the normal clearly defined brainstem in a different patient for comparison (Fig. 6.28*D*).

Summary

An automated, water-delay ultrasonic instrument rapidly produces high quality reproducible images of the intracranial contents in infants and children up to the age of 2 years. The examinations are not dependent upon the presence of acoustic windows such as open fontanelles or sutures. Each slice encompasses the entire cranium at that level, giving a panoramic view comparable to that obtained with CT. This optimizes orientation to normal and pathologic anatomy both for the diagnostic imager and the referring clinician.

This technique is particularly useful in defining fluid-filled lesions such as hydrocephalus, Dandy-Walker cysts, arachnoid cysts, porencephalic cysts and subdural fluid collections. Follow-up examinations in patients with intraventricular hemorrhage can signal the early onset of hydrocephalus well before increasing head circumference or bulging fontanelles is noted.

Frequent ultrasonic examinations after ventriculoperitoneal shunting in hydrocephalic neonates and children demonstrate the results of the treatment, detect shunt failure on a time basis and alert the neurosurgeon to any complications such as subdural fluid collections or mantle collapse. Congenital anomalies and some solid tumors are also readily demonstrable.

Acknowledgment. The author thanks Dr. Janice R. Smith, Laura E. Jasso, and Mary E. Giroux for their valuable assistance.

References

1. Howry DH, Bliss WR. Ultrasonic visualization of soft tissue structures of the body. J Lab Clin Med 1952; 40:579–592.
2. Holmes JH et al. The ultrasonic visualization of soft tissue structures in the body. Trans Am Clin Climat Assoc 1954; 66:208–225.
3. Jellins J et al. Ultrasonic visualization of the breast. Med J Aust 1971; 1:305–307.
4. Kossoff G et al. *Ultrasound in Medicine*, Vol 2, White D, Barnes (eds). New York: Plenum, 1976; 333–339.
5. Garrett W et al. *Ultrasound in Medicine*, Vol 2, White D, Barnes (eds). New York: Plenum, 1976; 341–349.
6. Haber K et al. Ultrasonic evaluation of intracranial pathology in infants: a new technique. Radiology 1980; 134:173–178.
7. Garrett WI, Kossoff G, Warren PS. Cerebral ventricular size in children: a two-dimensional ultrasonic study. Radiology 1980; 136:711–715.
8. Grant EG et al. The ultrasonic appearance of intraventricular hemorrhage. Presented at 66th Scientific Assembly of Radiological Society of North America, 1980.
9. Bejar R et al. Diagnosis and follow-up of intraventricular and intracerebral hemorrhage by ultrasound studies of infant's brain through the fontanelles and sutures. Pediatrics 1980; 66: 661–673.
10. Horbar ID et al. Ultrasound detection of changing ventricular size in posthemorrhagic hydrocephalus. Pediatrics 1980; 66:674–678.
11. Duffy P et al. Neonatal brain echography—the value of sagittal, parasagittal and occipital sections. Presented at 66th Scientific Assembly of Radiological Society of North America, Nov. 1980.
12. Howry DH. A brief atlas of diagnostic ultrasonic radiologic results. Radiol Clin North Am 1965; 3:433–452.
13. Holmes JH, Howry DH. Ultrasonic diagnosis of abdominal disease. Am J Dig Dis 1963; 8: 12–32.

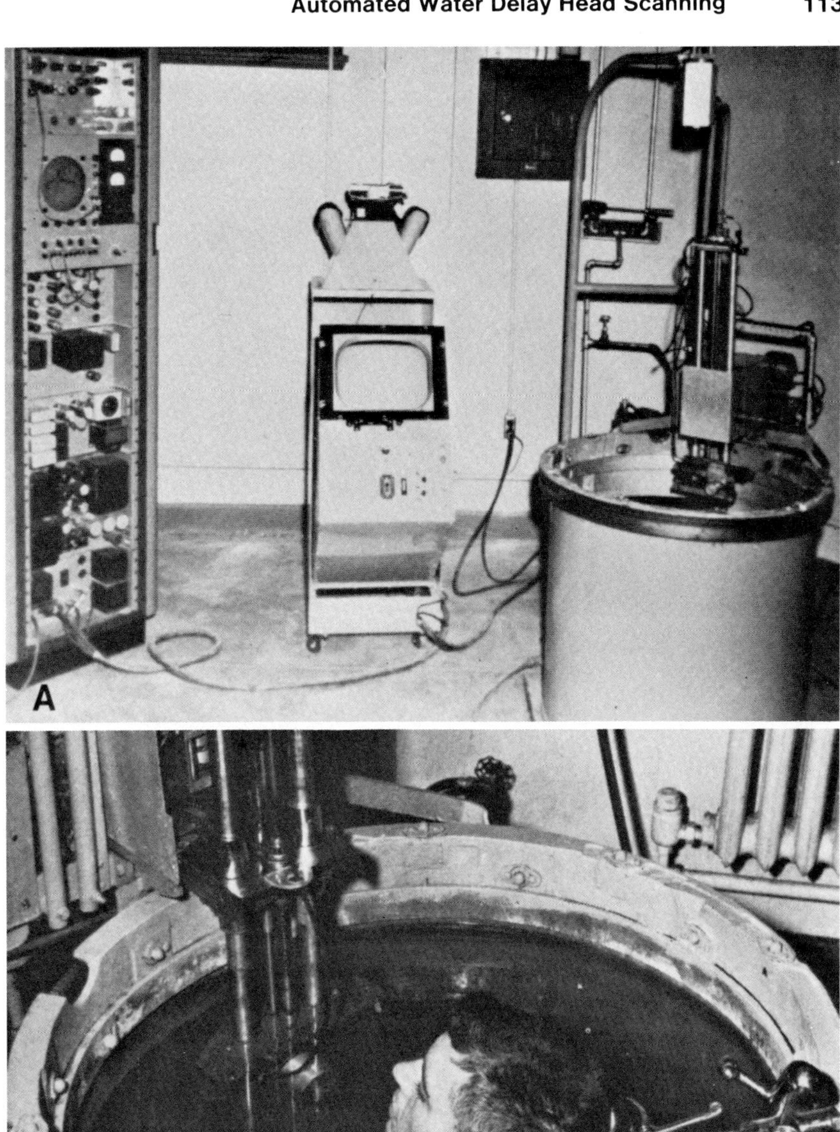

Figure 6.1 The Somascope (*A*) was first water-delay ultrasonic instrument developed in 1950 by Howry, Bliss, and Holmes.[1,2] (*B*) Patient was submerged in water tank while transducer traveled around tank on horizontal track. (Reproduced with permission from D. H. Howry: *Radiologic Clinics of North America*, *3:* 433–452, 1965.[12])

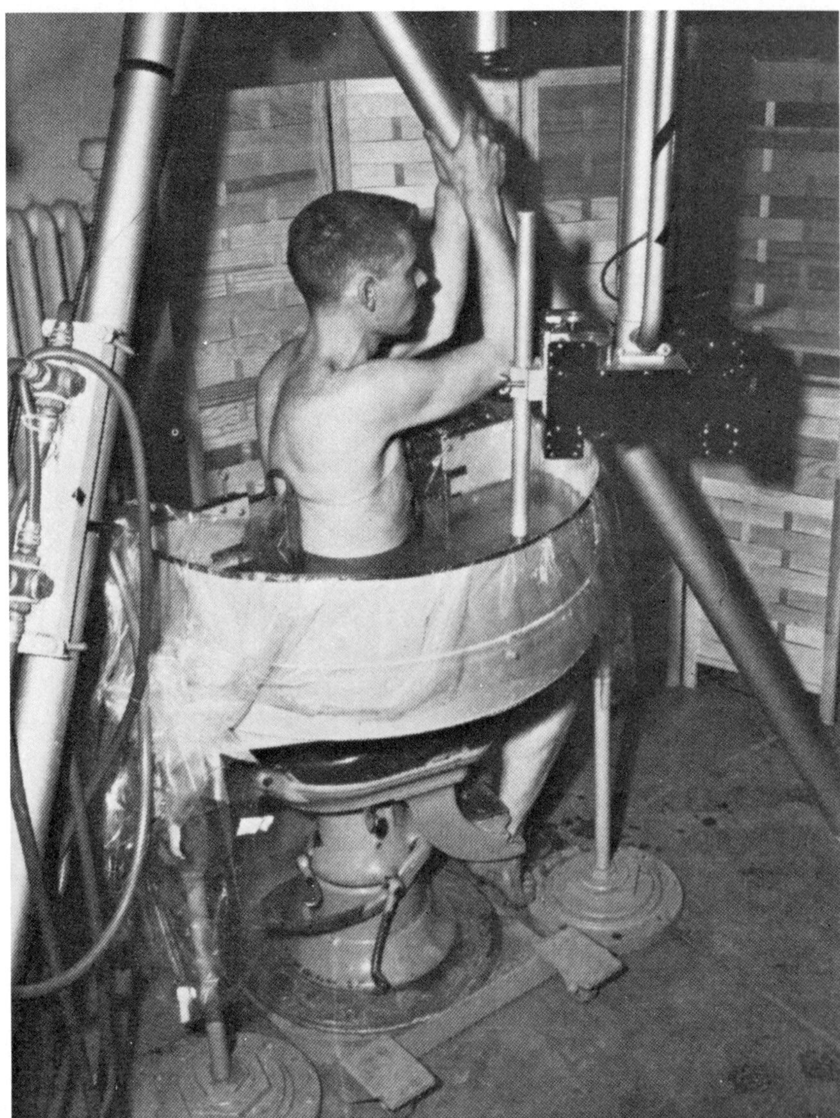

Figure 6.2 Half-pan water path ultrasound scanner allowed patient to sit outside water tank with body part being examined indenting plastic membrane acting as dam. (Reproduced with permission from J. H. Holmes and D. H. Howry: *American Journal of Digestive Diseases*, *8:*12–32, 1963.[13])

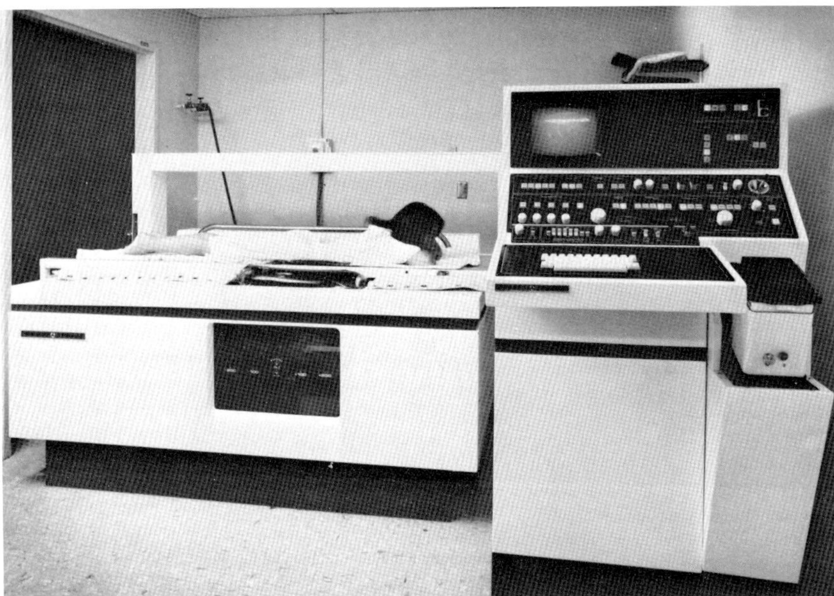

Figure 6.3 This automated, programmable, water path ultrasonic instrument is called the Octoson. In this figure, patient is lying supine upon plastic membrane while abdomen is being examined.

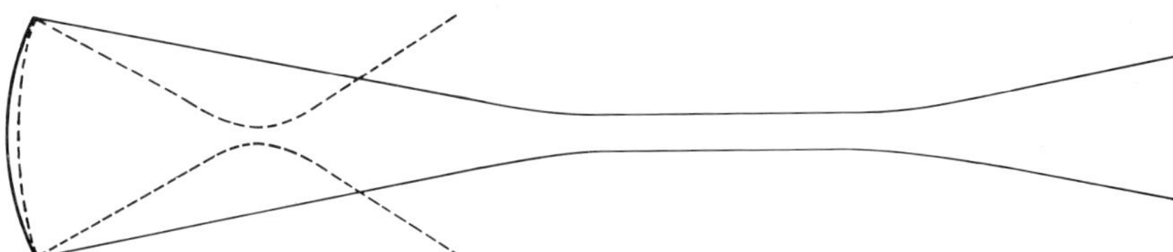

Figure 6.4 Large aperture (55 mm diameter) transducer and water path used in Octoson results in reasonably long focal zone (*solid lines*) which is not in acoustically complex near-field. Utilizing transducer of this size in contact instrument not practical because large curved surface would be in poor contact with body part examined and because of very narrow focal zone (*dotted lines*).

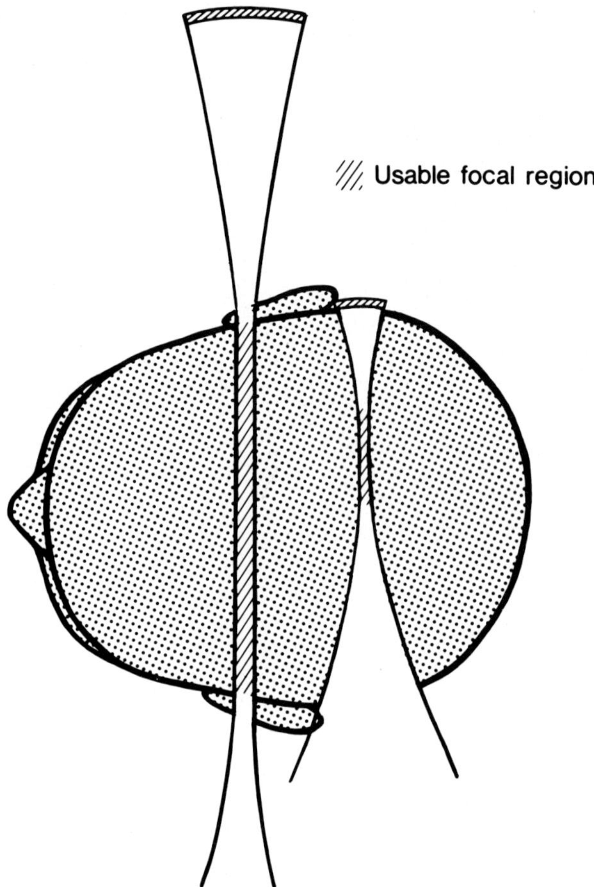

Figure 6.5 Large aperture transducer yields longer usable focal zone than smaller diameter of standard contact transducer. Note that the smaller the focal point (zone) the more rapidly the beam widens in far field.

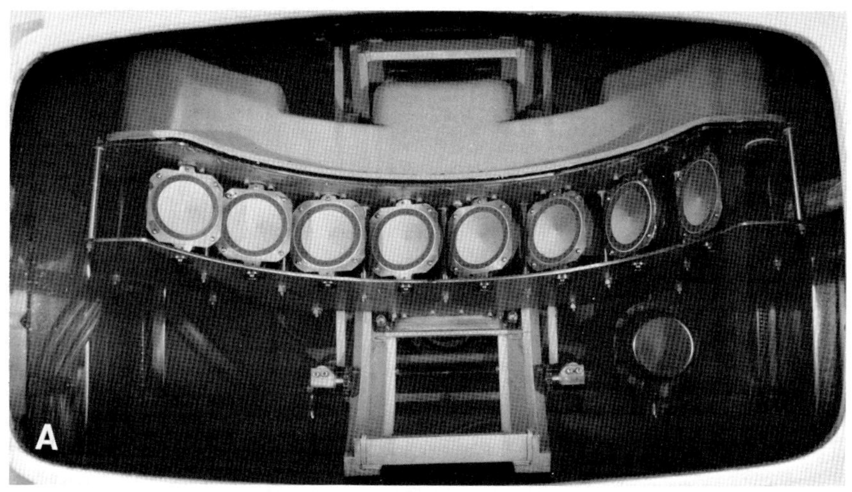

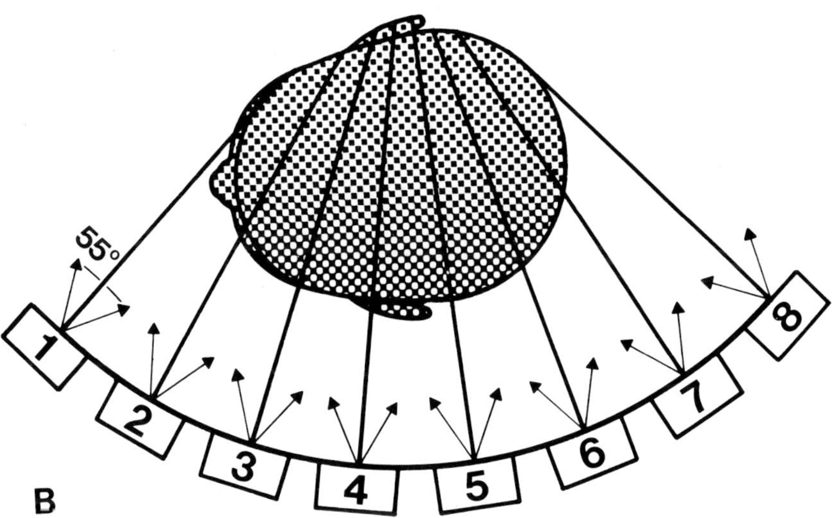

Figure 6.6 (A and B) Eight transducers each scan through arc of 55° yielding panoramic image of entire circumference of calvarium and intracranial contents.

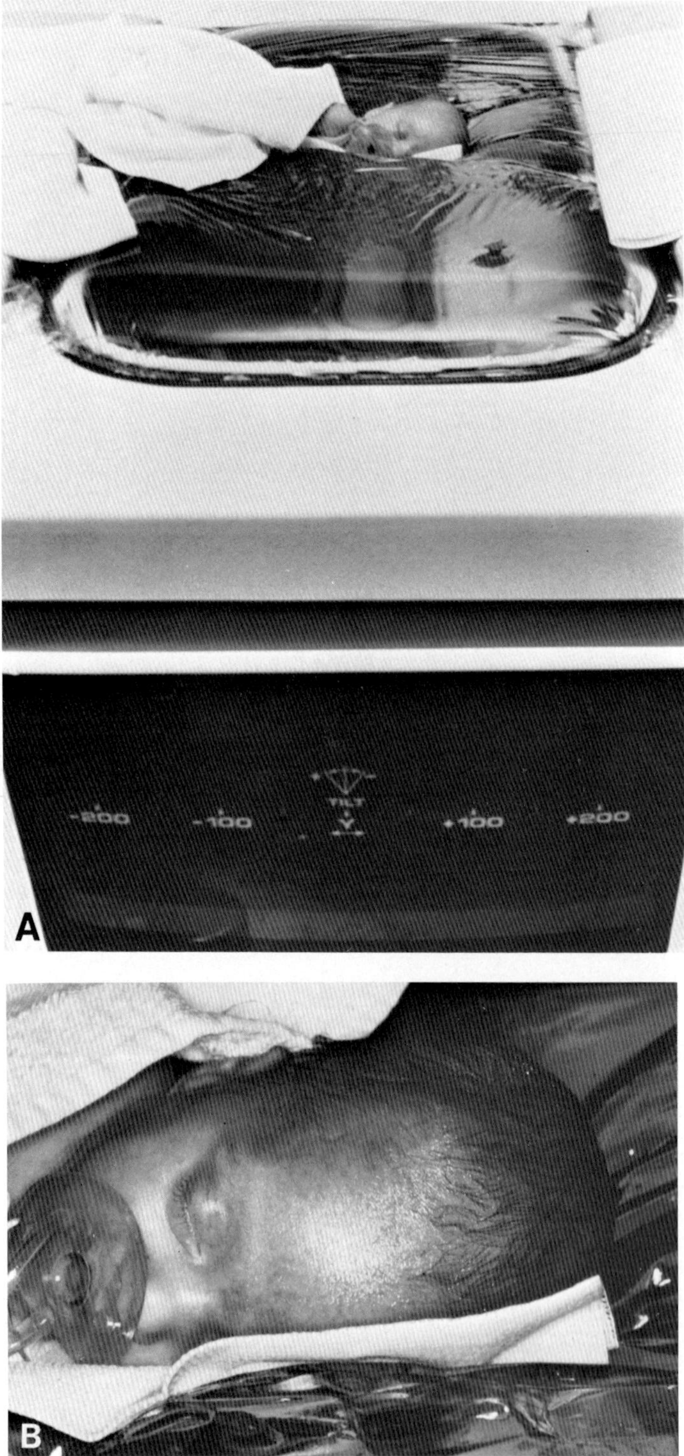

Figure 6.7 (A and B) Position of infant on membrane covering water tank of Octoson. Note gauze pad placed under anterior portion of infant's face to prevent mineral oil from entering eye.

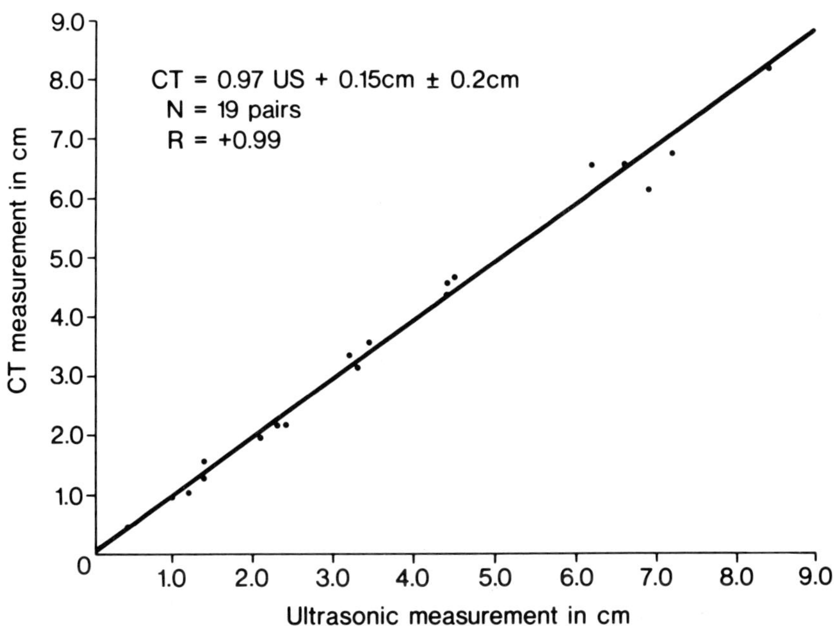

Figure 6.8 Linear regression analysis of measurements of fluid-containing normal and abnormal structures in 19 patients studied by CT and Octoson. (Reproduced with permission from K. Haber et al: *Radiology*, *134*:173–178, 1980.[6])

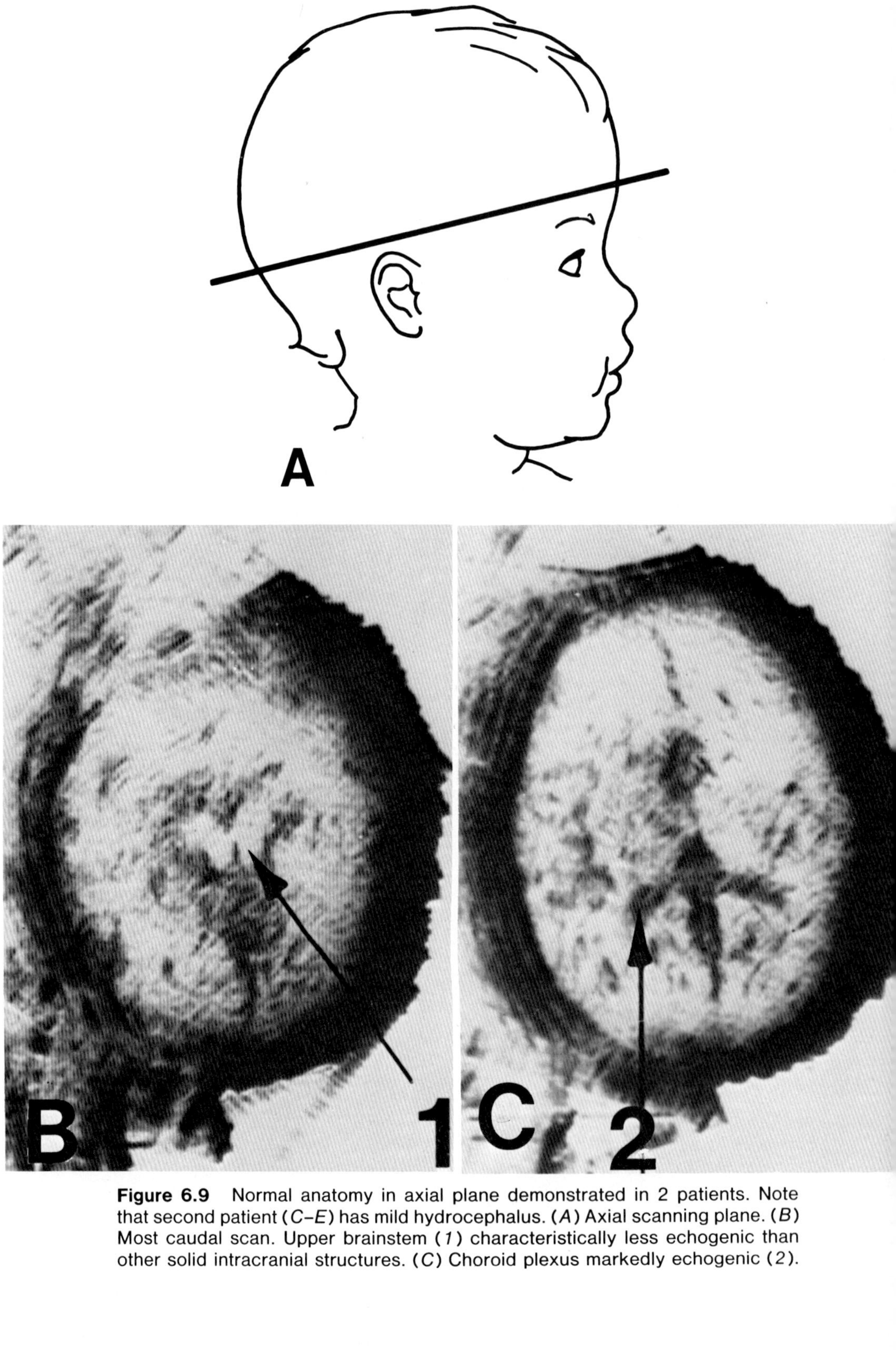

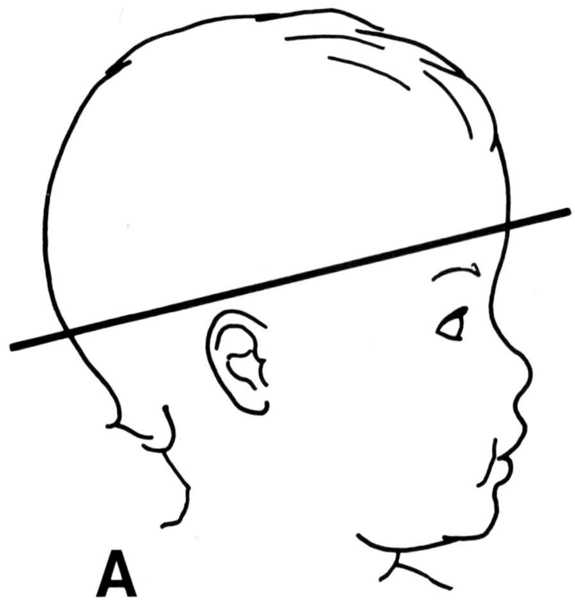

Figure 6.9 Normal anatomy in axial plane demonstrated in 2 patients. Note that second patient (*C–E*) has mild hydrocephalus. (*A*) Axial scanning plane. (*B*) Most caudal scan. Upper brainstem (*1*) characteristically less echogenic than other solid intracranial structures. (*C*) Choroid plexus markedly echogenic (*2*).

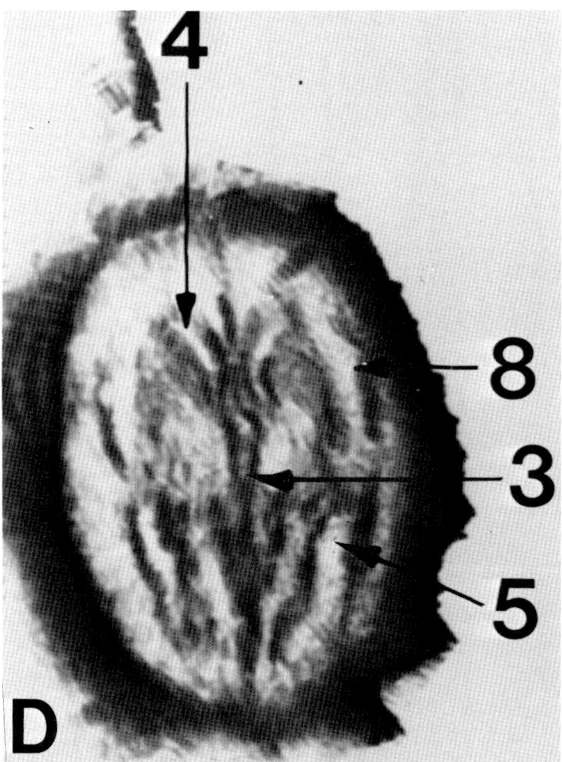

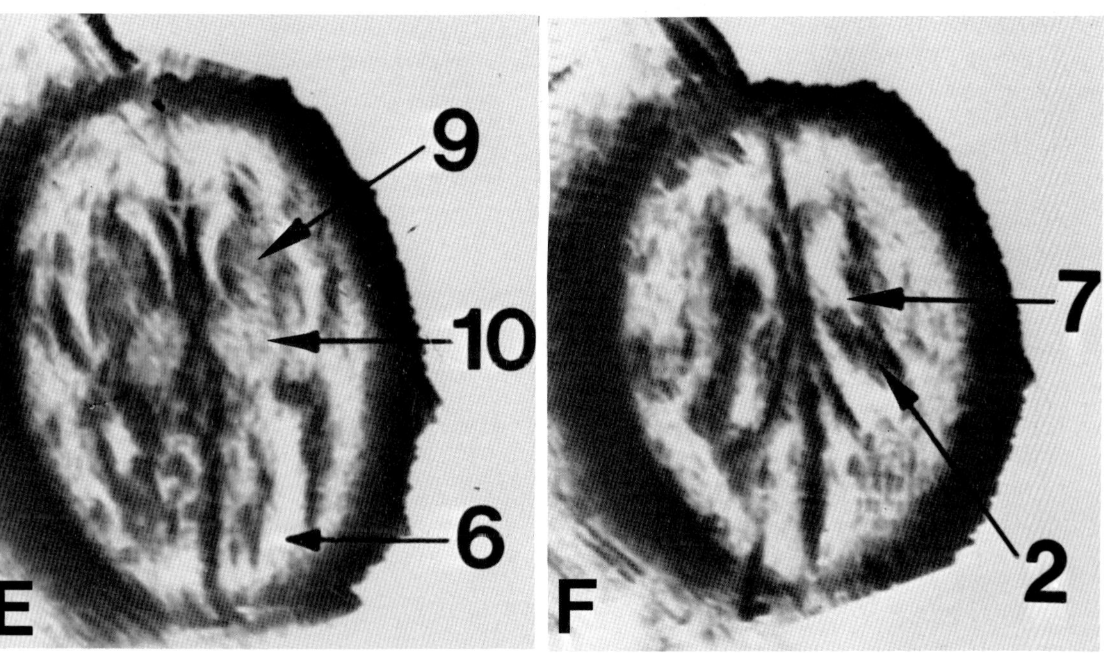

(*D–F*) Normally noted fluid-filled structures include third ventricle (*3*), lateral ventricles frontal horn (*4*), atrium (*5*), occipital horn (*6*), body (*7*), and circular sulcus (*8*). Also note clearly outlined head of caudate nucleus (*9*) and thalamus (*10*).

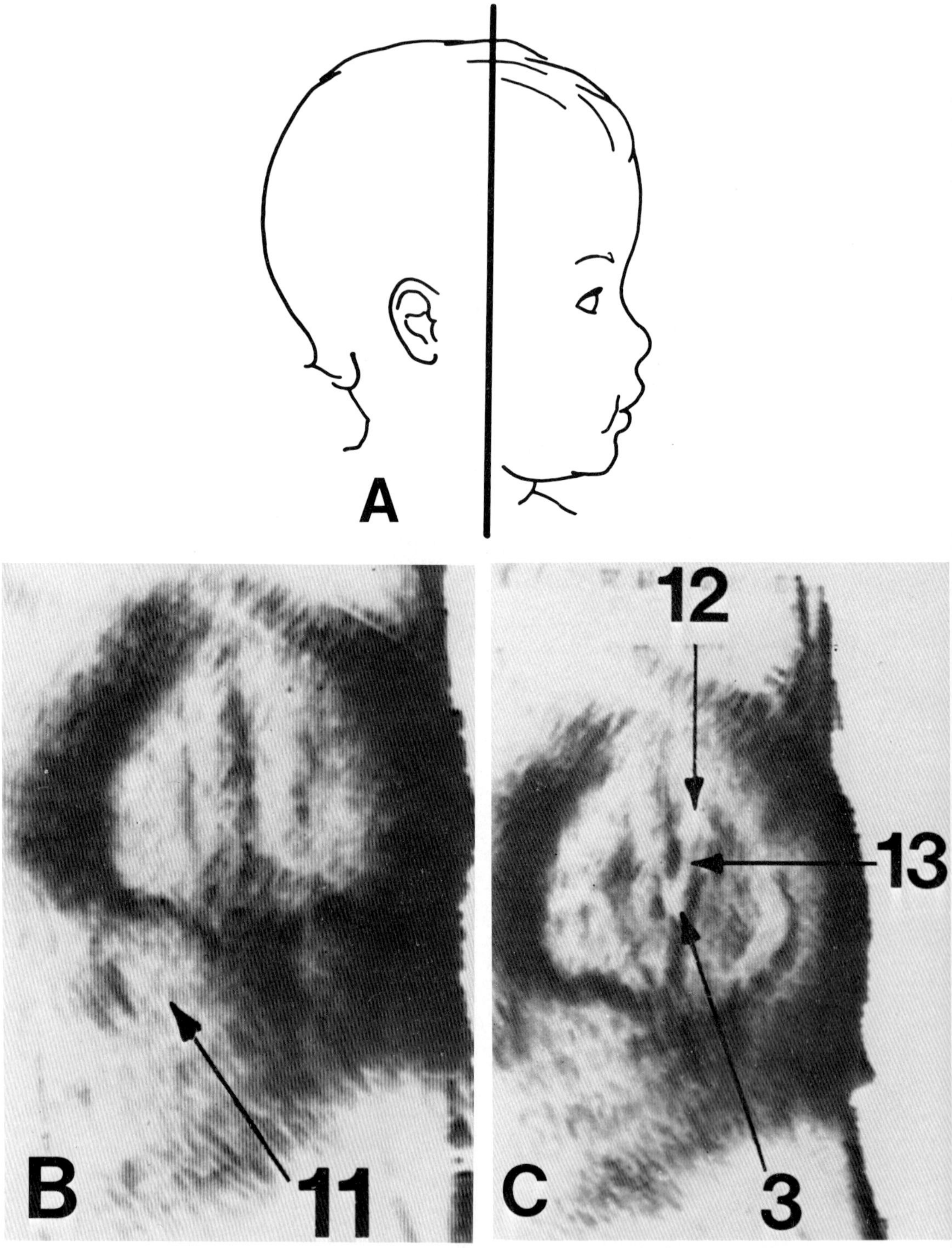

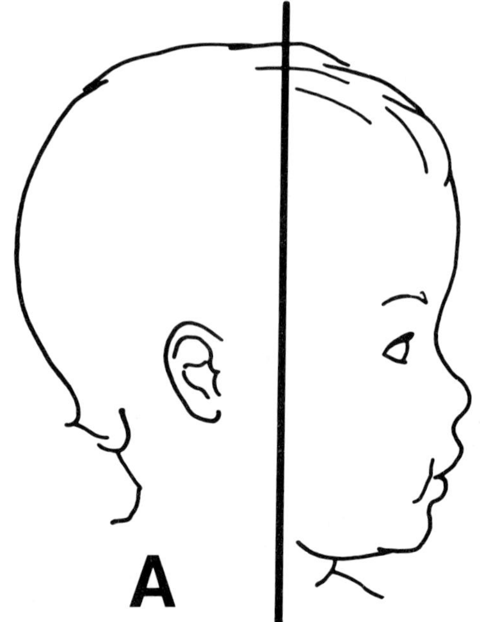

Figure 6.10 Normal anatomy demonstrated in coronal plane. (*A*) Coronal scanning plane. (*B*) Anterior slice shows right orbit (*11*). (*C*) The third (*3*) and lateral ventricles (*12*) seen at level of foramen of Monro (*13*). (*D*) Thalamus (*10*) and circular sulcus (*8*) again imaged. (*E*) Body (*7*) of lateral ventricle, thalamus

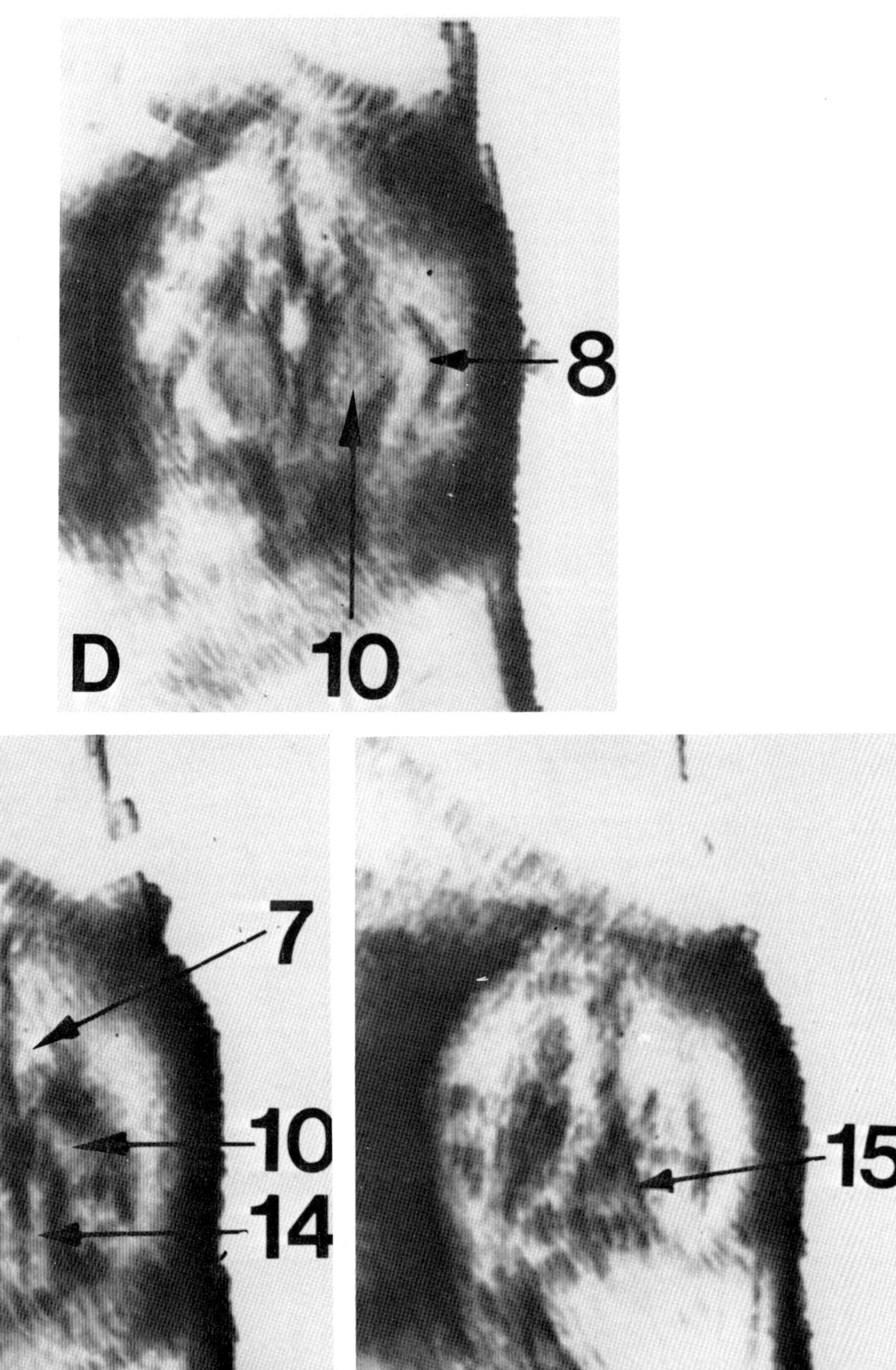

(*10*) and brainstem (*14*) sectioned. Note echogenic choroid plexus (*2*) on floor of lateral ventricular body (*7*). Further posteriorly (*F*), portion of tentorium cerebelli (*15*) seen.

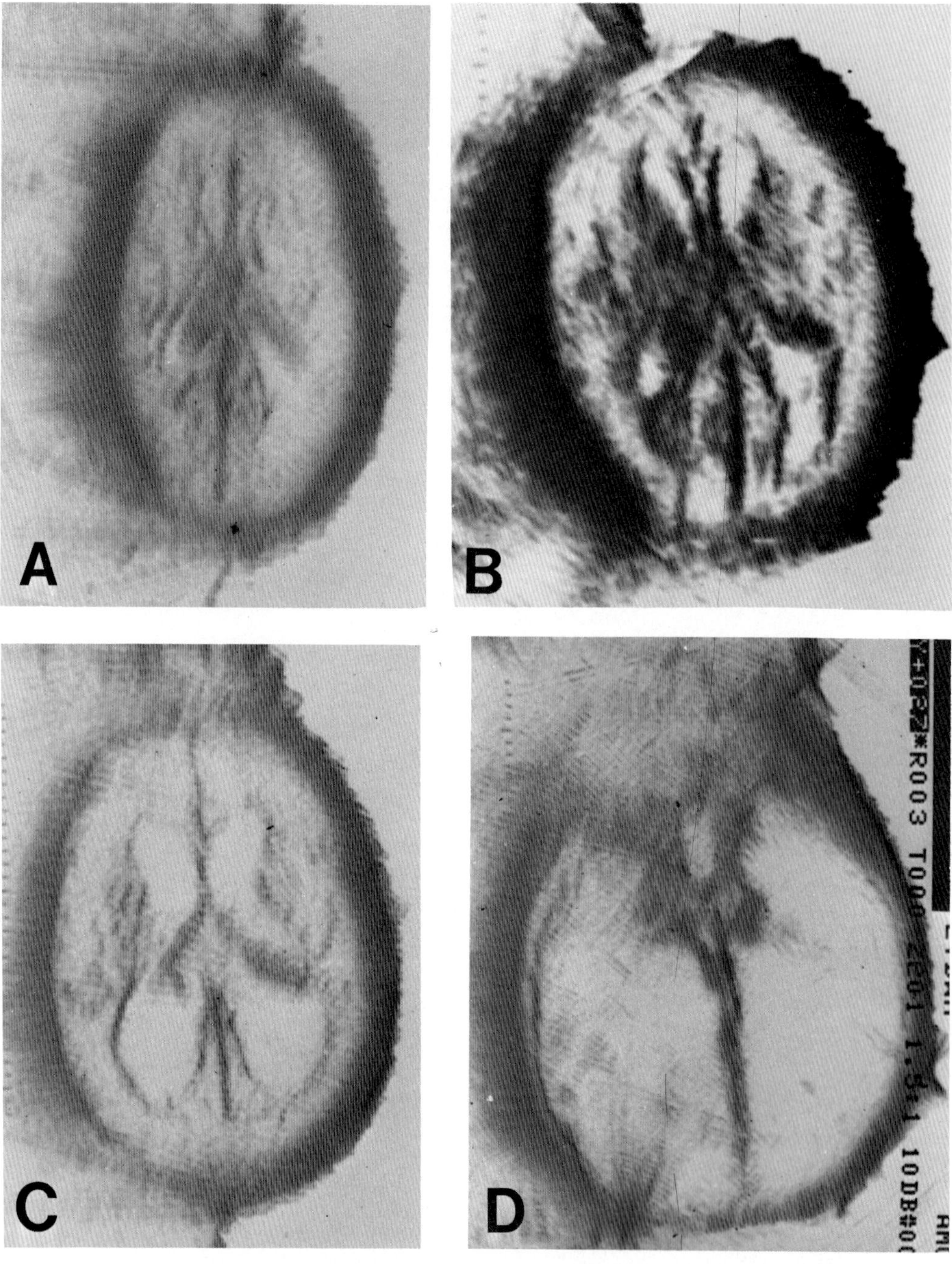

Figure 6.11 Ventricular system normally contains so little fluid that ventricles are either slitlike potential spaces or very thin fluid-containing structures (*A*). Mild (*B*) and moderate (*C*) hydrocephalus contrasted to severe (*D*) distention of ventricular system.

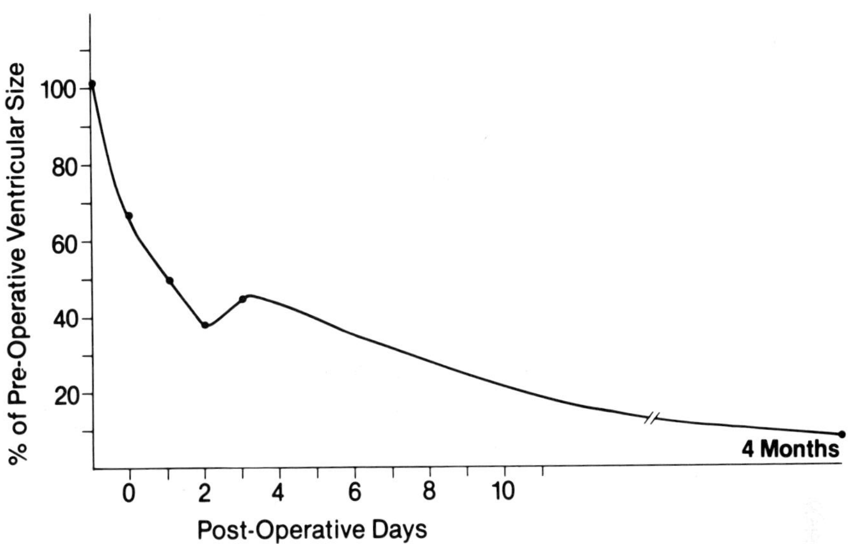

Figure 6.12 Time course of ventricular decompression after ventriculoperitoneal shunt placement in child who is neurologically normal at age 2 years.

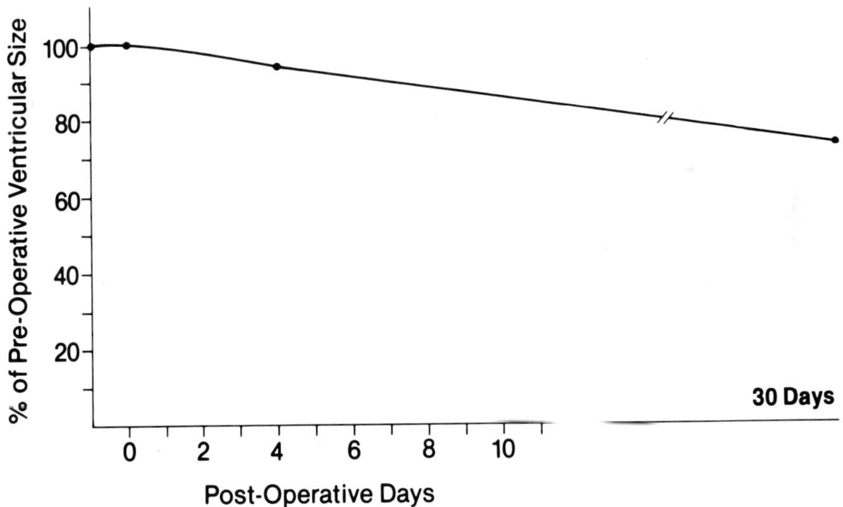

Figure 6.13 Time course of poor response of hydrocephalus to shunting in child who is significantly retarded at 20 months of age.

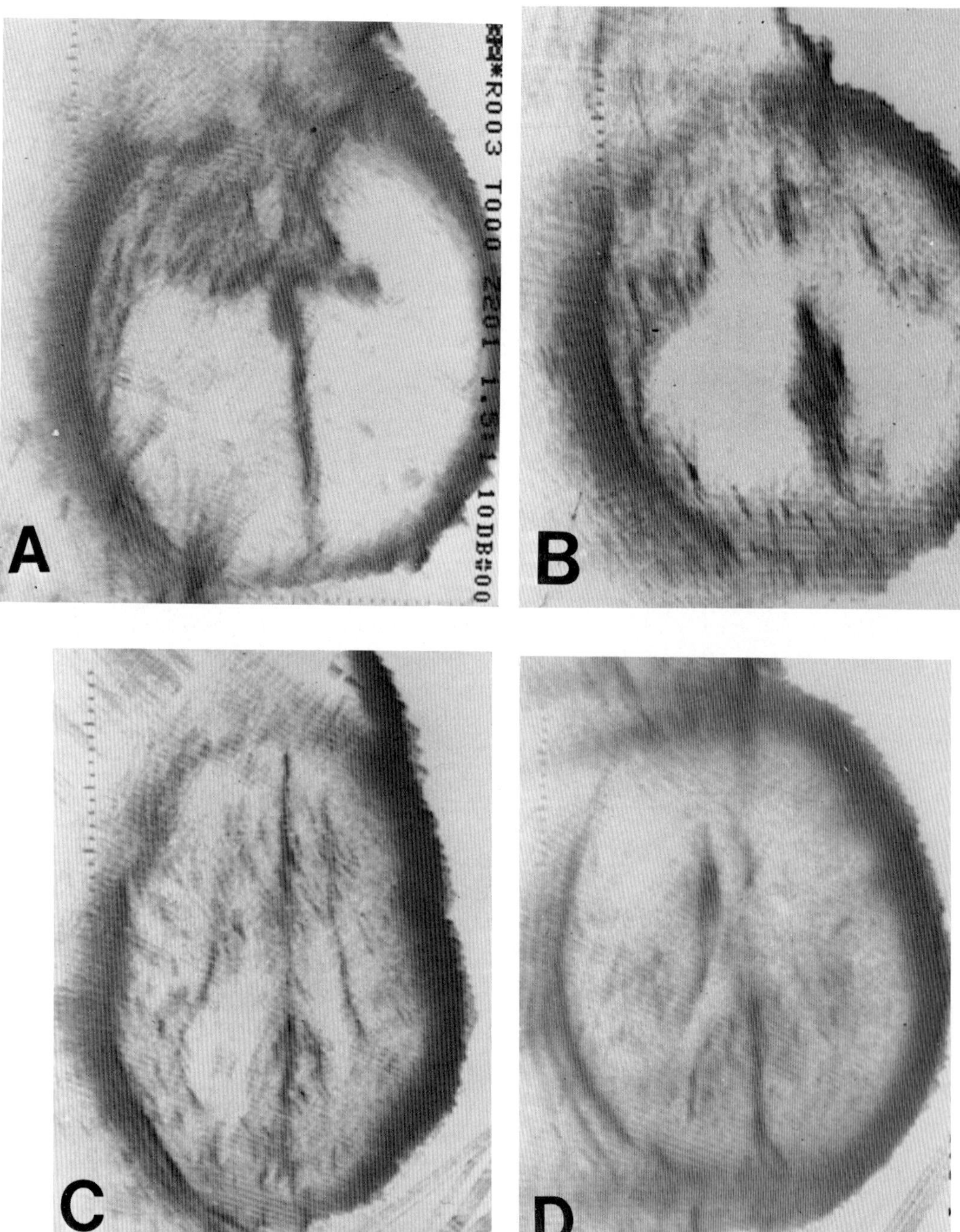

Figure 6.14 Newborn, full-term infant with severe congenital hydrocephalus. Marked ventricular dilatation and thin cortical mantle are demonstrated on axial sonogram made shortly after birth (*A*). Note dramatic response 2 days (*B*) and 4 days (*C*) after shunt placement. Follow-up examination at 6 months (*D*) normal.

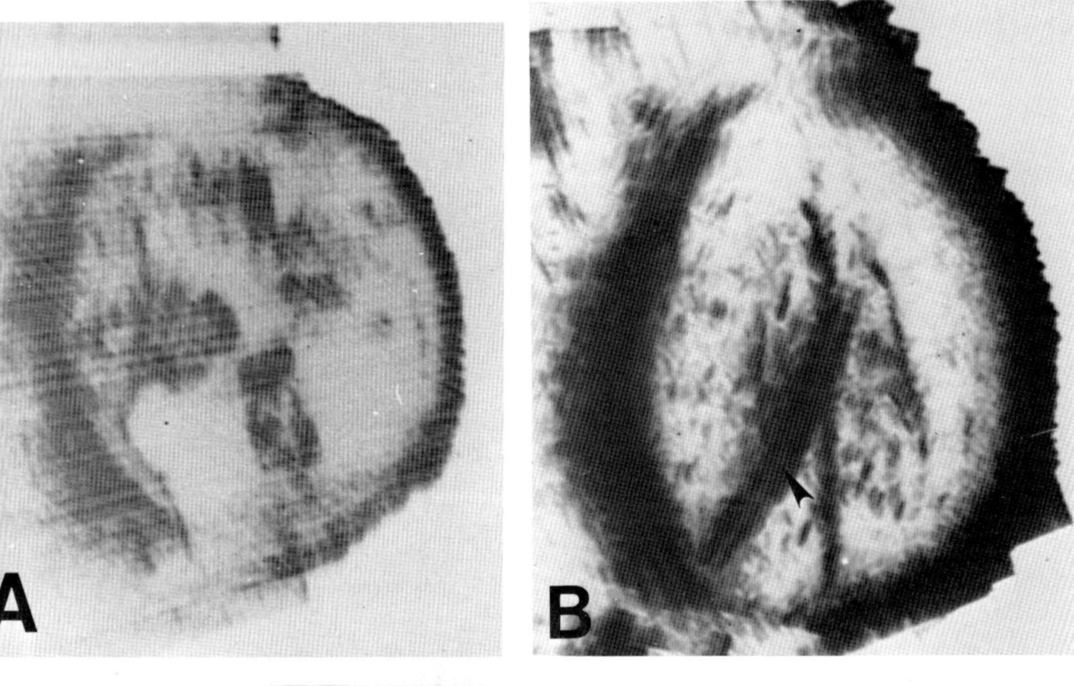

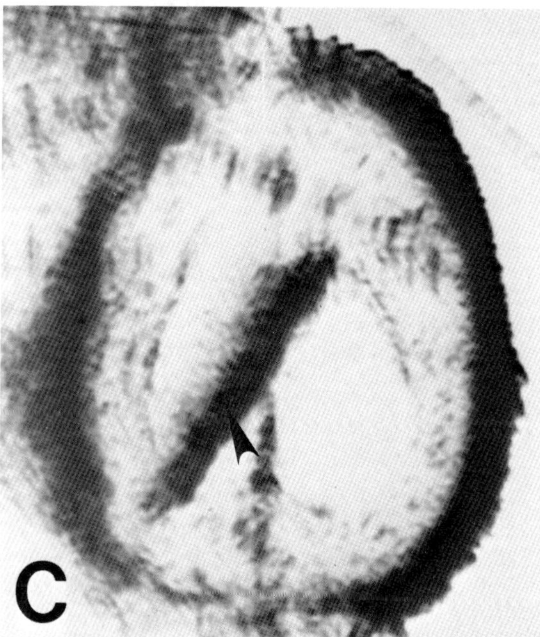

Figure 6.15 Twin premature infant developed hydrocephalus shortly after birth (*A*). Response to shunting (*arrow*) was excellent (*B*). Two months later (*C*) shunt failed and hydrocepahlus returned.

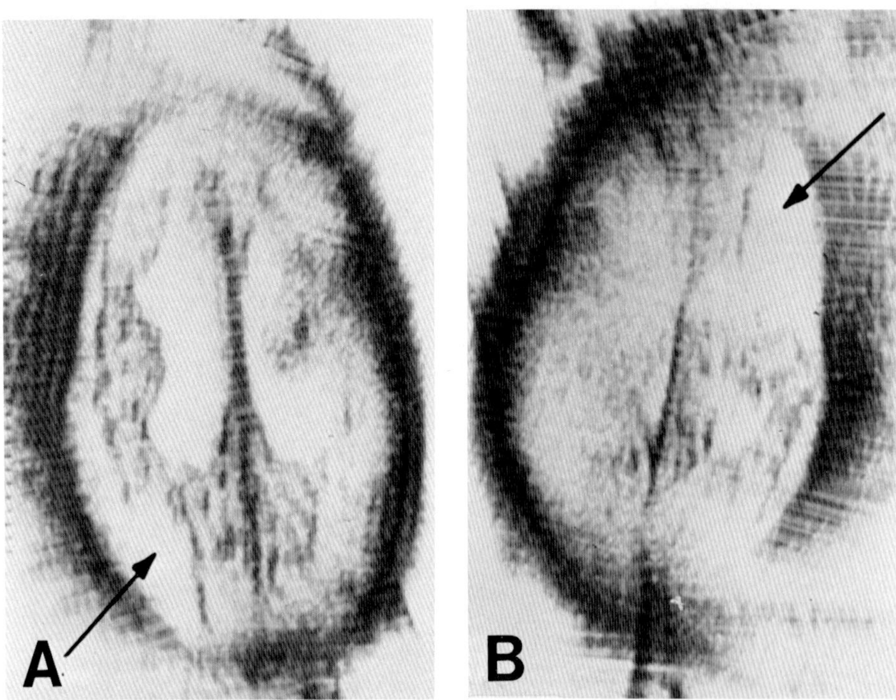

Figure 6.16 Five-week-old infant with hydrocephalus underwent surgical placement of ventriculoperitoneal shunt. Examination made 2 days postoperatively shows left occipital (*A*) and right frontal (*B*) hygroma (*arrows*) as result of localized cerebral mantle collapse.

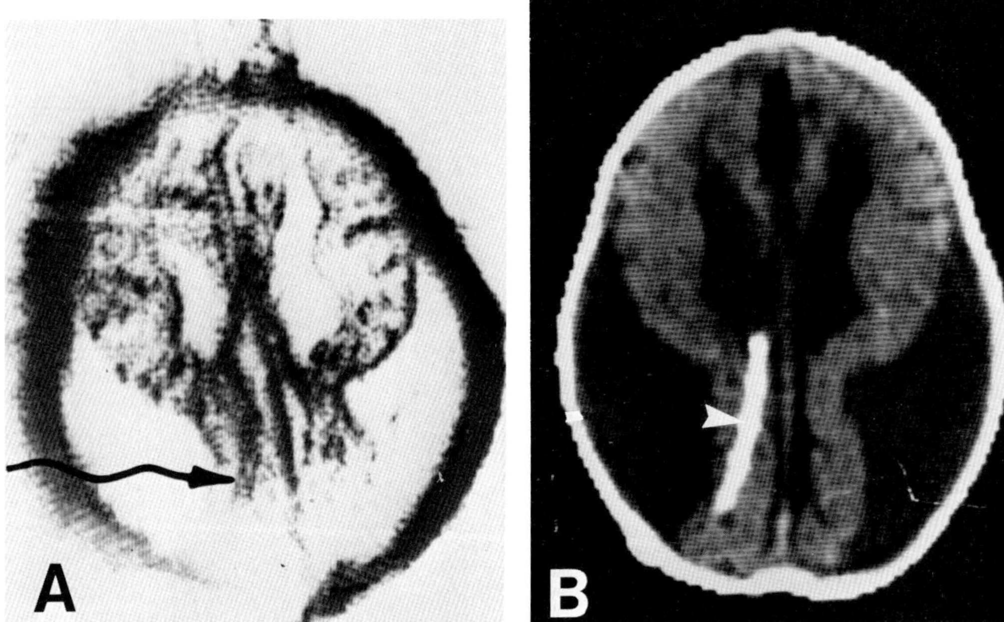

Figure 6.17 Severe bilateral parieto-occipital mantle collapse occurred after shunt (*arrows*) placement in 7-week-old patient with congenital hydrocephalus. Note that panoramic Octoson image (*A*) is comparable to CT study (*B*) made on same day.

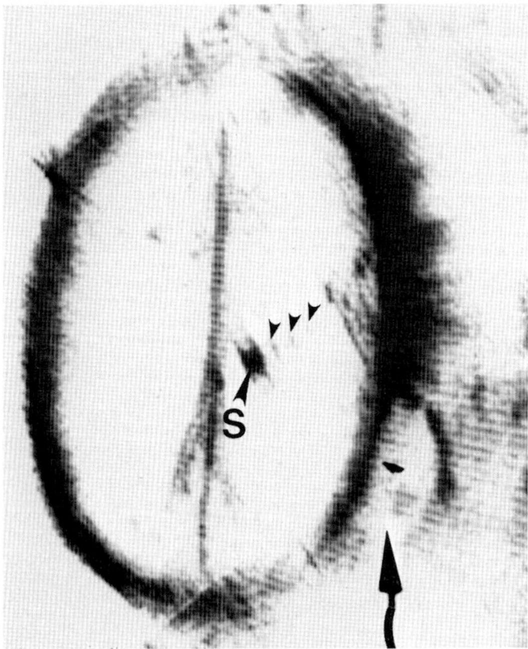

Figure 6.18 Example of shunt leak into subgaleal space (*arrow*) in postoperative infant with severe hydrocephalus. Note reverberation echoes (*arrowheads*) from portion of shunt (*S*) which is in scanning plane.

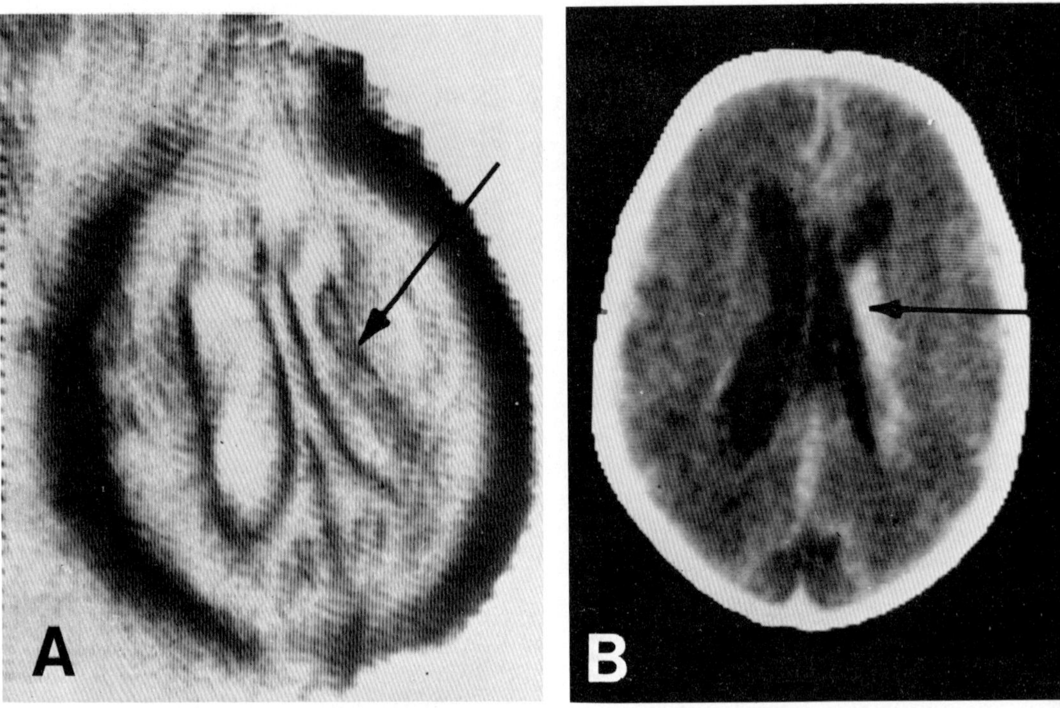

Figure 6.19 Premature infant with echogenic subependymal hemorrhage in left germinal matrix region (*arrows*) and mild hydrocephalus. Note identical information displayed on Octoson study (*A*) as imaged on CT exam (*B*).

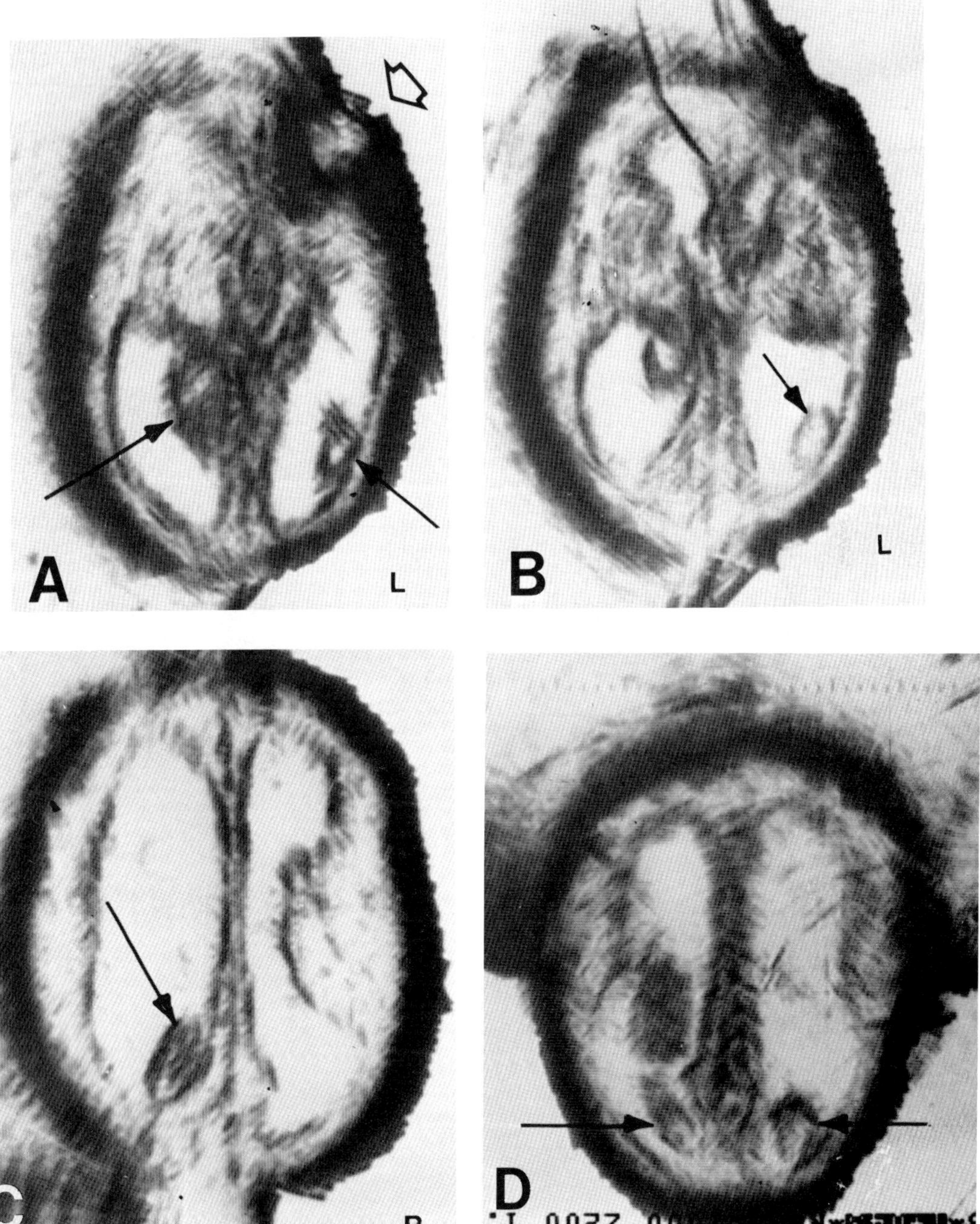

Figure 6.20 Mildly premature infant with moderate hydrocephalus and bilateral blood casts (*arrows*) in lateral ventricles. Note dramatic shift of casts within each ventricle with changes in patient position. Slices made with left side down (*A* and *B*) are lower than one made with right side down (*C*). Occiput down position illustrated in *D*. *Open arrow* in *A* points to left orbit.

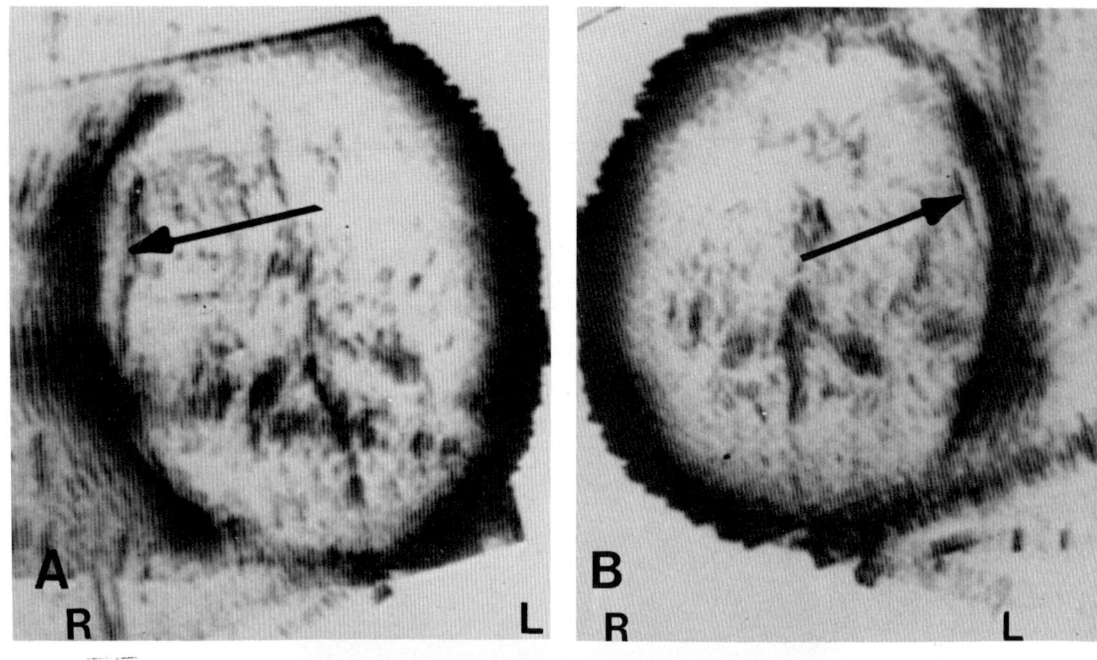

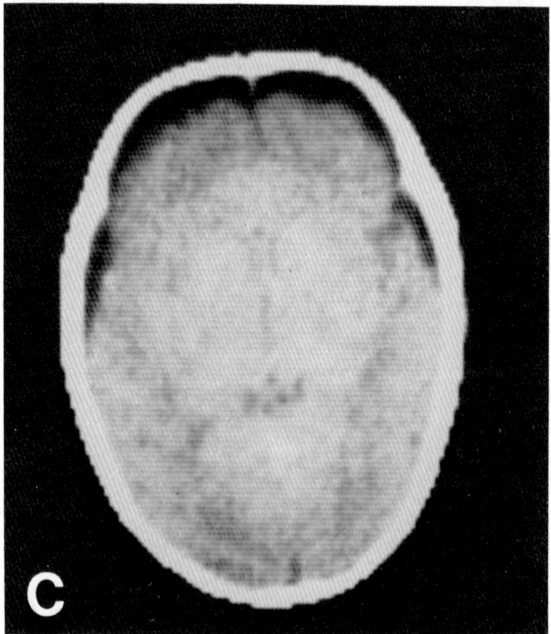

Figure 6.21 Changing patient's position and examining head with both right and left sides down proved diagnostic in 6-week-old with bilateral frontal subdural fluid collections. Left side down axial (*A*); right side down axial (*B*). Fluid imaged only on side opposite transducers because of strong echoes of calvarium on near side and dependent position of brain. On CT (*C*), dependent position of brain with infant supine helps to accentuate bilateral frontal fluid collections.

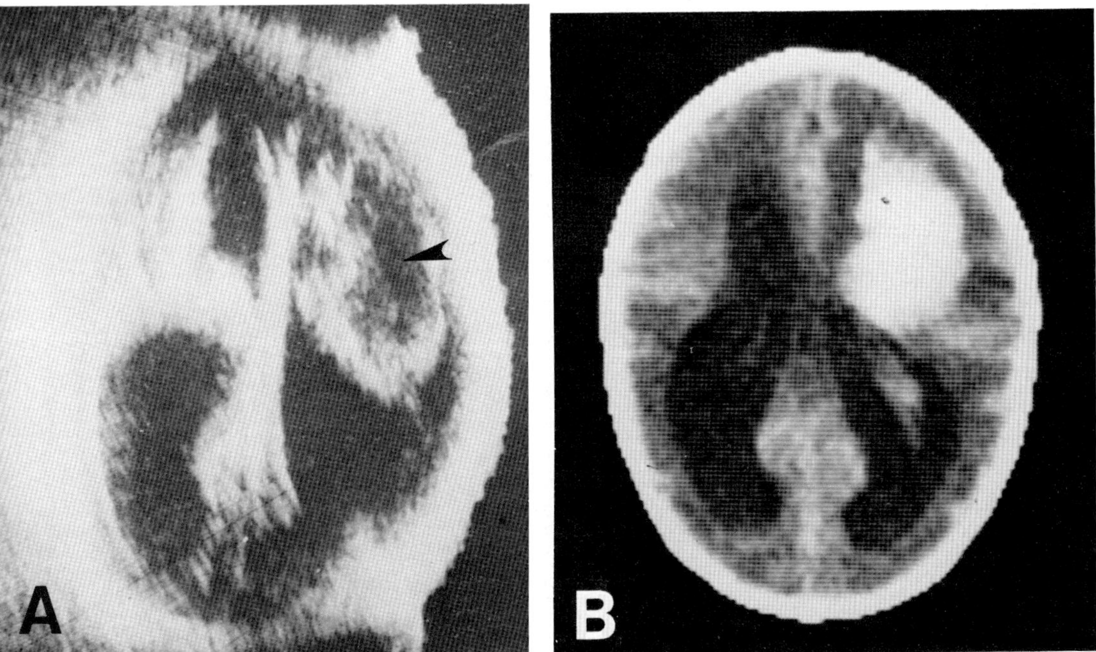

Figure 6.22 Newborn premature with intracerebral hemorrhage in left frontal region. Note that ultrasound examination (*A*) shows central liquefaction (sonolucent area—*arrowhead*), whereas CT study (*B*) made on same day does not.

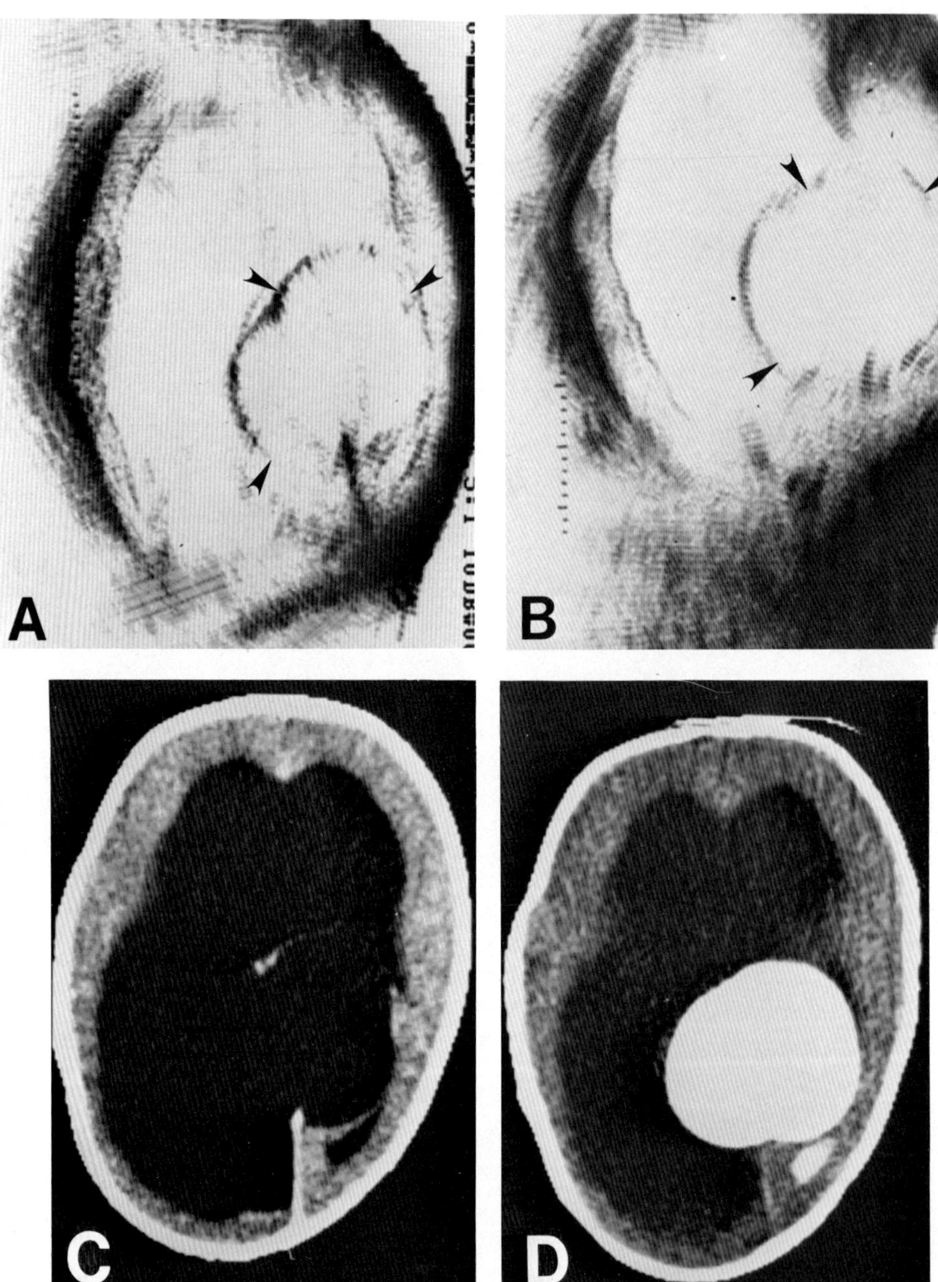

Figure 6.23 Full-term infant with congenital hydrocephalus shunted immediately after birth. Shunt was effective (image not shown) for first postoperative month, at which time shunt failed. Arachnoid cyst (*arrows*) felt to be complication of initial shunting procedure readily demonstrated on Octoson examination (*A* and *B*), but was not appreciated on nonenhanced CT study (not shown) and not well imaged on enhanced CT study (*C*). (*D*) shows CT image after percutaneous injection of metrizamide.

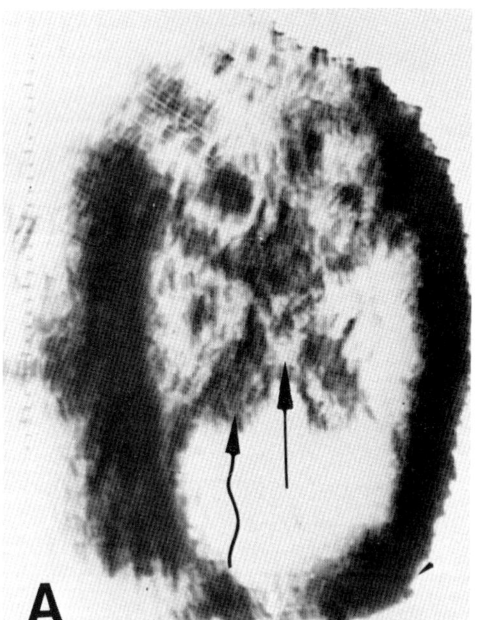

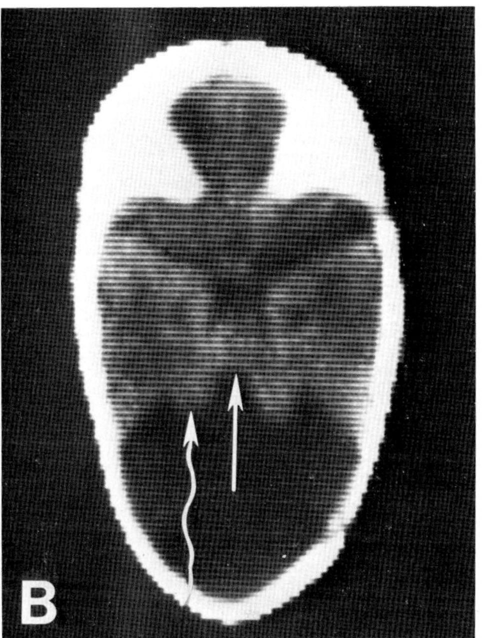

Figure 6.24 Newborn infant with Dandy-Walker malformation. Octoson (*A*) and CT (*B*) axial scans give strikingly similar images of posterior fossa cyst and hypoplastic cerebellum (*curved arrow*) with increased echogenicity compared to brainstem (*straight arrow*).

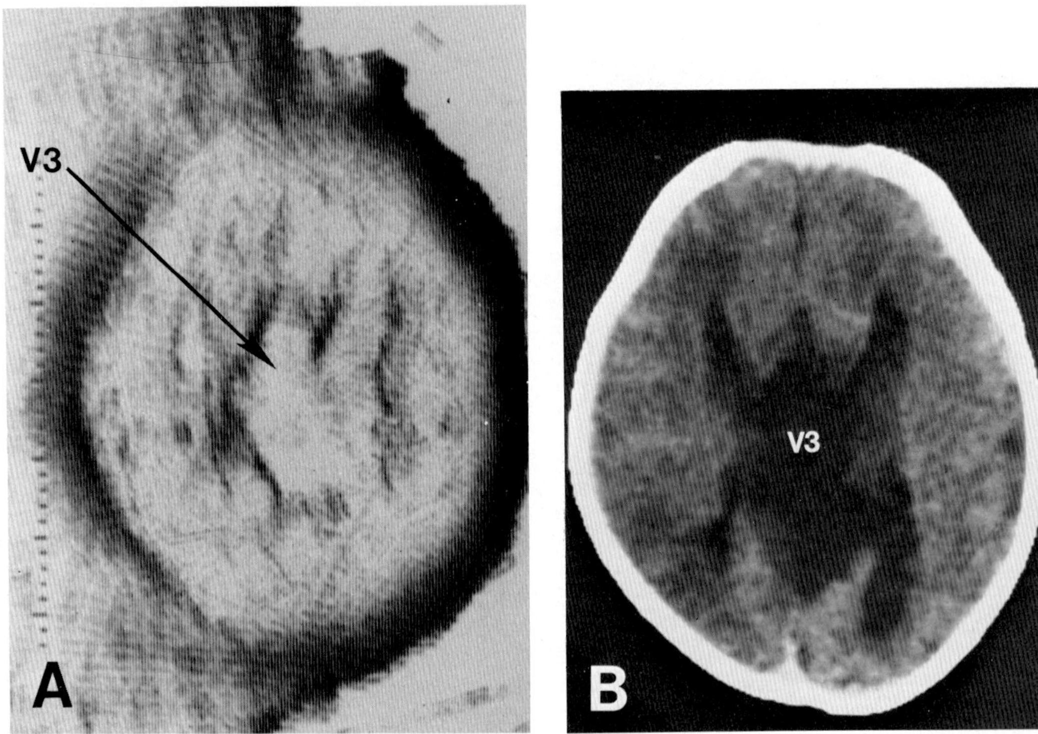

Figure 6.25 Agenesis of corpus callosum. Axial ultrasound (*A*) and CT (*B*), show lateral ventricles separated by high positioned third ventricle (*V3*).

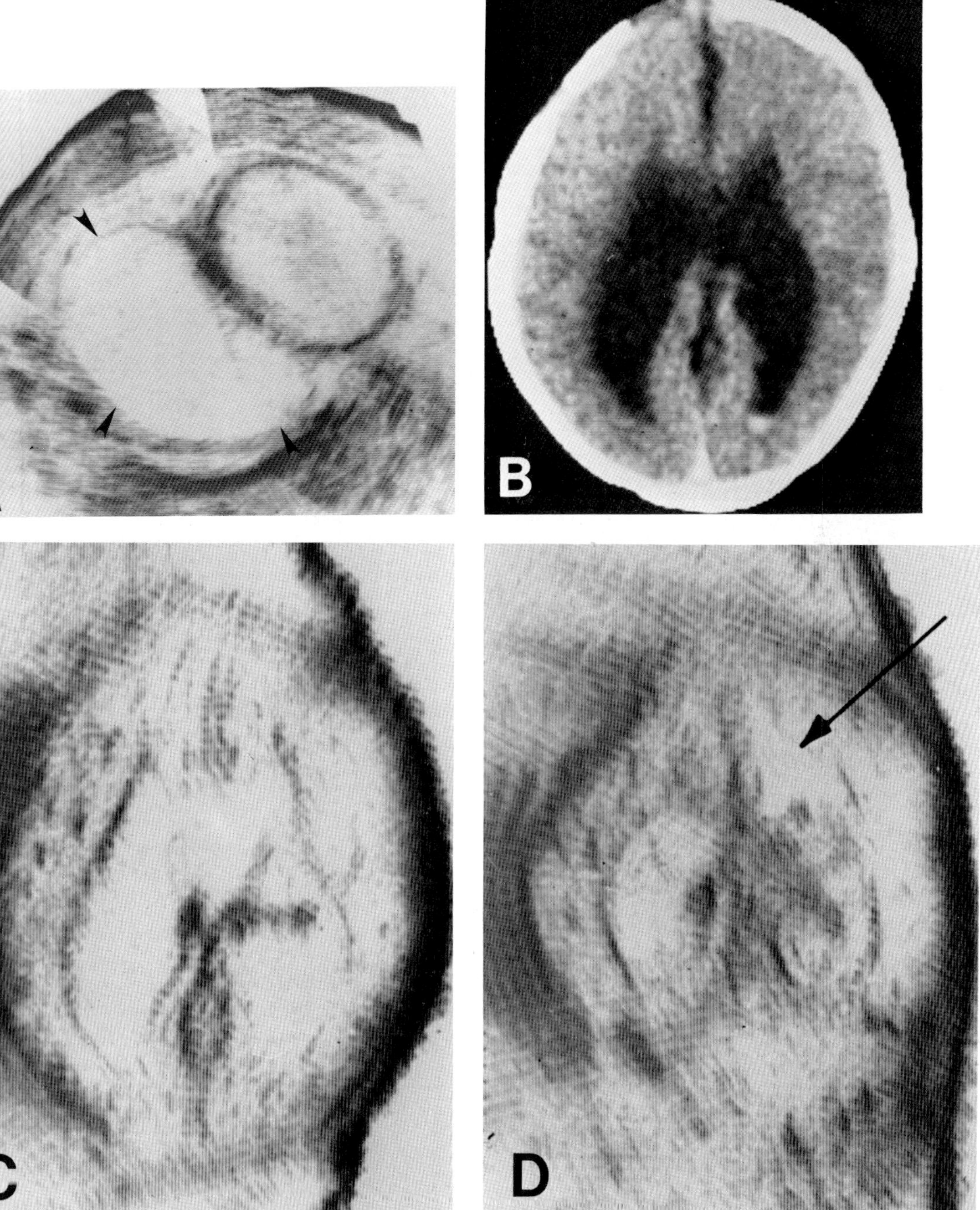

Figure 6.26 Patient with encephalocoele (*arrowhead*) detected in utero (*A*). Postoperative axial CT (*B*) and sonogram (*C*) shows hydrocephalus and pointed shape of frontal horns indicating dysgenesis of corpus callosum with high positioned third ventricle. Coronal Octoson image (*D*) demonstrates connection between left lateral ventricle and area from which encephalocoele was removed (*arrow*).

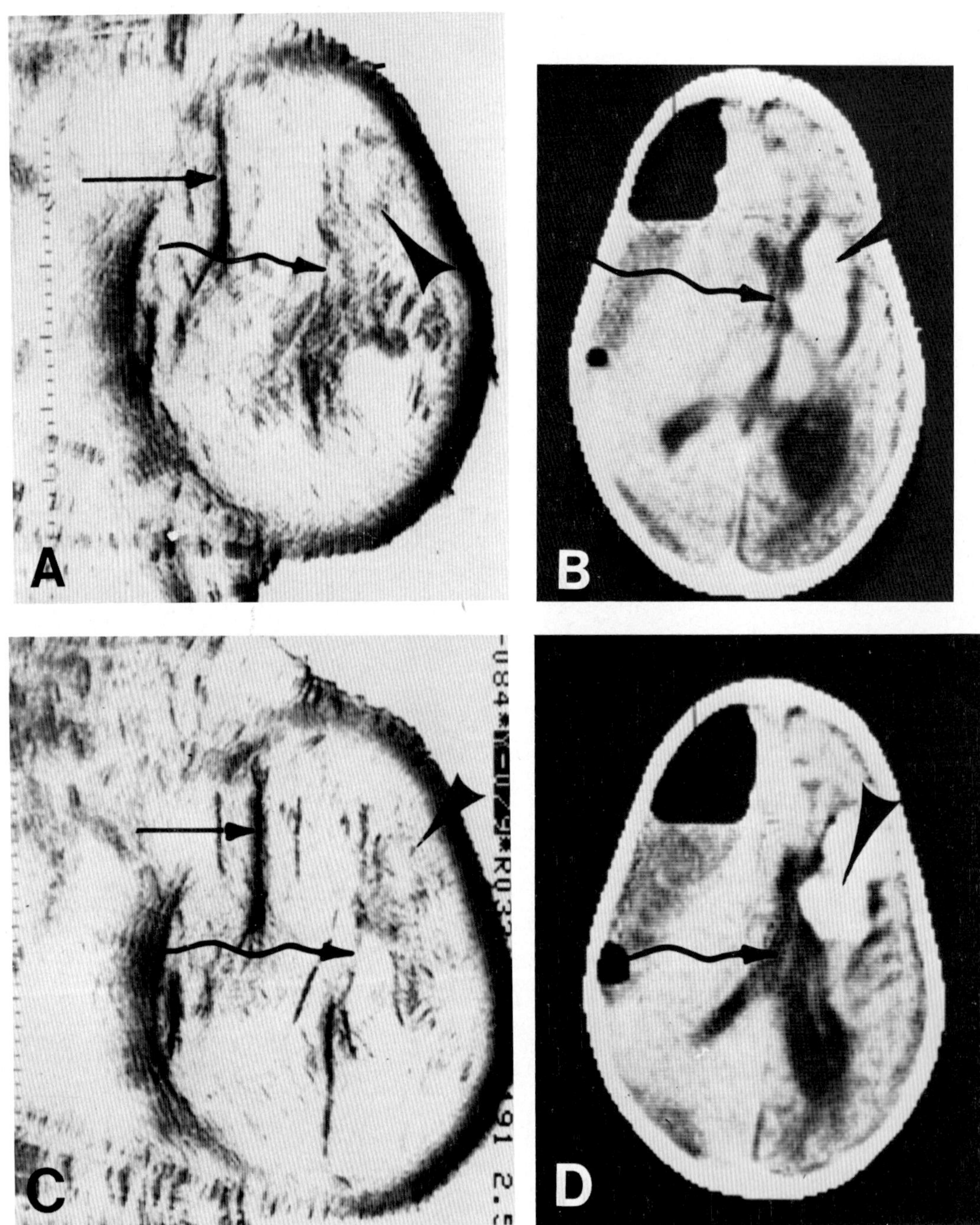

Figure 6.27 Postoperative ultrasound (*A* and *C*) and CT (*B* and *D*) slices in 4-year-old with Wiskott-Aldrich syndrome and primary CNS lymphoma (*arrowhead*). Air introduced into right subdural fluid collection by recent surgical procedure layers (*straight arrow*) in different planes on two studies because of differences in patient position. (Octoson—left side down, CT—occiput down.) Note shifted midline (*curved arrow*) to left due to subdural fluid, and left hemispheric mass (*arrowhead*).

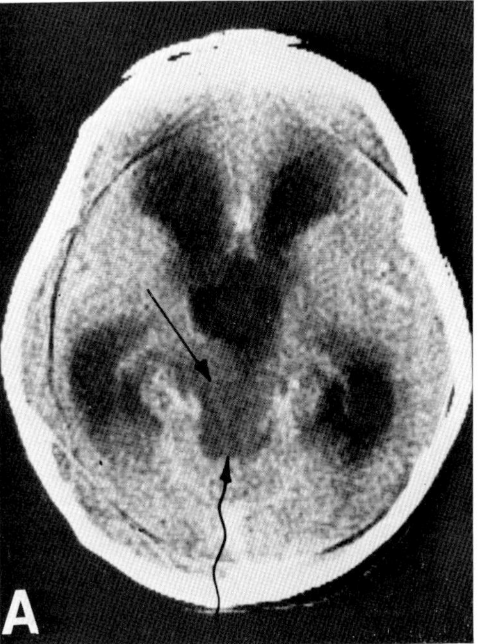

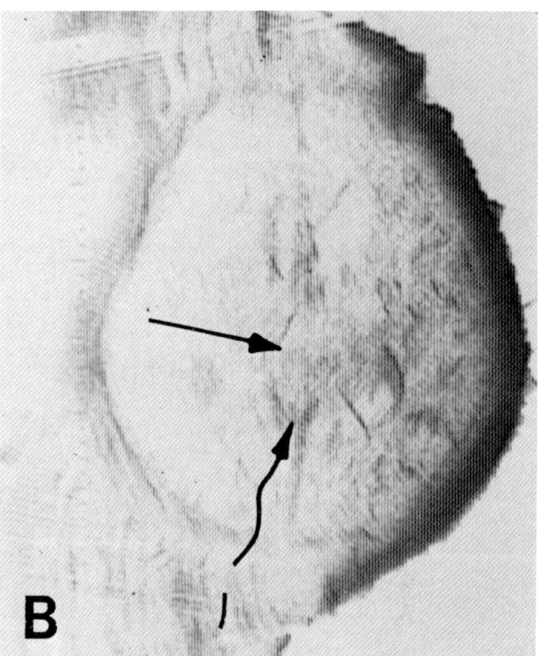

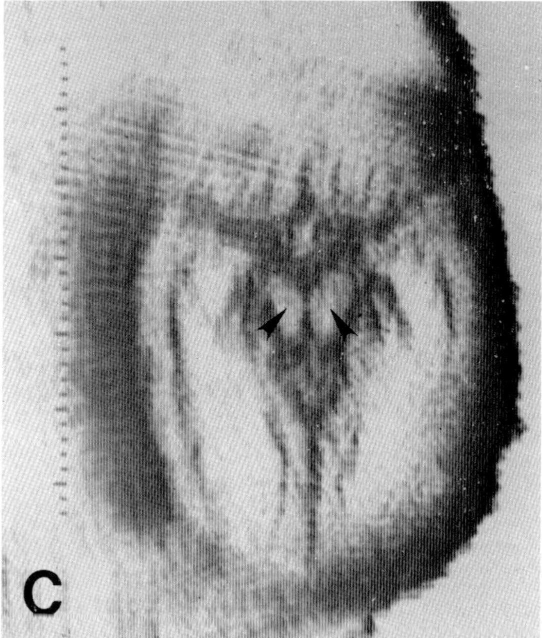

Figure 6.28 Three-year-old child with brainstem glioma. CT examination (*A*) made before shunt placement shows hydrocephalus and brain stem mass (*arrows*). Postshunt ultrasound examination (*B*) showns brain stem mass and decrease in ventricle size. Compare to appearance of normal brainstem (*arrowheads*) in another patient (*C*) with hydrocephalus.

CHAPTER 7

Meningomyelocele Patients and the Chiari II Malformation

The Chiari II (Arnold-Chiari) malformation is a congenital abnormality of the brain with elongation of the pons and fourth ventricle and downward displacement of the medulla and fourth ventricle into the cervical spinal canal with a relatively small posterior fossa.[1–3] The cerebellum may wrap around the pons laterally and anteriorly and may herniate superiorly through the tentorial hiatus. The tectum is prolonged upward and forms a beak at the colliculi. Infants with the Chiari malformation often present after birth or in early infancy with hydrocephalus of varying degree. This malformation is always associated with some form of spinal dysraphism, usually a meningomyelocele. A meningomyelocele is always associated with the Chiari malformation, however a simple meningocele may not be. Many of the abnormal findings that have previously been demonstrated on cranial computerized tomography (CT) and ventriculographic examinations[4–7] can also be demonstrated on cranial ultrasound examination.[8]

Hydrocephalus

In patients examined shortly after birth the size of the lateral ventricles can be normal, mildly-to-moderately (Fig. 7.1), or markedly dilated (Fig. 7.2). The ventricular size has been shown to gradually increase on serial examinations until a shunt procedure is performed. After shunting, the ventricles decrease in size but may not return to normal.

The lateral ventricles are frequently asymmetric (Fig. 7.2). The occipital horns and atria tend to be more dilated than the frontal and temporal horns (Fig. 7.3). This has been noted in congenital hydrocephalus from other etiologies as well and is likely related to the ease of separation of the bones and sutures in this area of the skull. The cerebral mantle is thinnest over the occipital horns (Fig. 7.3).

Configuration of Lateral Ventricles

On axial view, a characteristic anterior pointing and medial concavity of the frontal horns can frequently be demonstrated[4] (Fig. 7.4).

Inferior pointing of the frontal horns resulting from prominence of the caudate nuclei which bulge medially into the lateral walls of the lateral ventricles has been described on ventriculography[2] and can frequently be seen with ultrasound (Fig. 7.5).

Evaluation of Septum Pellucidum

The septum pellucidum is frequently completely or partially absent (Figs. 7.4, 7.7, and 7.11). A cavum septi pellucidi, or visible separation between the leaves of the septum pellucidum, can sometimes be seen but is not related to the Chari II malformation (Fig. 7.6); it is a normal structure frequently seen in newborn infants.

Third Ventricle Abnormalities

The third ventricle is frequently mildly dilated, it may become large in some patients (Fig. 7.7).

The massa intermedia has been described as being unusually enlarged in 82–90% of Chiari II brains.[1] The massa intermedia can be demonstrated easily on sagittal views and a prominent massa intermedia can be identified (Figs. 7.7 and 7.8) and appears to lie unusually close to the foramen of Monro in these patients.

A prominent anterior commissure has been described by ventriculography and can be identified occasionally on ultrasound (Fig. 7.8*A*). Herniation of the third ventricle into the parasellar cistern (Fig. 7.8*B*) and an enlarged suprapineal recess (Fig. 7.8, *A* and *B*) are occasionally seen in these patients. Most of the abnormalities of the third ventricle can be identified only on sagittal views.

Tentorial-Cerebellar Pseudomass

The posterior fossa abnormalities in the Chiari II malformation include downward displacement of the cerebellum, medulla, and fourth ventricle, with a relatively small posterior fossa. On coronal scans the tentorium cerebelli appears relatively low in position with a small posterior fossa (Fig. 7.9). The fourth ventricle is not identified in these patients, probably because of its low position in the posterior fossa or cervical spinal canal and because it is not dilated in this malformation.

The tentorial-cerebellar pseudomass which has been described on CT examinations[4, 6] can be seen on low axial ultrasound views (Fig. 7.10). On axial scans the leaves of the tentorium come together to form a sharp angle posteriorly, producing a V-shaped configuration rather than a normal U-shape. The tentorium is hypoplastic with a wide incisura through which the cerebellum bulges upward, producing the heart-shaped or bullet-shaped tentorial-cerebellar pseudomass.

Interhemispheric Fissure

The interhemispheric fissure may be prominent in these patients and associated with hydrocephalus (Fig. 7.11). It has been postulated that communicating hydrocephalus with distal block at the foramen magnum may result in simultaneous dilatation of both the ventricles and the interhemispheric fissure. It has been noted that the interhemispheric fissure enlarges when the ventricles decrease in size after ventricular shunting.

Summary

Meningomyelocele patients with Chiari II malformation show a variety of findings on cranial CT and ventriculographic examinations which can also be demonstrated on cranial ultrasound examination. Ultrasonography has the advantage of being a rapid, safe, and less expensive method for studying these patients with no radiation exposure with repeated examinations. This is particularly important for following ventricular size and shunt function, which will be discussed further in Chapter 13. The need for deep sedation and anesthesia is also avoided. Ultrasonography has one disadvantage in that only patients with open sutures can be evaluated by this method.

References

1. Peach B. Arnold-Chiari malformation. Anatomic features of 20 cases. Arch Neurol 1965; 12:613–621.
2. Gooding CA, Carter A, Hoare RD. New ventriculographic aspects of the Arnold-Chiari malformation. Radiology 1967; 89:626–632.
3. Harwood-Nash DC, Fitz CR. *Neuroradiology in Infants and Children.* St. Louis: C. V. Mosby 1976; 1000–1014.
4. Zimmerman RD, Breckbill D, Dennis MW, David DO. Cranial CT findings in patients with meningomyelocele. AJR 1979; 132:623–629.
5. Naidich TP, Pudlowski RM, Naidich JB, Gornish M, Rodriguez FJ. Computed tomographic signs of the Chiari II malformation. Part I: Skull and dural partitions. Radiology 1980; 134: 65–71.
6. Naidich TP, Pudlowski RM, Naidich JB, Gornish M, Rodriguez FJ. Computed tomographic signs of the Chiari II malformation. Part II: Midbrain and cerebellum. Radiology 1980; 134:391–398.
7. Naidich TP, Pudlowski RM, Naidich JB, Gornish M, Rodriguez FJ. Computed tomographic signs of the Chiari II malformation. Part III: Ventricles and cisterns. Radiology 1980; 134: 657–663.
8. Babcock DS, Han BK. Cranial ultrasound findings in patients with meningomyelocele. AJNR 1980; 1:493–499 and AJR 1981; 136:563–569.
9. Babcock DS, Farruggia S. Cavum septi pellucidi: its appearance and incidence with cranial ultrasonography in infancy. Radiology 1981; 139:147–150.

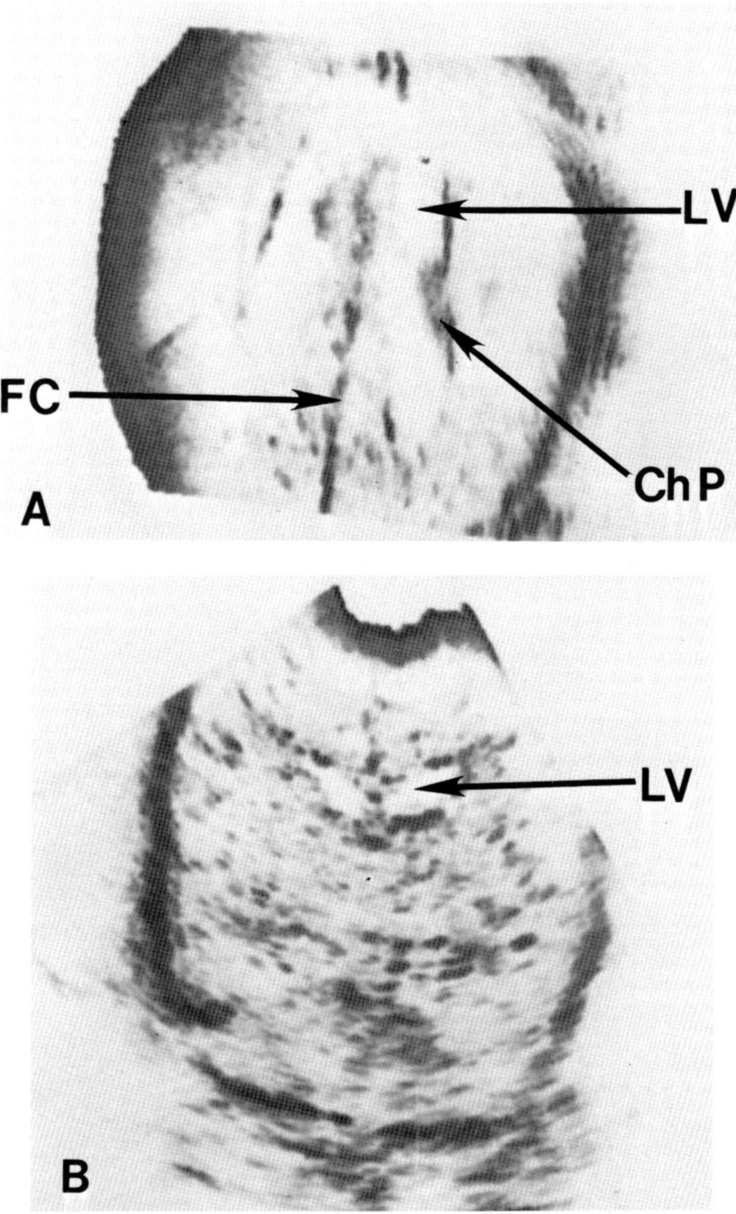

Figure 7.1 Mild hydrocephalus. (*A*) Axial and (*B*) coronal scans. Mild dilatation of lateral ventricles (*LV*). *FC*, falx cerebri; *ChP*, choroid plexus. (Reproduced with permission from D. S. Babcock and B. K. Han: *American Journal of Neuroradiology*, *1*:493–499, 1980.[8])

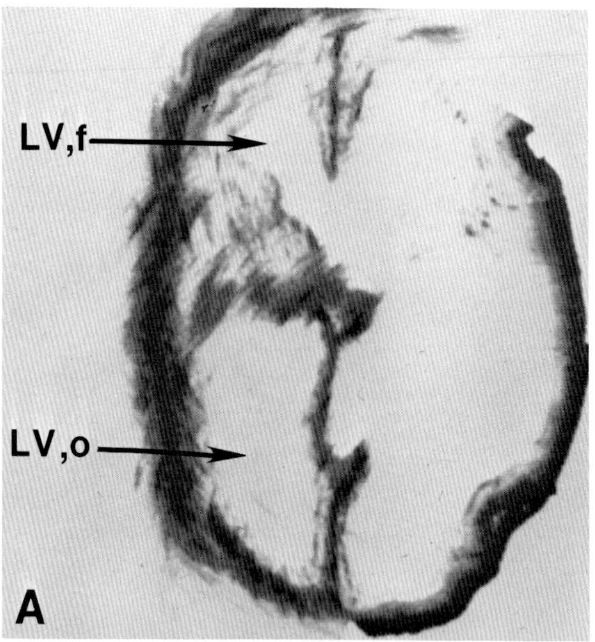

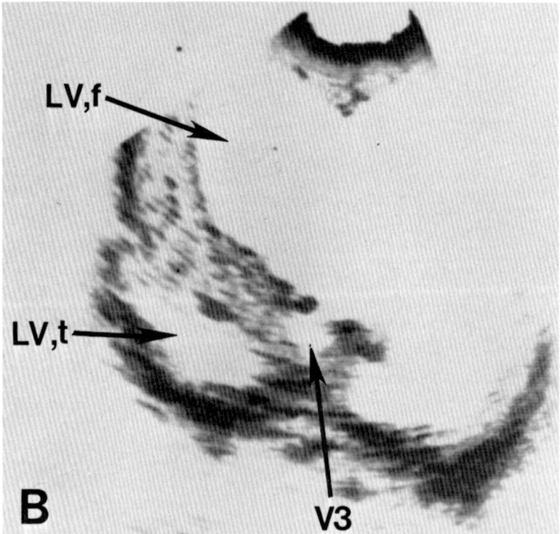

Figure 7.2 Asymmetric, marked hydrocephalus. (*A*) Axial and (*B*) coronal scans showing asymmetric dilatation of the lateral ventricles. *LV,f*, frontal horn; *LV,t*, temporal horn; *LV,o*, occipital horn. (Reproduced with permission from D. S. Babcock and B. K. Han: *American Journal of Neuroradiology*, *1*:493–499, 1980.[8])

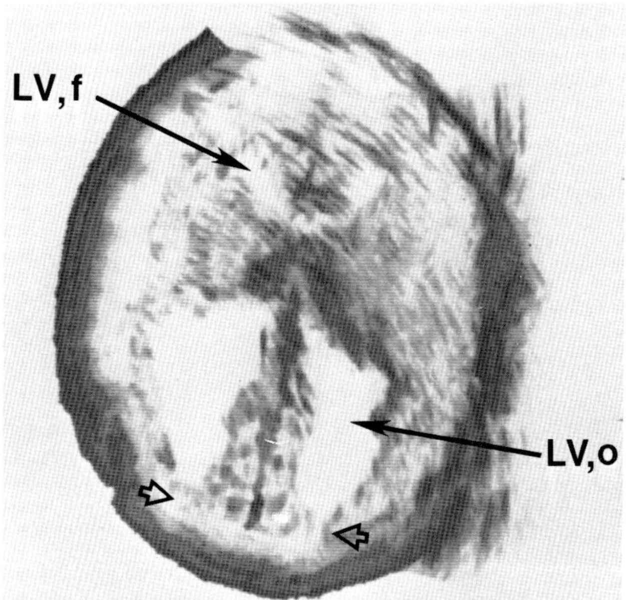

Figure 7.3 Lateral ventricles. Axial scan showing more dilatation of atria and occipital horns (*LV,o*) than frontal horns (*LV,f*) and thinnest cerebral mantle over occipital horns (*open arrows*). (Reproduced with permission from D. S. Babcock and B. K. Han: *American Journal of Neuroradiology*, *1*:493–499, 1980.[8])

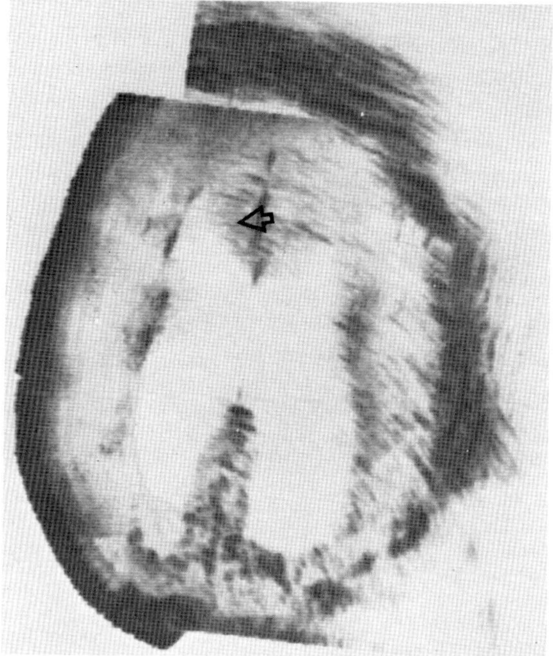

Figure 7.4 Lateral ventricles. Axial scan showing characteristic anterior pointing and medial concavity of frontal horns (*arrow*). (Reproduced with permission from D. S. Babcock and B. K. Han: *American Journal of Neuroradiology*, *1*:493–499, 1980.[8])

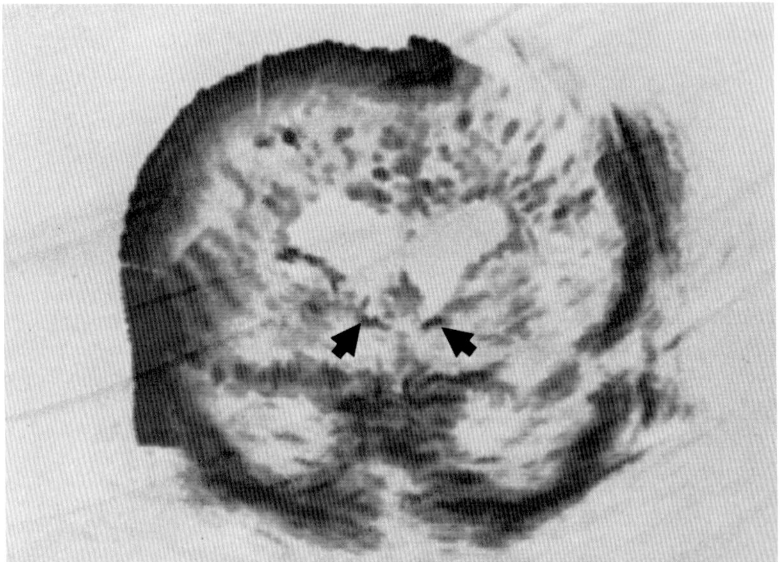

Figure 7.5 Lateral ventricles. Coronal scan through frontal horns of lateral ventricles showing inferior pointing of frontal horns (*arrows*). (Reproduced with permission from D. S. Babcock and B. K. Han: *American Journal of Neuroradiology*, *1*:493–499, 1980.[8])

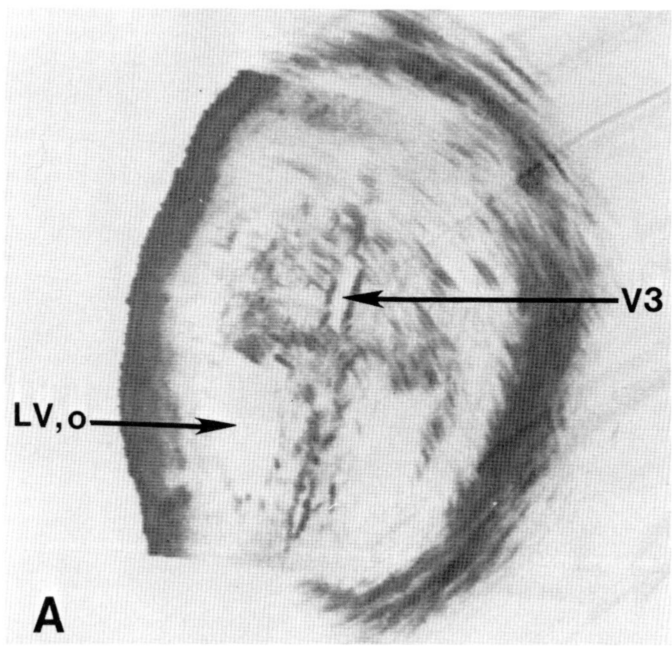

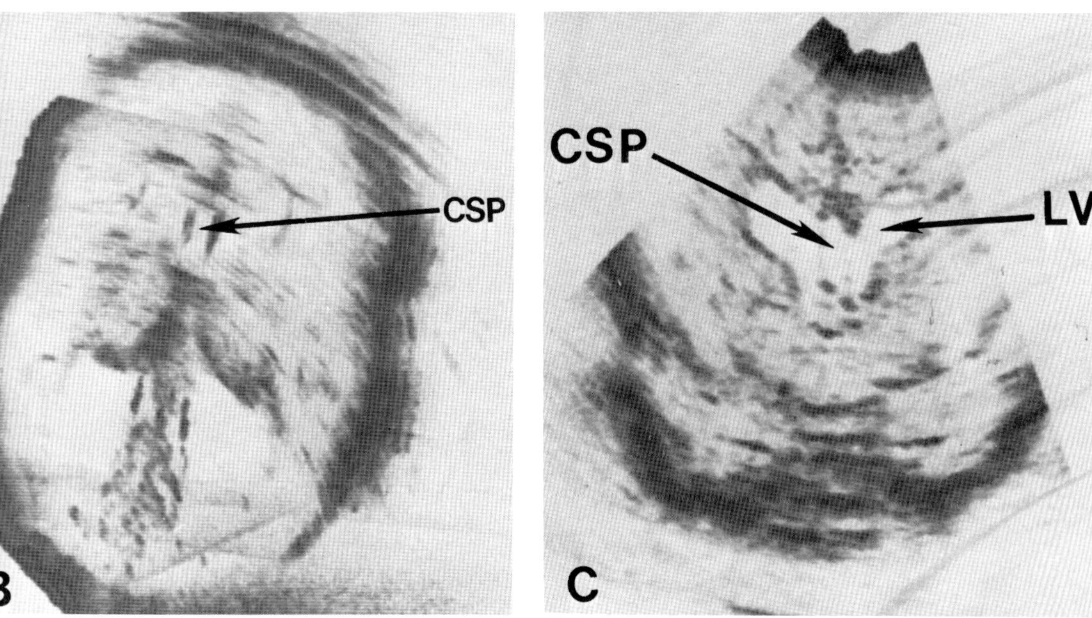

Figure 7.6 Cavum septi pellucidi. (*A*) Axial scan through lower thalamus and (*B*) higher axial scan. Cavum septi pellucidi (*CSP*) and third ventricle (*V3*) are seen on different levels. Dilated occipital horns of lateral ventricles (*LV,o*). (Reproduced with permission from S. Farruggia and D. S. Babcock: *Radiology*, 139:147–150, 1981.[9] (*C*) Coronal scan. Cavum septi pellucidi between dilated frontal horns of lateral ventricles (*LV*). (Reproduced with permission from D. S. Babcock and B. K. Han: *American Journal of Neuroradiology*, *1*:493–499, 1980.[8])

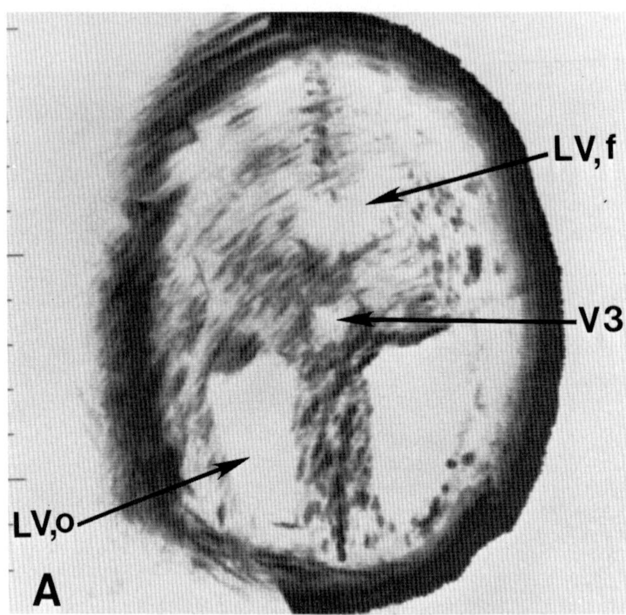

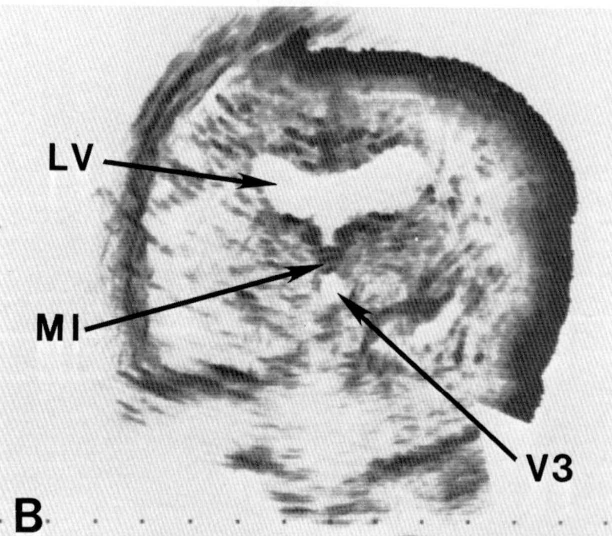

Figure 7.7 Absent septum pellucidum. Dilated third ventricle with prominent massa intermedia. (*A*) Axial and (*B*) coronal scans showing absent septum pellucidum and moderate dilatation of lateral and third ventricles (*V3*). Occipital horns (*LV,o*) more dilated than frontal horns (*LV,f*). *MI*, massa intermedia. (Reproduced with permission from D. S. Babcock and B. K. Han: *American Journal of Neuroradiology*, *1*:493–499, 1980.[8])

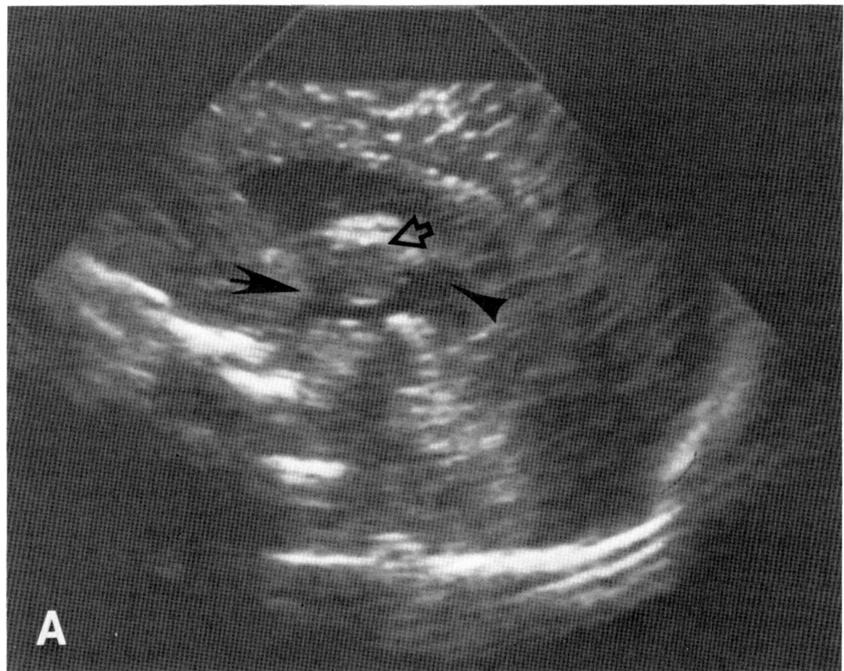

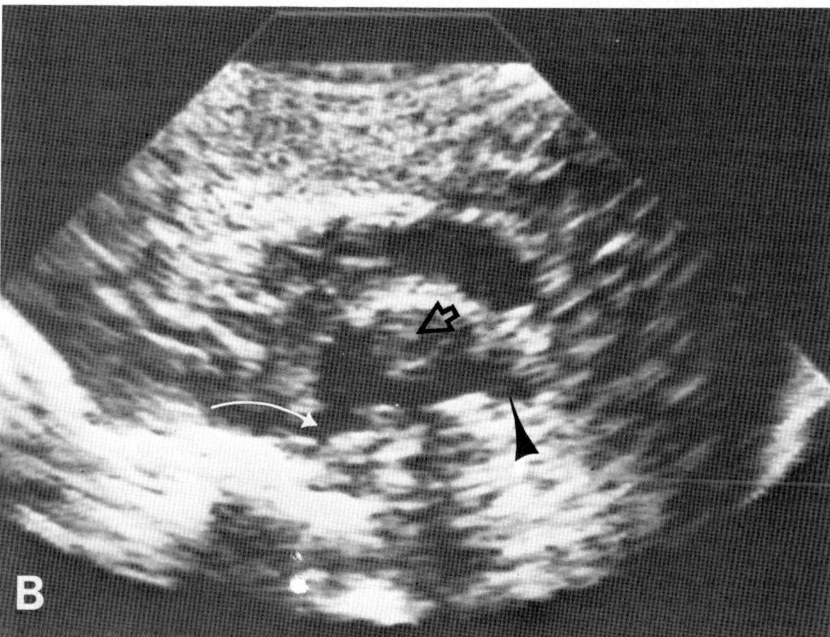

Figure 7.8 Third ventricle abnormalities. (*A* and *B*) Midline sagittal scans on two different patients showing enlarged massa intermedia (*open arrows*), prominent anterior commissure (*black arrow*), herniation of third ventricle into the parasellar cistern (*white arrow*), and enlarged suprapineal recess (*arrowheads*). (Reproduced with permission from D. S. Babcock and B. K. Han: *American Journal of Neuroradiology*, *1*:493–499, 1980.[8])

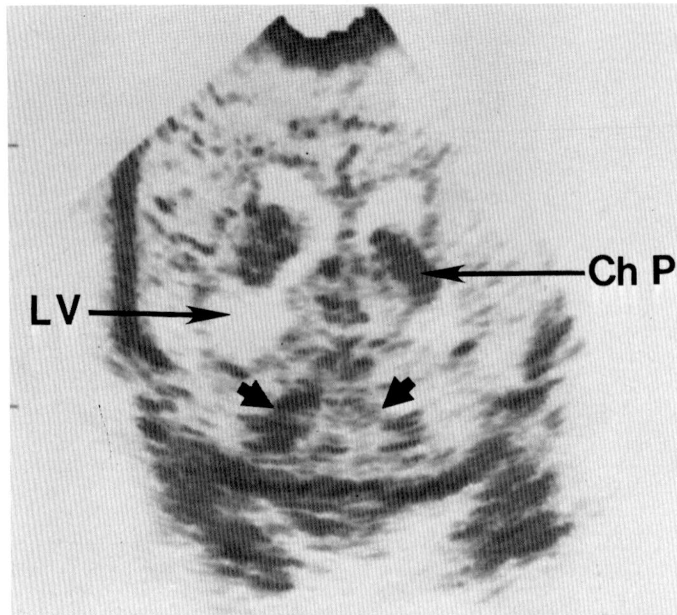

Figure 7.9 Low position of tentorium cerebelli. Coronal scan. Relatively low position of tentorium cerebelli (*arrows*) is shown with small posterior fossa. Dilated lateral ventricles with choroid plexuses (*ChP*). (Reproduced with permission from D. S. Babcock and B. K. Han: *American Journal of Neuroradiology*, *1*: 493–499, 1980.[8])

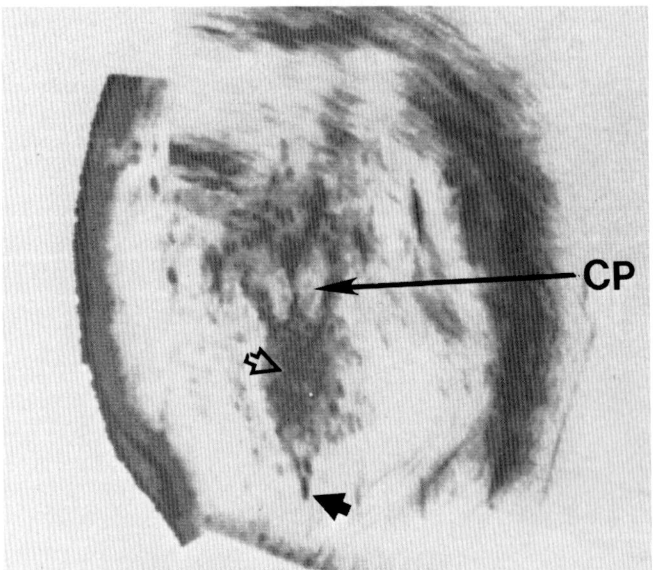

Figure 7.10 Tentorial-cerebellar pseudomass. Low axial scan showing heart-shaped tentorial-cerebellar pseudomass (*open arrow*) and V-shaped tentorium cerebelli posteriorly (*arrow*). *CP*, cerebral peduncles. (Reproduced with permission from D. S. Babcock and B. K. Han: *American Journal of Neuroradiology*, *1*: 493–499, 1980.[8])

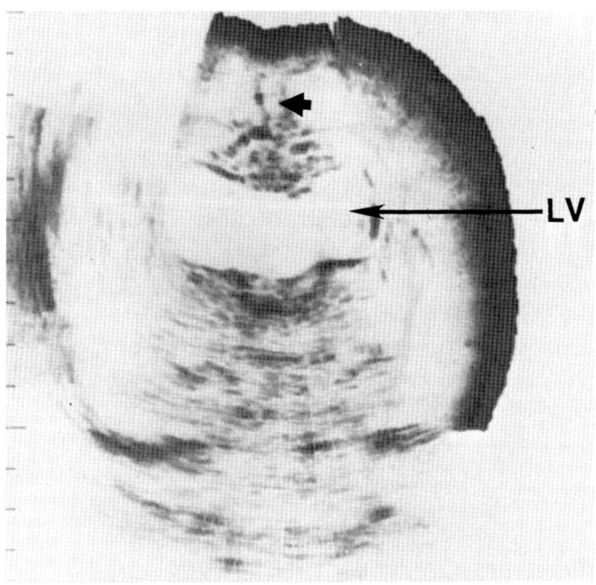

Figure 7.11 Prominent interhemispheric fissure. Coronal scan showing prominent interhemispheric fissure (*arrow*) and moderate dilatation of lateral ventricles with absence of septum pellucidum. (Reproduced with permission from D. S. Babcock and B. K. Han: *American Journal of Neuroradiology*, *1*:493–499, 1980.[8])

CHAPTER 8

Intracranial Cystic Abnormalities

Intracranial fluid collections such as the ventricles or cysts are particularly well demonstrated by ultrasonography because of the impedance mismatch between the brain and fluid. Harwood-Nash[1] has described an intracranial cyst as a well-circumscribed fluid containing cavity that exhibits a mass effect and displaces normal structures. It may communicate with and enlarge by pressure or a pulsatile force from a hydrocephalic ventricle or the subarachnoid space, respectively. Cysts can be divided into four categories: cysts containing cerebrospinal fluid (CSF) (e.g., an arachnoid or a porencephalic cyst), a viscous high-protein fluid (cystic tumor), pus (abscess), or parasitic fluid (hydatid cyst). This chapter deals with cerebrospinal fluid-containing cysts and demonstrates how ultrasonography can be used to establish the geography and character of the cyst and sometimes to demonstrate communication with the normal CSF pathways.

Hydranencephaly and Severe Hydrocephalus

In both hydranencephaly and severe hydrocephalus there is severe loss of cerebral tissue and the head is largely filled with fluid. In hydranencephaly (Fig. 8.1) there is massive destruction of the cerebral hemispheres associated with intrauterine bilateral supraclinoid internal carotid arterial occlusion. That portion of the brain supplied by the internal carotid arteries is destroyed and only the brainstem and portion of the occipital lobes fed by the posterior cerebral arteries from the basilar artery are present. The falx is intact.[2]

We have seen one patient with unilateral absence of that portion of the brain supplied by the internal carotid artery (Fig. 8.2).

Severe hydrocephalus may be similar in appearance with replacement of cerebral tissue with fluid; however the remnant of occipital lobes are not present. Cerebral angiography and possibly computerized tomography (CT) are the only ways to differentiate between these possibilities.[2] In hydranencephaly, the supraclinoid internal carotid arteries are occluded, whereas with severe hydrocephalus the vessels are present but markedly stretched. With a huge subdural hygroma, which may also present with a large fluid collection, the normal vessels are present but displaced away from the skull.

Dandy-Walker Cyst

The Dandy-Walker syndrome is a congenital cystic dilatation of the fourth ventricle due to atresia of the foramen of Magendi, and possibly also the foramina of Luschka, associated with dysgenesis of the vermis of the cerebellum.[3] The cerebellum is small and the inferior vermis is commonly absent or rudimentary. Other associated cerebral malformations may be present such as an encephalocele, agenesis of the corpus callosum, or holoprosencephaly. Dilatation of the ventricles is present to varying degrees.

Ultrasonography (Figs. 8.3 and 8.4) demonstrates a large posterior fossa cyst continuous with a dilated fourth ventricle. The cerebellum is small and displaced anterolaterally. The lateral and third ventricles may be dilated to varying degree and the occipital horns of the lateral ventricles show a typical divergence due to displacement by the posterior fossa cyst and elevated tentorium. Sagittal and coronal views demonstrate enlargement of the posterior fossa and high position of the tentorium corresponding to the torcula/lambdoid inversion seen on the skull x-rays.[4]

Arachnoid Cysts

The arachnoid cyst is a CSF fluid collection which lies in contact with the surface of the brain. The cyst may be congenital due to abnormal mechanism of leptomeningeal formation or, more frequently, acquired as a result of the entrapment of subarachnoid or cisternal space by arachnoid adhesions and the unidirectional inward flow of CSF. Arachnoid cysts frequently communicate with the subarachnoid space on pneumoencephalography and are most common within the cisterns, around the sella (Fig. 8.5) and the posterior third ventricle, and the posterior fossa. They occur less commonly in the middle fossa and over the hemispheres. Arachnoid cysts differ from enlarged cisterns because their mass effect displaces normal structures and sometimes causes obstruction of the ventricular system.

Ultrasonography of an arachnoid cyst (Fig. 8.5) demonstrates a fluid-containing space displacing adjacent structures and sometimes causing obstruction of the ventricles. In our case with the suprasellar arachnoid cyst, the third ventricle is compressed and displaced superiorly and posteriorly. The lateral ventricles are dilated due to obstruction at the third ventricle, foramen of Monro, or aqueduct. A characteristic appearance similar to the head of a "bunny" (rabbit) has been described on axial CT scans with dilated lateral ventricles.[5]

Porencephalic Cysts

A porencephalic cyst is a CSF-containing cavity of the brain and may be associated with hydrocephalus. It may communicate with the ventricle but is not lined by true ependyma. The etiology of the cyst may be congenital, due to failure of development of the cerebral mantle, or, more commonly, the cystic defect results from destruction of cerebral tissue by cerebral vascular occlusion, intracranial infection, intracranial hemorrhage, or trauma.[1]

Ultrasonography demonstrates a fluid-containing mass communicating with dilated ventricles. Figure 8.6 shows scans of a premature infant with intraventricular hemorrhage who had multiple transcerebral ventricular taps which led to dilatation of the needle track and formation of a porencephalic cyst.[6]

Figure 8.7 is a patient with porencephalic cyst secondary to trauma and brain necrosis in an area of hematoma.

Encysted Ventricle

Encystment of a ventricle by occlusion of its CSF outlet can occur due to adhesions after intraventricular infection or hemorrhage, or due to pressure effect by an extrinsic mass lesion. It results in enlargement of the ventricle which becomes an intracranial mass lesion and requires separate shunting.

Ultrasonography demonstrates a fluid-filled mass in the area of the ventricle which may or may not resemble a ventricle (Fig. 8.8). Encystment of a lateral ventricle is more common and results from occlusion of the foramen of Monro producing a symmetric enlargement of the lateral ventricle (Fig. 13.2, Chapter 13).

Enlargement of Normal Cisterns

The cisterns about the brain are not normally identified on ultrasound scans; however, occasionally a prominent cistern is seen as a fluid-filled space. The cisterna magna varies in size and, when prominent, can be identified as a fluid-filled space in the posterior fossa surrounding the cerebellum (Fig. 8.9).

Enlarged cisterns can be seen with communicating hydrocephalus when hemorrhage, infection, or tumor cause obstruction of the CSF flow over the convexities to the arachnoid granulations resulting in progressive dilatation of the ventricular system and enlargement of the cisterns proximal to the obstruction. Figure 8.10 is the scan of a baby with a prominent quadrigeminal cistern posterior to the third ventricle and communicating hydrocephalus.

Summary

A variety of intracranial cystic abnormalities can be demonstrated by cranial ultrasonography.[7] The exact pathogenesis and nature of the fluid cannot always be determined; however, the geography and probable histologic type can be established. The relationship of the cyst to the ventricles and CSF pathways can frequently be determined and is important since some cysts require separate shunting and decompression, whereas others are treated with the standard ventricular shunting.

References

1. Harwood-Nash DC, Fitz CR. *Neuroradiology in Infants and Children.* St. Louis: C. V. Mosby, 1976; 965–997.
2. Dublin AB, French BN. Diagnostic image evaluation of hydranencephaly and pictorially similar entities with emphasis on computed tomography. Radiology 1980; 137:81–91.
3. Raimondi AJ. *Pediatric Neuroradiology.* Philadelphia: W. B. Saunders, 1972; 275.
4. LeQuesne GW. Ultrasonic diagnosis of the Dandy-Walker malformation. Presented at 25th Annual Meeting of American Institute of Ultrasound in Medicine; New Orleans, Sept. 15–19, 1980.

5. Marali R, Epstein F. Diagnosis and treatment of suprasellar arachnoid cyst. Report of three cases. J Neurosurg 1979; 50:515–518.
6. Grainger RG, Lorber J. Development of ventricular diverticula following ventricular puncture in hydrocephalic infant. Acta Radiol 1963; 1:569–576.
7. Mack LA, Rumack CM, Johnson ML. Ultrasound evaluation of cystic intracranial lesions in the neonate. Radiology 1980; 137:451–455.
8. Swischuk, L. *Radiology of the Newborn and Young Infant*, Ed. 2, Baltimore: Williams & Wilkins, 1980; 771.
9. Babcock DS, Han BK. The accuracy of high resolution real-time ultrasonography of the head in infancy. Radiology 1981; 139:665–676.

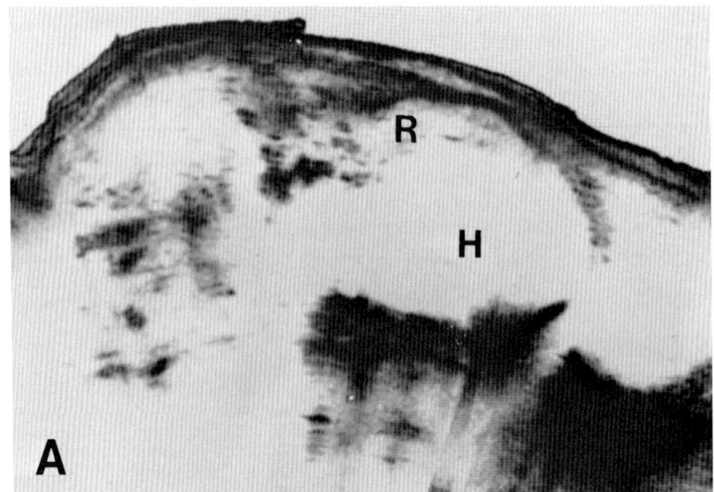

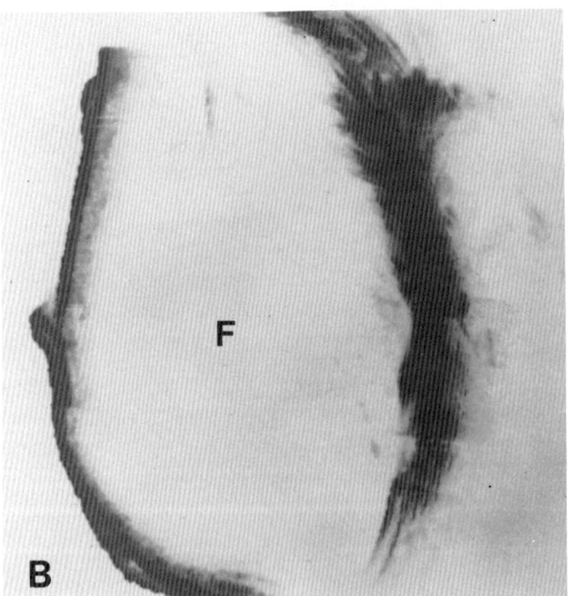

Figure 8.1 Hydranencephaly. (*A*) Prenatal ultrasound examination during labor shows single intrauterine fetus with abnormally large, fluid-filled head (*H*). Artifactual reverberations (*R*) seen in anterior portion of head. (*B*) High axial, (*C*) Coronal scans, and (*D*) CT scan show brainstem and thalamus (*Th*) in mid lower portion of head. Remainder of head filled with fluid (*F*) and no cerebral mantle identified (Reproduced with permission from D. S. Babcock and B. K. Han: *Radiology*, *139:*665–676, 1981.[9])

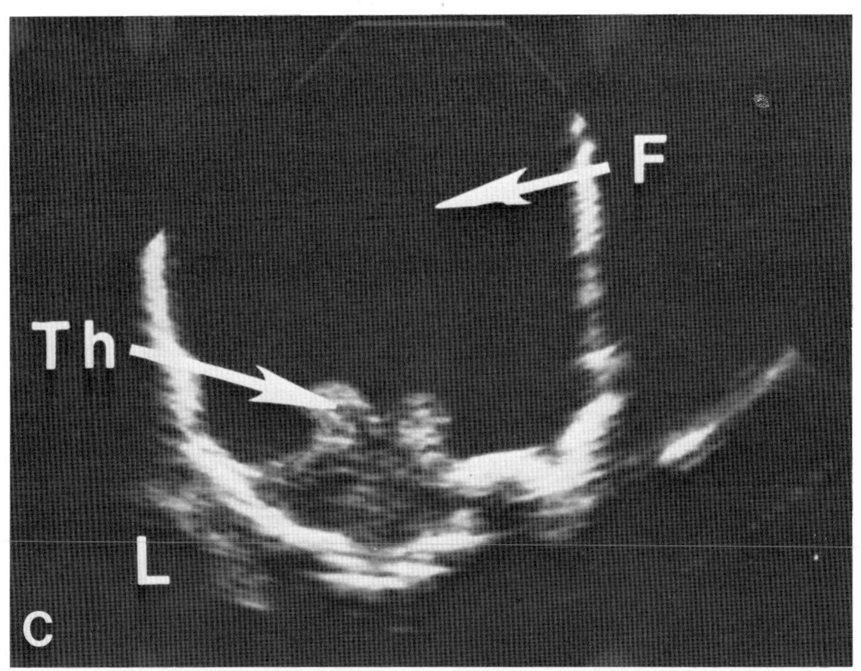
F
Th
L
C

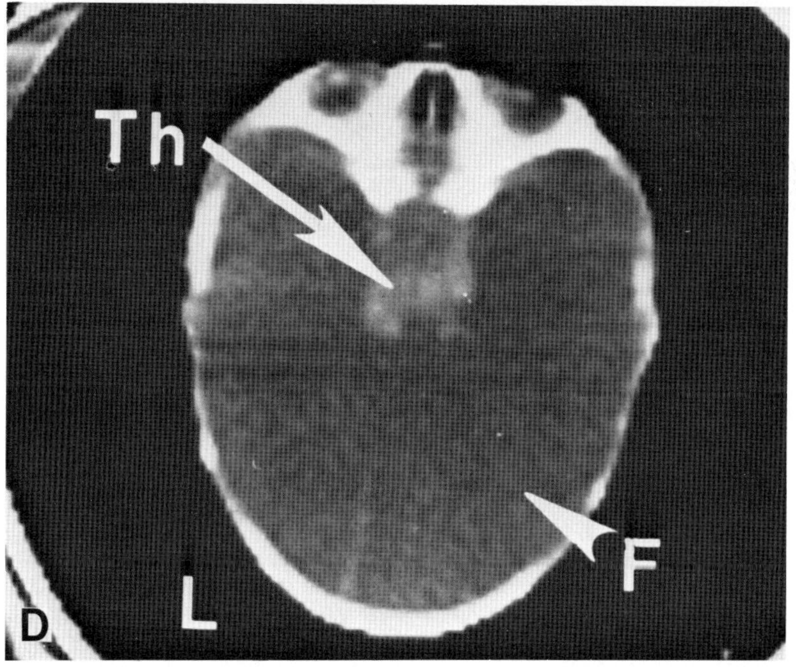
Th
F
L
D

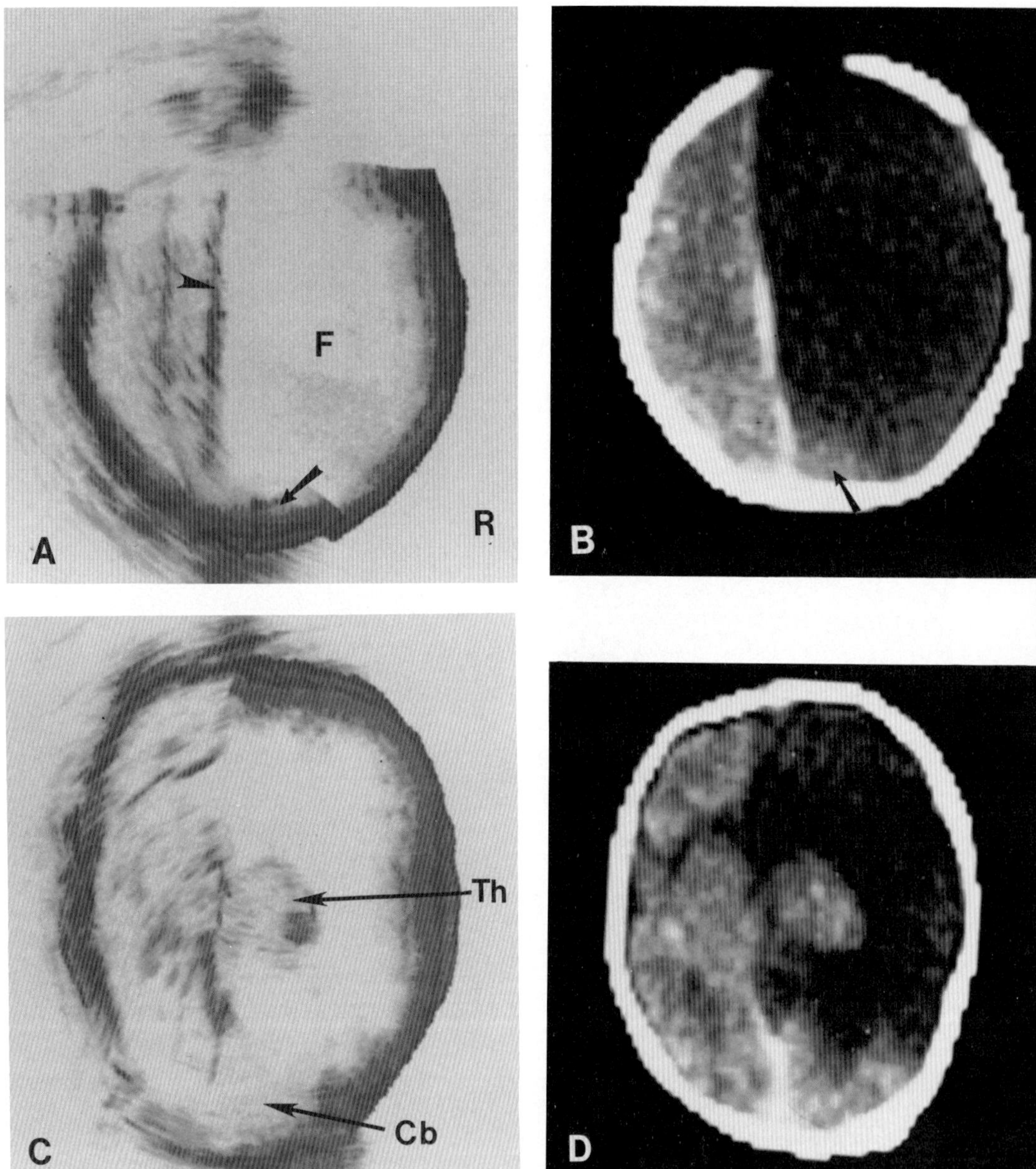

Figure 8.2 Hemihydranencephaly. Premature infant, 34 weeks gestation, who developed apnea, bradycardia, and seizures on second day after traumatic delivery. History of trauma to mother in fourth month of pregnancy. (*A*) High axial scan and (*B*) corresponding CT scan. Right side of head filled with fluid (*F*) with small occipital lobe seen posteriorly (*arrows*). Left cerebral hemisphere smaller than normal and falx displaced to left (*arrowhead*). (*C*) Low axial scan, (*D*) corresponding CT scan, and (*E*) coronal scan. Normal midbrain, thalamus (*Th*) and cerebellum (*Cb*) identified on right. (*F* and *G*) Pneumoencephalography.

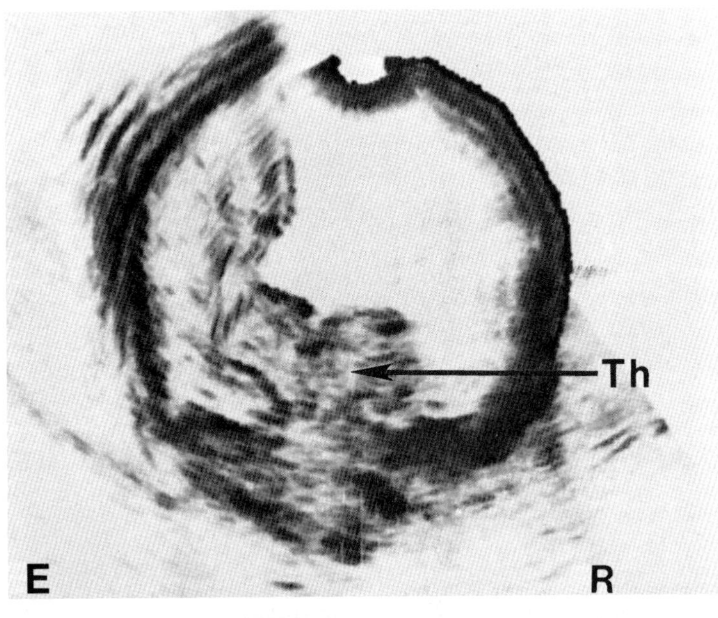
Th
E
R

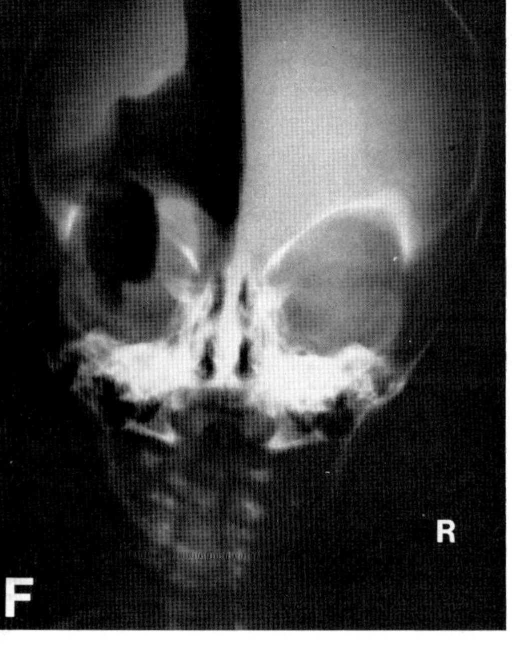
R
F

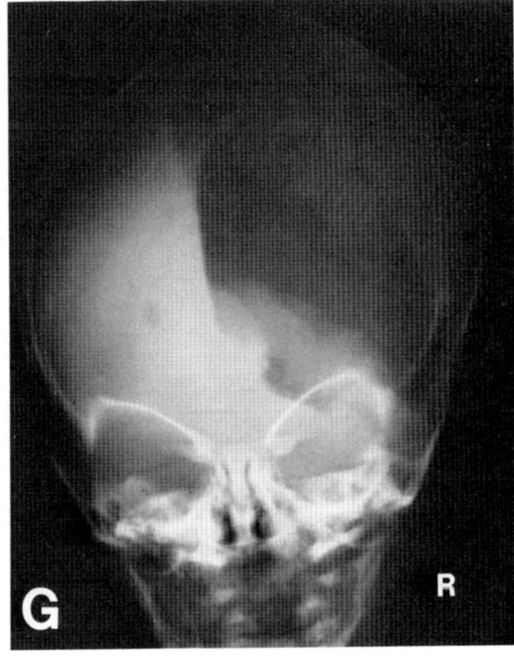
G
R

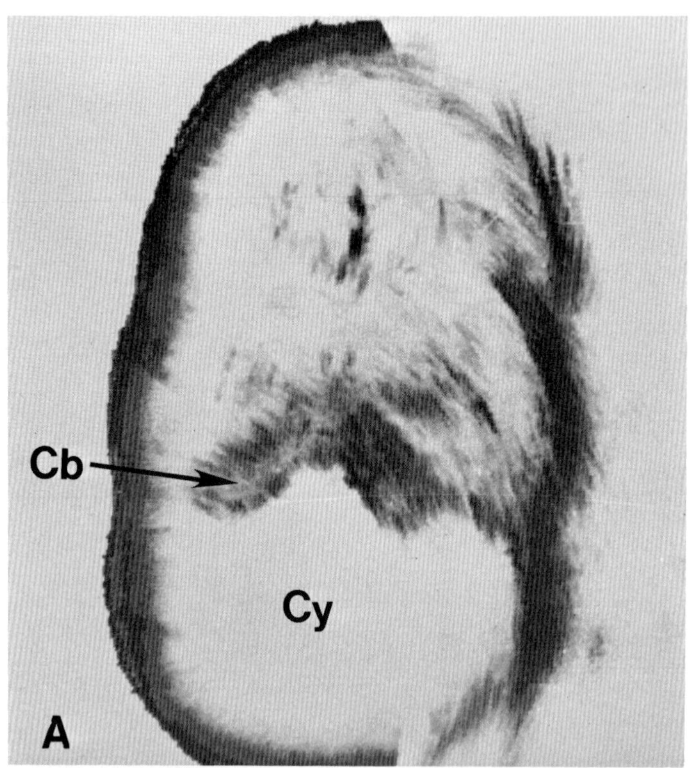

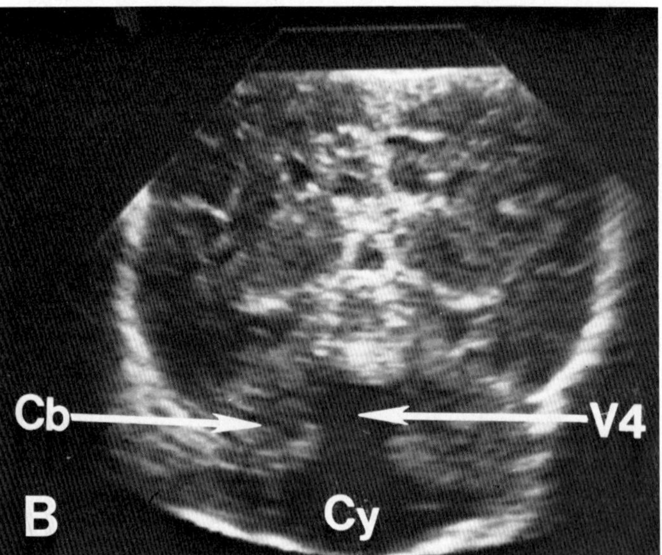

Figure 8.3 Dandy-Walker cyst. Two-day-old infant with dysmorphic features and increasing head size with prominent fontanelles. (*A*) Axial, (*B*) coronal, (*C*) posterior coronal, (*D*) sagittal, and (*E*) posterior fossa scans show large cyst (*Cy*) in posterior fossa tapering anteriorly into fourth ventricle (*V4*). Hypoplastic cerebellum (*Cb*) seen laterally and anteriorly. Slight dilatation of lateral and third ventricles present with unusually high position of tentorium cerebelli (*TC*). ((*A*) Reproduced with permission from L. E. Swischuk: *Radiology of the Newborn and Young Infant*, ed. 2, p. 771, 1980.[8] ((*B–D*) Reproduced with permission from D. S. Babcock and B. K. Han: *Radiology*, *139:*665–676, 1981.[9])

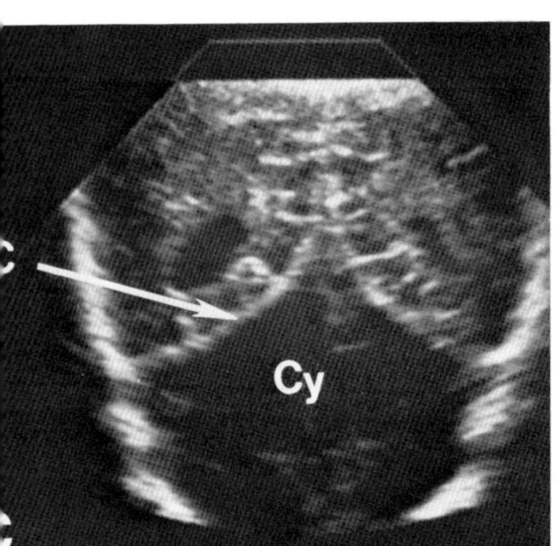
Cy

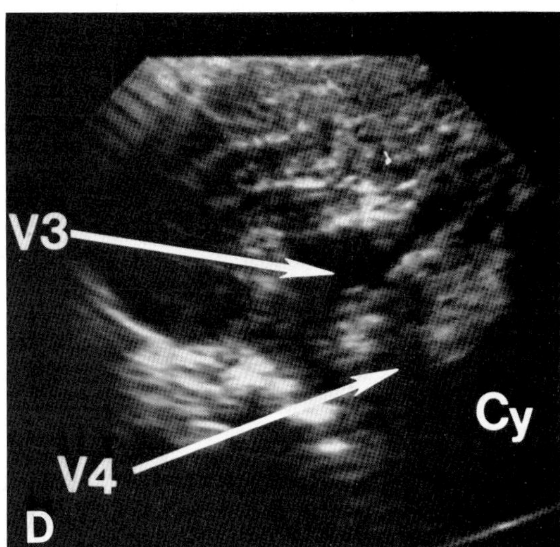
V3
V4
Cy
D

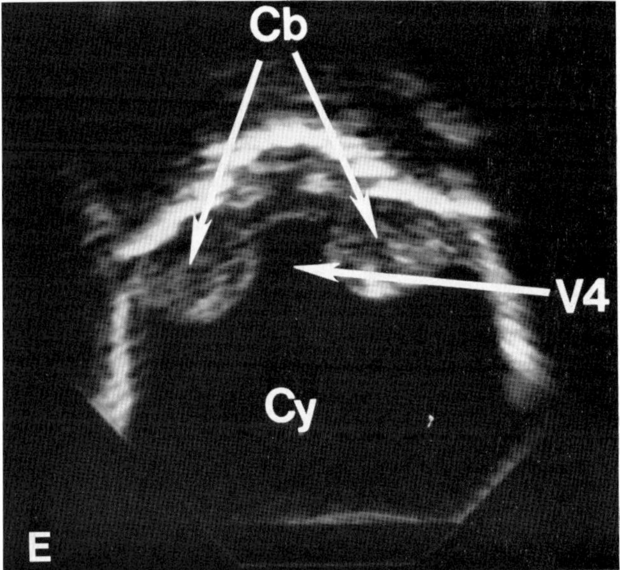
Cb
V4
Cy
E

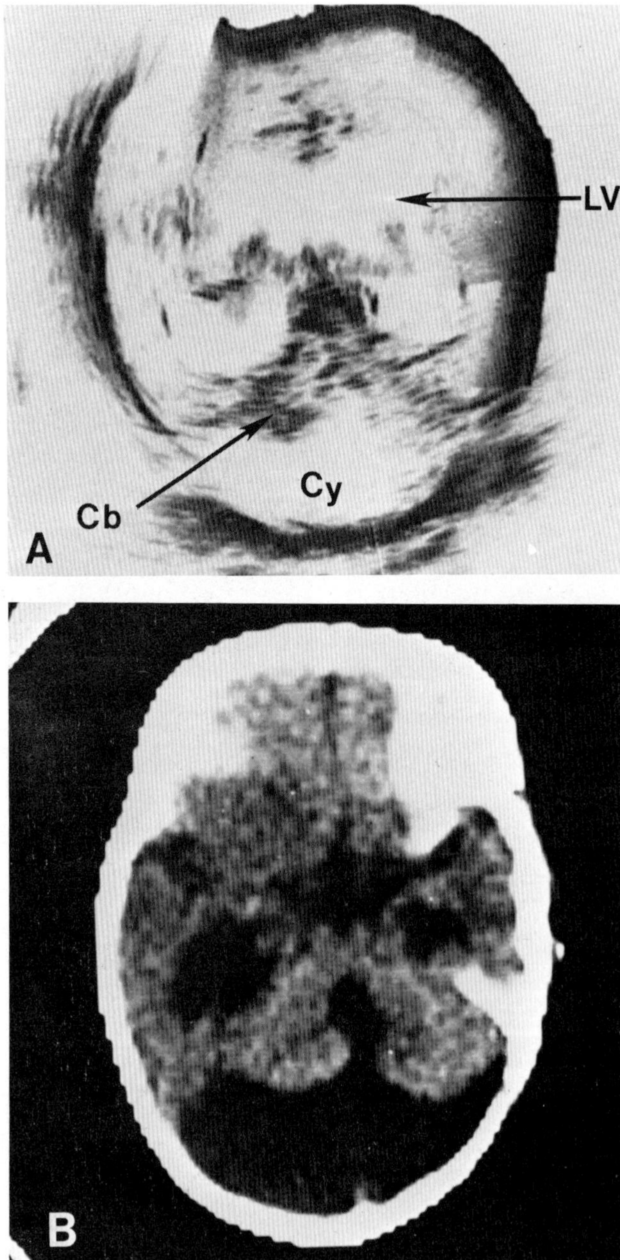

Figure 8.4 Dandy-Walker cyst. Three month old baby with macrocrania and enlarging head. (*A*) Coronal ultrasound scan and (*B*) axial CT scan. Large cyst (*Cy*) in posterior fossa continuous with dilated fourth ventricle. Hypoplastic cerebellum (*Cb*) seen anteriorly. Both lateral ventricles moderately dilated.

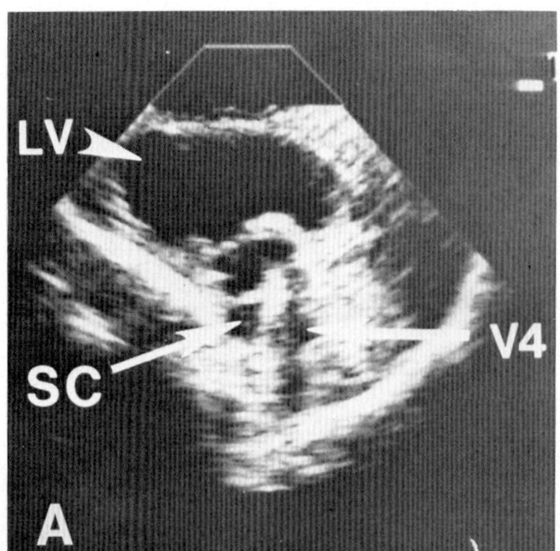

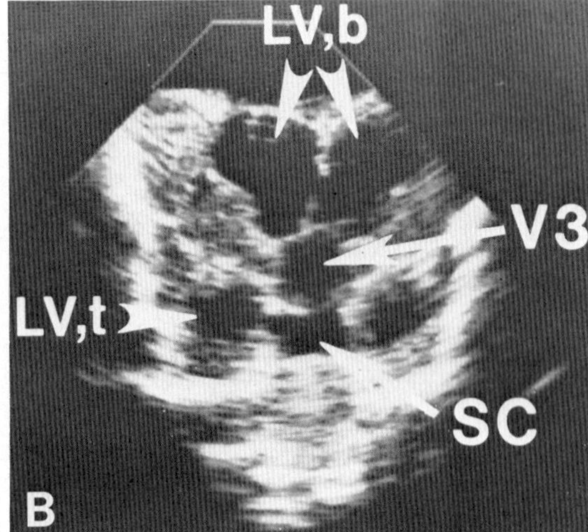

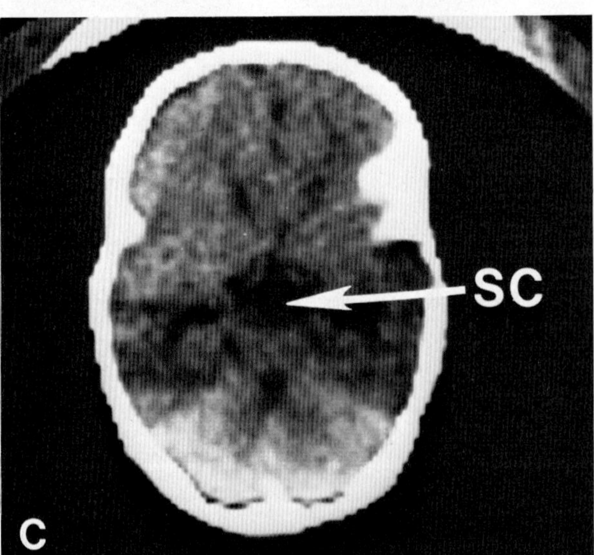

Figure 8.5 Suprasellar arachnoid cyst. A 17-month-old infant with multiple problems including large head. (*A*) Sagittal, (*B*) coronal scans, and (*C*) axial CT scan show moderate dilatation of lateral and third ventricles and small suprasellar cyst (*SC*). Ventriculoperitoneal shunt inserted. Five months later he presented with vomiting and increased irritability. (*D*) Sagittal and (*E*) coronal scans. Lateral ventricles diminished, although still moderately enlarged. Further enlargement of suprasellar arachnoid cyst shown. (*F*) CT scan shows characteristic appearance of head of a "bunny" (rabbit). Suprasellar arachnoid cyst removed surgically. (Reproduced with permission from D. S. Babcock and B. K. Han: *Radiology*, *139:*665–676, 1981.[9])

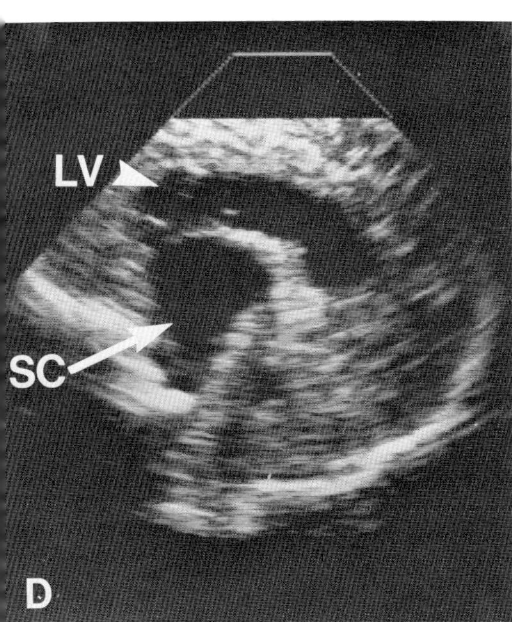
LV
SC
D

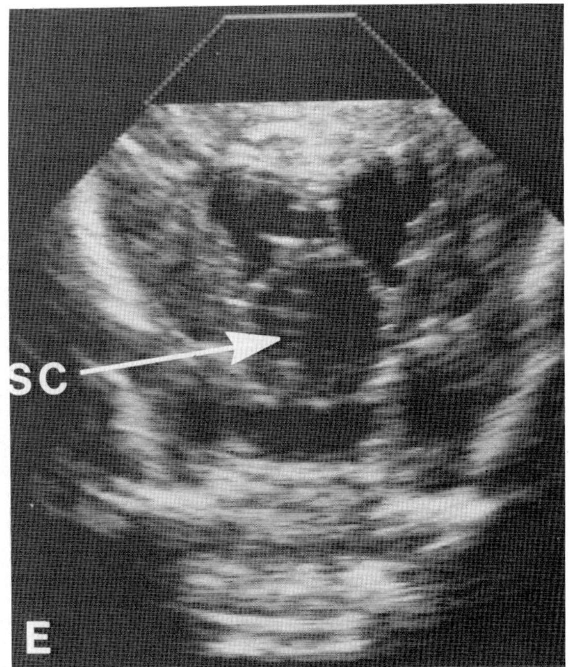
SC
E

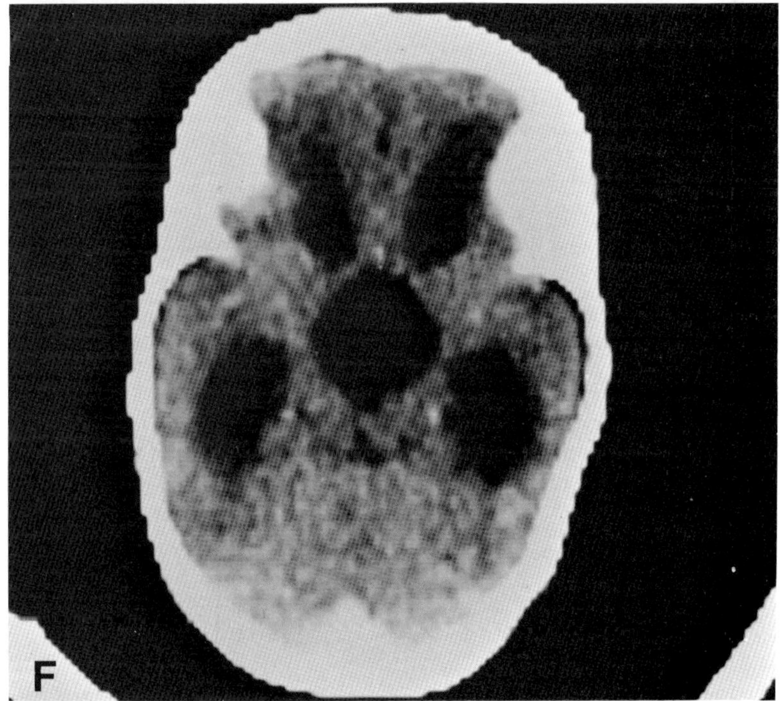
F

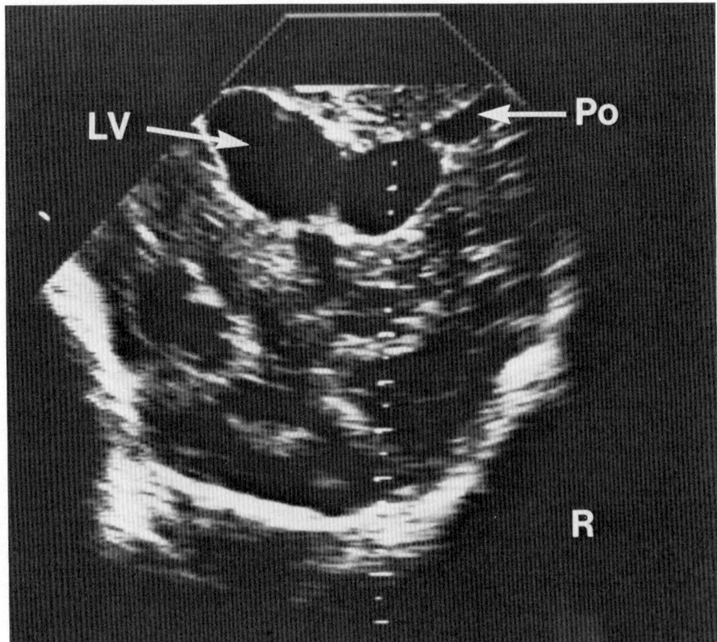

Figure 8.6 Porencephalic cyst secondary to repeated ventricular taps. Premature infant with moderate hydrocephalus secondary to previous intraventricular hemorrhage. Repeated ventricular taps performed in right frontal area. Coronal scan shows moderate panhydrocephalus and small porencephalic cyst (*Po*) in right frontal area. *LV*, lateral ventricle.

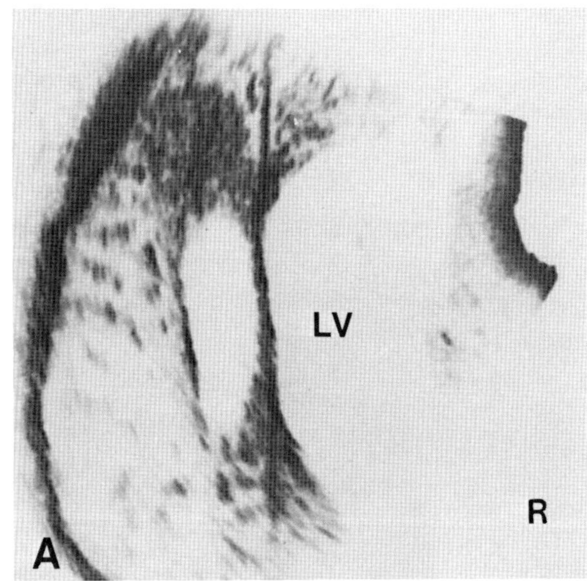

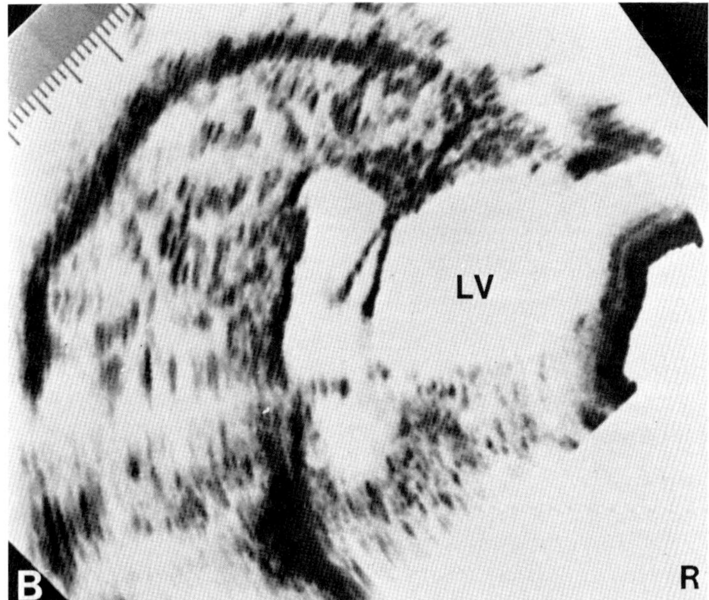

Figure 8.7 Porencephalic dilatation of right lateral ventricle due to previous trauma. Nine-year-old boy with head trauma at 2 years of age with removal of portion of crushed right brain. (*A*) Axial and (*B*) coronal scans obtained through right parietal craniotomy defect. Marked dilatation of right lateral ventricle (*LV*) seen with thinning of brain over ventricle laterally indicating porencephaly. Moderate dilatation of left lateral ventricle also seen.

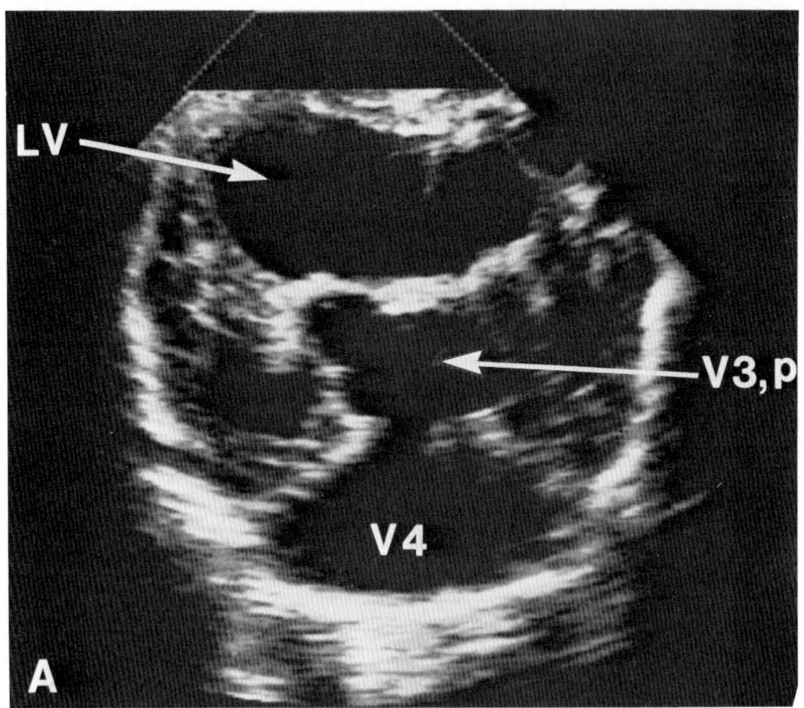

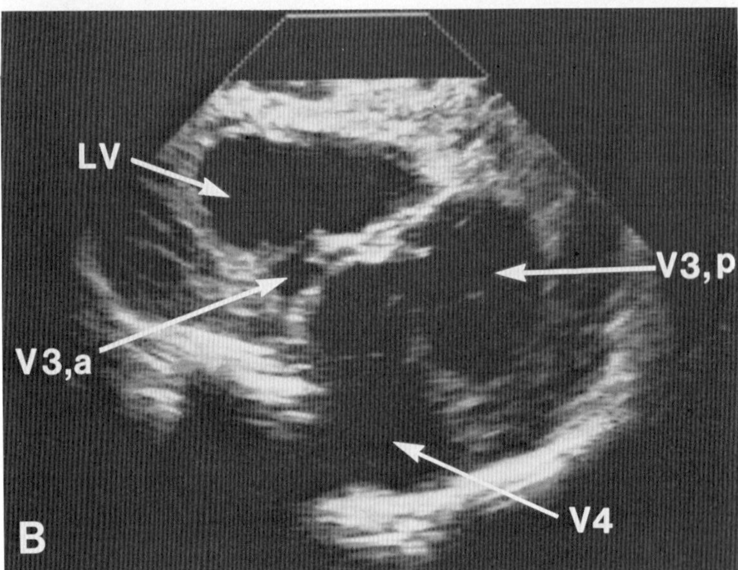

Figure 8.8 Encysted ventricles. Premature infant, 29 weeks gestation, with hydrocephalus from previous massive intraventricular hemorrhage presented with possible malfunctioning shunt. (*A*) Coronal and (*B*) midline sagittal scans show moderate asymmetric enlargement of lateral ventricles (*LV*) and slight dilatation of anterior third ventricle (*V3,a*). Large cystic structure in posterior fossa seen in midline extending up to supratentorial region thought to be dilated fourth (*V4*) and posterior third (*V3,p*) ventricles. Malfunctioning shunt in lateral ventricle revised. (*C*) Coronal and (*D*) sagittal scans. Lateral ventricles now collapsed and slitlike. Persistent enlargement of posterior third and fourth ventricles due to arachnoidal adhesions found at operation.

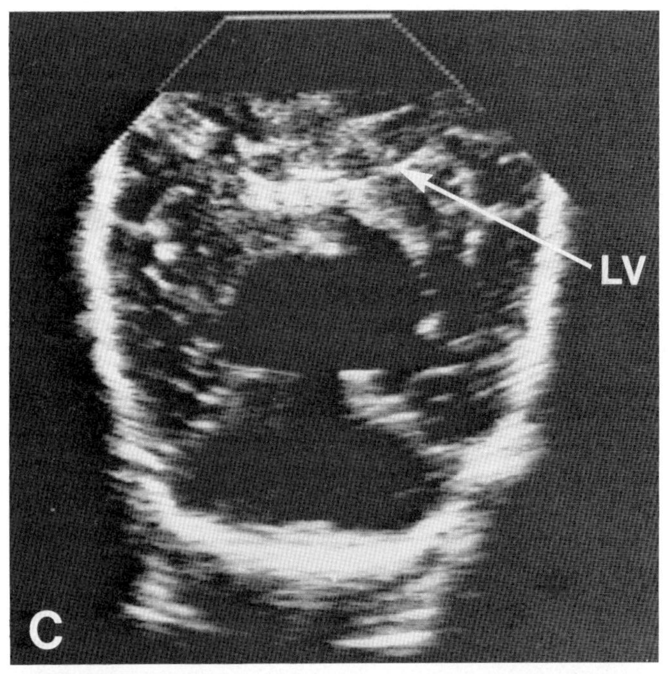
LV
C

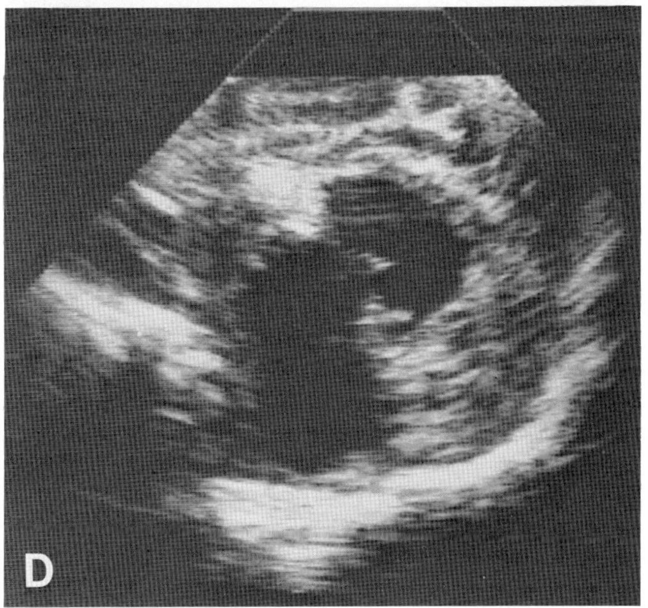
D

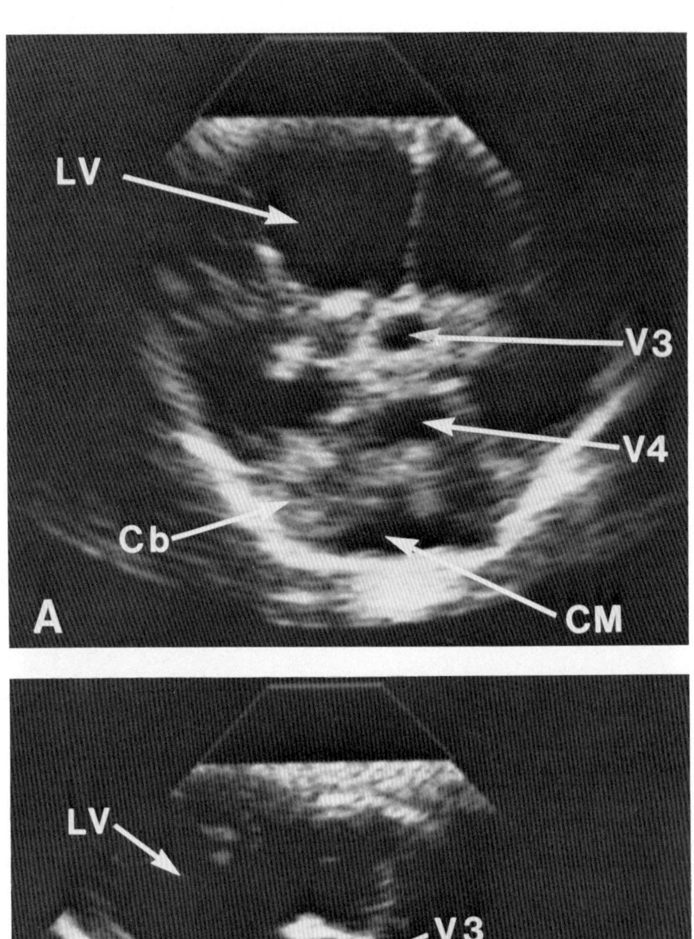

Figure 8.9 Panhydrocephalus with enlarged cisterna magna. Five-month-old infant with macrocrania. (*A*) Coronal and (*B*) midline sagittal scans show moderate dilatation of all ventricles. Cisterna magna (*CM*) also enlarged. (*C*) CT scan and (*D*) higher CT scan show hydrocephalus and enlarged cisterna magna. *LV*, lateral ventricle; *Cb*, cerebellum; *V3* and *V4*, third and fourth ventricle, respectively.

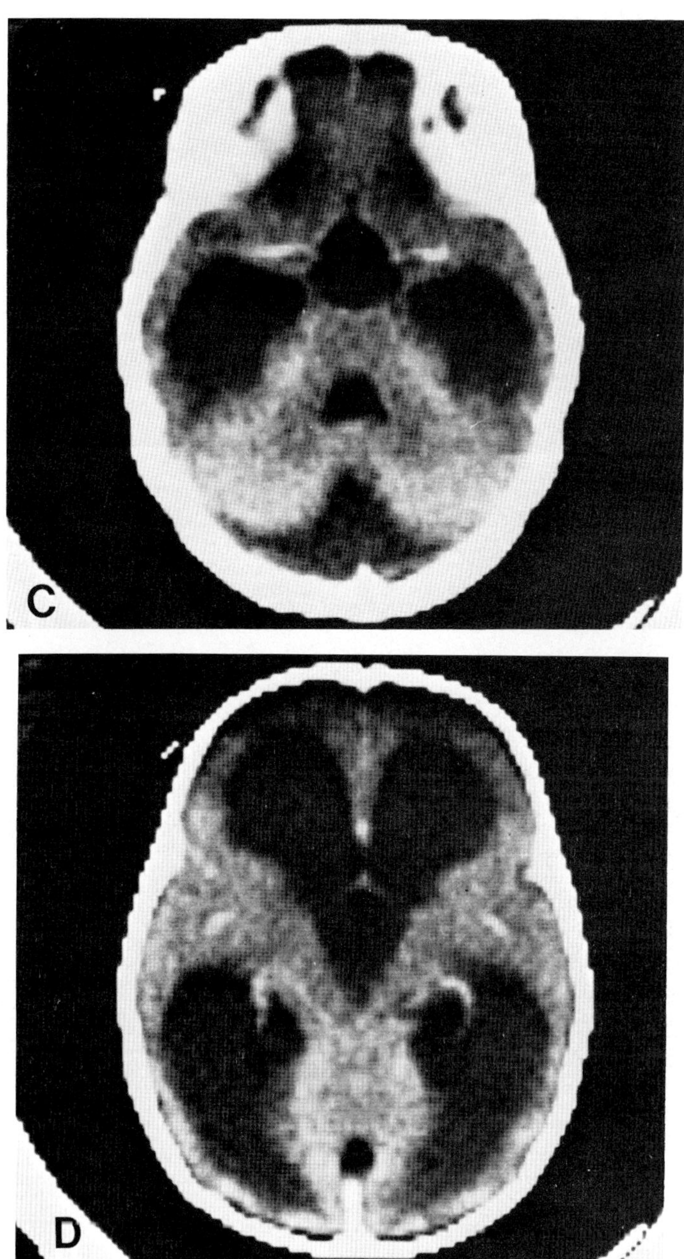
C
D

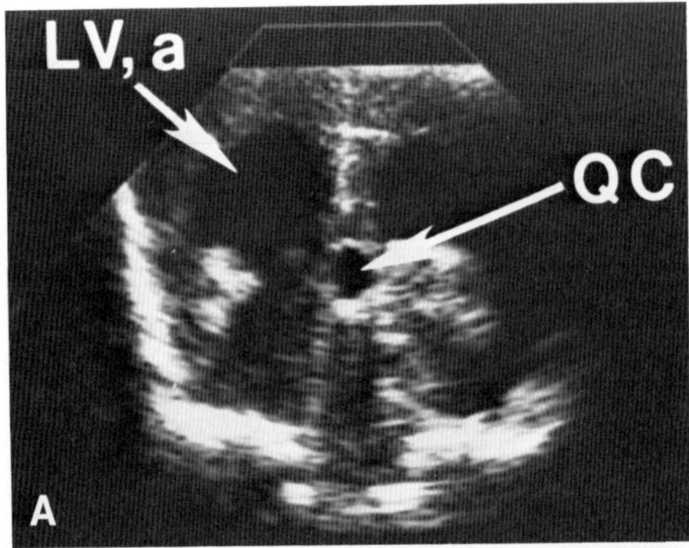

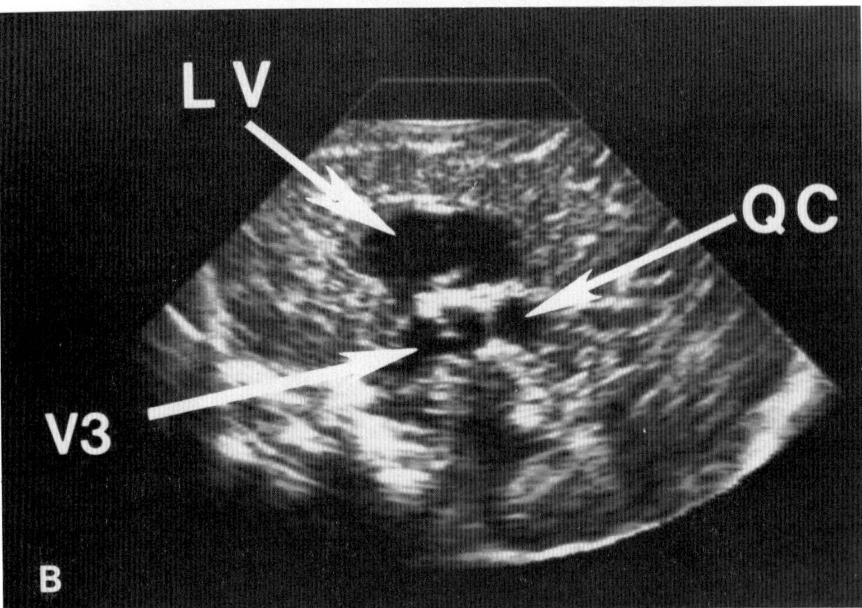

Figure 8.10 Cyst of quadrigeminal cistern. Premature infant with respiratory distress syndrome, sepsis, patent ductus arteriosus, and necrotizing enterocolitis. At 8 months of age, tense fontanelle noted. (*A*) Posterior coronal and (*B*) sagittal scans. Moderate hydrocephalus involving lateral (*LV, LV,a*), third (*V3*), and fourth ventricles demonstrated. Also present, small cyst of quadrigeminal cistern (*QC*) posterior to third ventricle. ((*B*) Reproduced by permission from L. E. Swischuk: *Radiology of the Newborn and Young Infant*, Ed. 2, p. 788, 1980.[8])

CHAPTER 9

Other Congenital Malformations

Ultrasonography has proven useful in evaluating congenital malformations of the brain which have altered macroscopic morphology. The Chiari II malformation is discussed in Chapter 5 and the Dandy-Walker cyst in Chapter 6. We will discuss other gross malformations in this chapter. Disorders at the molecular level of anatomy and mild disorders at the macroscopic level are not identifiable by ultrasonography.

Agenesis of the Corpus Callosum

The corpus callosum is the principal tract connecting the right and left cerebral hemispheres. Absence of the corpus callosum may be complete due to embryonic agenesis, or may be partial due to acquired intrauterine encephalomalacia. It may be associated with other intracranial malformations such as microcephaly, hydrocephalus, porencephaly, or a Chiari malformation.[1] It may be entirely asymptomatic.

Ultrasonography demonstrates similar findings to those observed on pneumoencephalography. There is separation of the lateral ventricles with increased angulation of the roofs of the lateral ventricles in the region of the frontal horns and bodies (Fig. 9.1). The third ventricle is dilated and herniates superiorly between the lateral ventricles. The septum pellucidum is absent. The lateral ventricles may be quite bulbous and there is medial convexity resulting from the rearranged longitudinal callosal bundles.

Macrocrania can be seen with this malformation and is usually due to hydrocephalus secondary to associated malformations such as aqueductal stenosis, a large midline arachnoid cyst, or the Chiari or Dandy-Walker malformations. The dilatation and upward extension of the third ventricle is variable and may form a large midline cyst occupying the interhemispheric fissure and extending to the bony calvaria (Fig. 9.2). Differential diagnosis includes a midline arachnoid cyst.

Holoprosencephaly

Holoprosencephaly, or the formation of a holospheric cerebrum, results from a disorder of diverticulation of the fetal brain. The cerebral hemispheres and lateral ventricles develop between the 4th and 8th weeks of fetal life as two paired vesicles arising laterally from the prosencephalon to form a telencephalon (cerebral hemispheres) and a diencephalon (thalamus, hypothalamus). A defect in midline cleavage of this prosencephalon causes failure of formation of the separate cerebral hemispheres. Variations of holoprosencephaly are determined by the degree of separation of the holosphere which is a thin, pancake-like primitive cerebrum.[1, 2]

The most severe form is the alobar holoprosencephaly in which there is a small amount of cerebral tissue peripherally with no division into cerebral hemispheres, a large horseshoe-shaped single ventricular cavity, and fused thalami (Fig. 9.3).

Lobar and semilobar holoprosencephaly have partial separation into cerebral hemispheres of varying degree, however the frontal horns are always fused and the cerebral sagittal falx is only partially developed (Fig. 9.4).

Arhinencephaly or absence of the rhinic lobe is the mildest form and we have not been able to identify this malformation with ultrasonography.

Holoprosencephaly may be associated with other abnormalities including maternal diabetes mellitus, toxoplasmosis, trisomy 13-15 syndrome, amino acid abnormalities, endocrine dysgenesis, or intrauterine rubella. Midline facial anomalies are often associated with these cerebral malformations. The most severe facial malformations—cyclopia, ethmocephaly, and cebocephaly—are associated with alobar holoprosencephaly and microcephaly. Cleft lip and cleft palate, hypotelorism, and trigonenocephaly are associated with alobar or lobar holoprosencephaly. Thus, skull radiographs on these patients may show microcephaly with varying degrees of hypoplasia of the ethmoid, sphenoid, nasal bones, and palate with hypoteleorism, trigonocephaly, absent crista galli, and cribriform plate.[1]

Arteriovenous Malformation

Our experience with arteriovenous malformations (AVM) occurring within the brain is very limited and we suspect that they are demonstrable by ultrasound only when relatively large or when there is an associated intracerebral hematoma.

Ultrasound demonstrates a mass displacing the normal structures (Fig. 9.5). The mass may be echogenic due to thrombosed blood or sonolucent due to liquid blood. Dilated ventricles may be present due to obstruction by the mass or a previous subarachnoid hemorrhage. AVM are difficult to distinguish from solid tumors and other fluid collections and angiography is necessary for diagnosis.

Summary

Ultrasonography is accurate for identifying congenital malformations of the brain which have altered macroscopic morphology. The findings are very similar to that seen on computerized tomography (CT) and pneumoencephalography. Ultrasound images can be obtained in multiple planes which is helpful in categorizing the malformation. These babies are sometimes clinically unstable, and ultrasound has the advantage of allowing a diagnosis to be made without moving the infant from the nursery.

References

1. Harwood-Nash, Fitz CR. *Neuroradiology in Infants and Children*. T. Louis: C. V. Mosby, 1976; 119–1030.
2. Byrd SE, Harwood-Nash DC, Fitz CR, Rogovitz DM. Computed tomography evaluation of holoprosencephaly in infants and children. J Comput Assist Tomogr 1977; 1:456–463.
3. Babcock DS, Han BK, LeQuesne GW. B-Mode gray scale ultrasound of the head in the newborn and young infant. AJR 1980; 134:457–468.

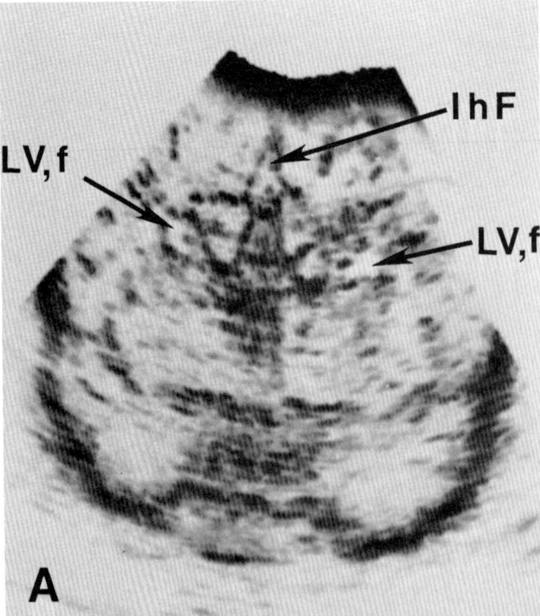

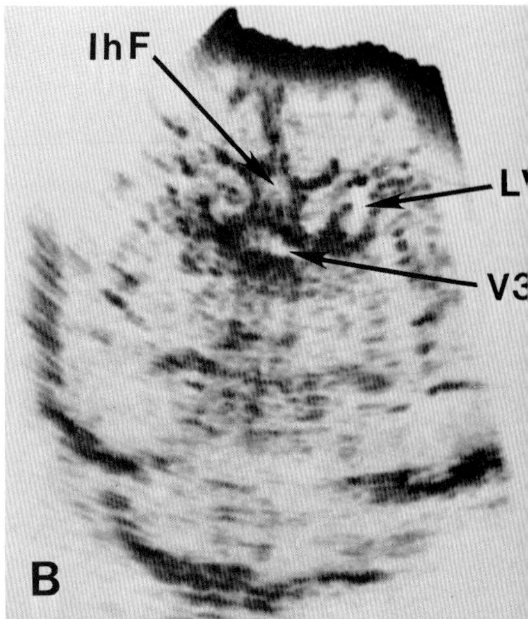

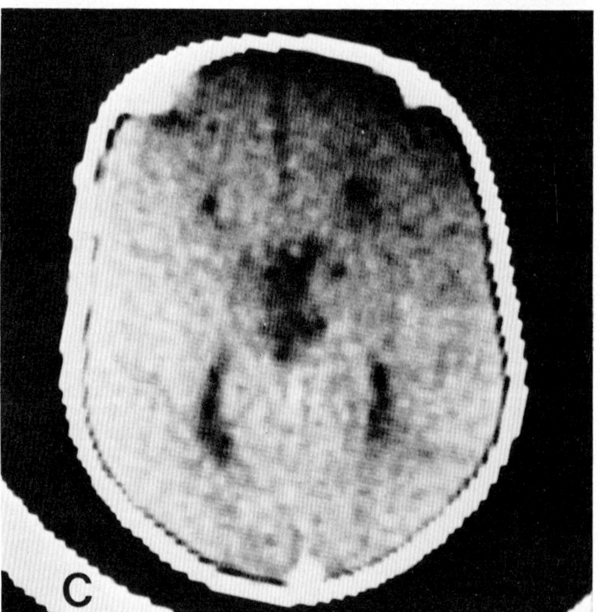

Figure 9.1 Agenesis of corpus callosum. Three-month-old infant with failure to thrive and abnormally increasing head size. (*A*) Coronal scan through frontal horns of lateral ventricles, (*B*) more posterior coronal scan through bodies of lateral ventricles, and (*C*) axial CT scan. Lateral ventricles (*LV*) abnormally separated with increased angulation of roofs. Third ventricle (*V3*) slightly enlarged and herniated superiorly between lateral ventricles. Interhemispheric fissure (*IhF*) mild-to-moderately prominent and extends down to upper margin of superiorly displaced third ventricle. *LV,f,* lateral ventricle, frontal horn.

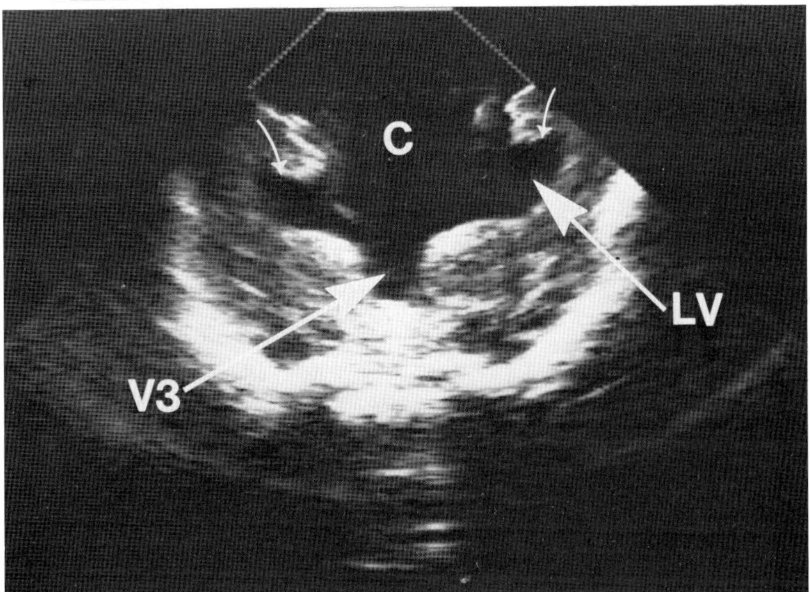

Figure 9.2 Midline cystic malformation with agenesis of corpus callosum. Dysmorphic infant, 2800 g, 37 weeks gestation. Hydrocephalus diagnosed in utero. Coronal scan on 8th day of life. Lateral ventricles (*LV*) abnormally separated with characteristic concave inner borders (*arrows*). Septum pellucidum absent. Third ventricle (*V3*) enlarged and displaced superiorly. Large midline cystic structure (*C*) communicates with lateral and third ventricles and extends into interhemispheric compartment with no visible corpus callosum.

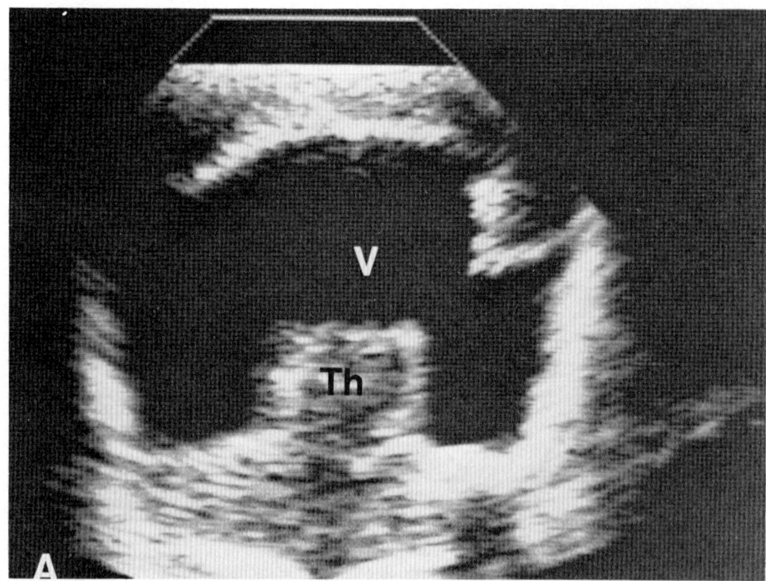

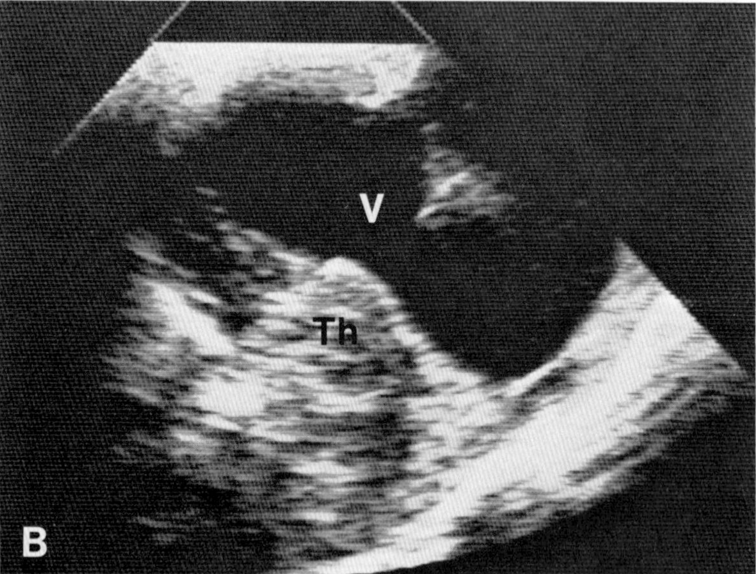

Figure 9.3 Alobar holoprosencephaly. Infant, 1600 g, 35 weeks gestation, with trisomy 13 and cebocephaly. (*A*) Coronal and (*B*) sagittal scans show large U-shaped single ventricle (*V*) and prominent fused thalami (*Th*). Patient died on first day of life. (*C*) Pathology specimen showing posterior aspect of brain. (*D*) Posterior view with cerebrum lifted forward. Brain is undivided, with no interhemispheric fissure. Thin rum of cerebral tissue covers single U-shaped ventricle (*V*). Thalamus is fused. Brainstem and cerebellum (*Cb*) appear normal.

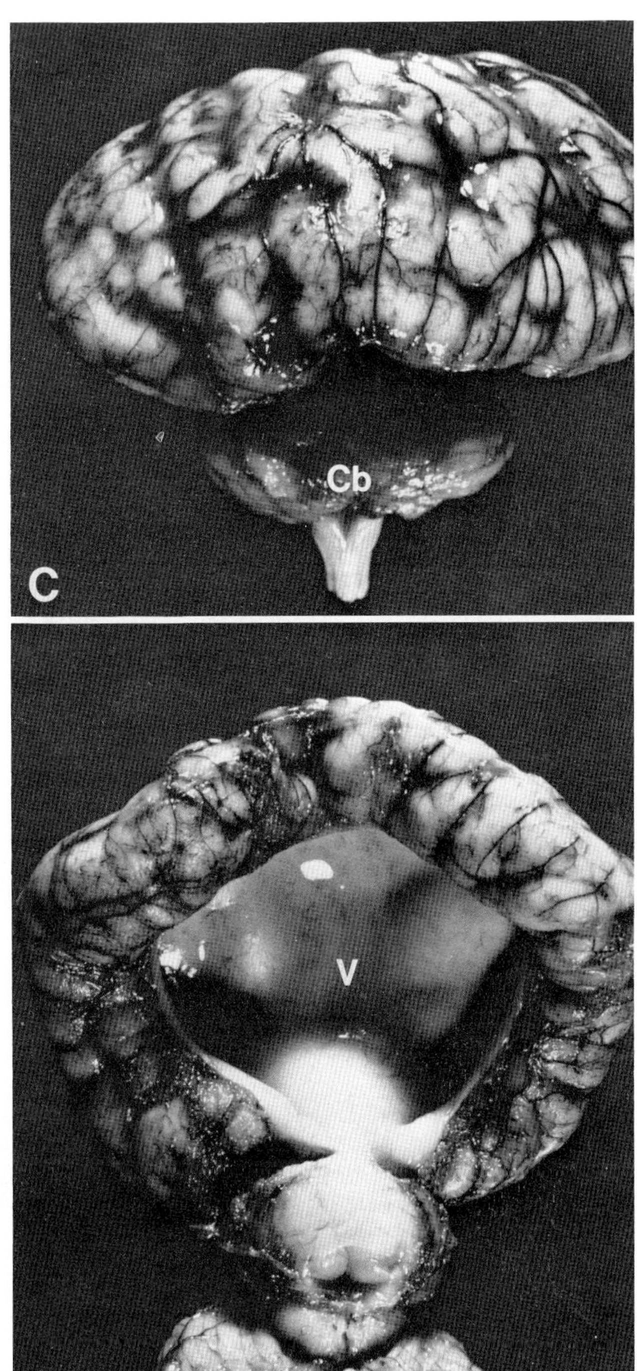
Cb
C
V
D

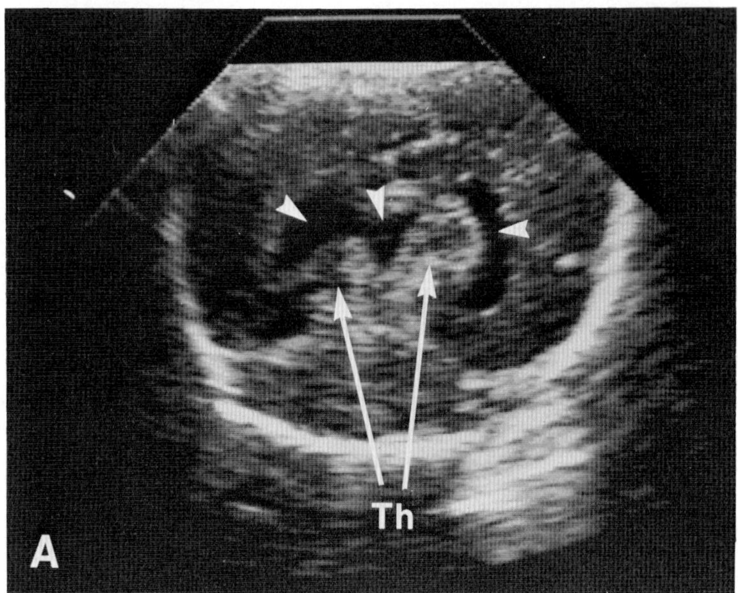

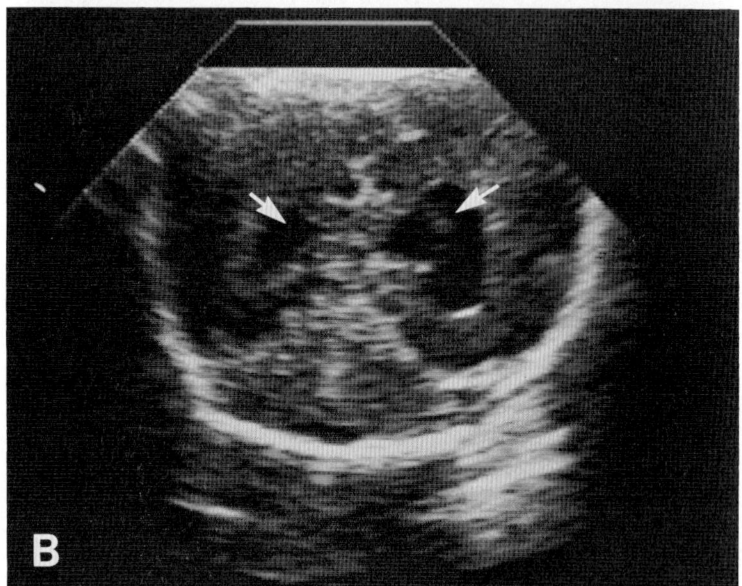

Figure 9.4 Semilobar holoprosencephaly. Newborn infant with multiple congenital anomalies including cleft palate, hypotelorism, and microcephaly. (*A*) Coronal scan through thalami (*Th*) and (*B*) more posterior coronal scan show single ventricular cavity (*arrowheads*) with attempt at formation of occipital horns (*arrows*). Fused thalami seen inferior to single ventricle. (*C*) Right parasagittal and (*D*) left parasagittal scans show anteriorly rotated thalami (*Th*) and single ventricle with attempt at formation of occipital horns (*arrows*), larger on right.

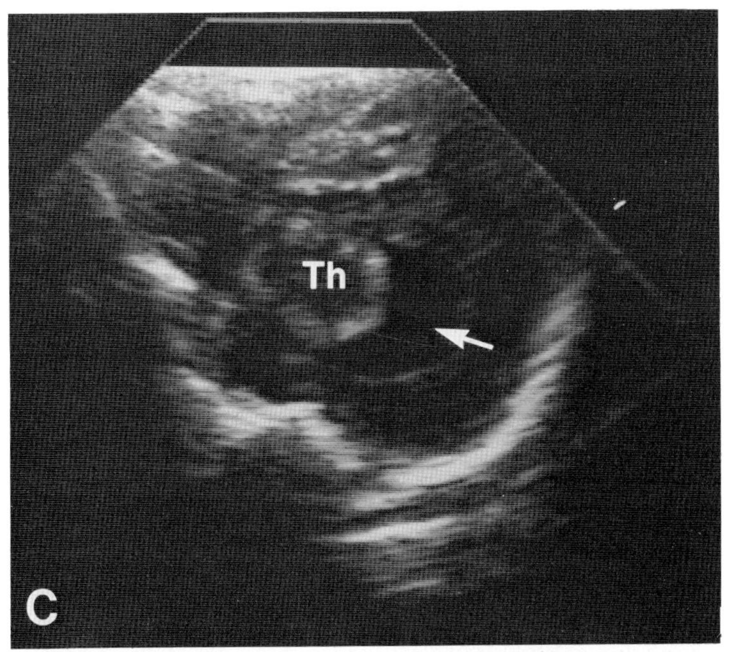
Th
C

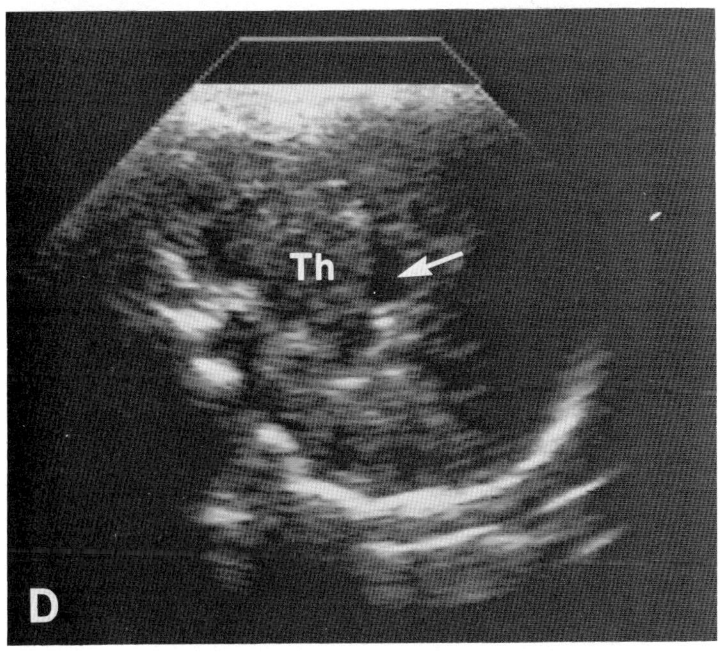
Th
D

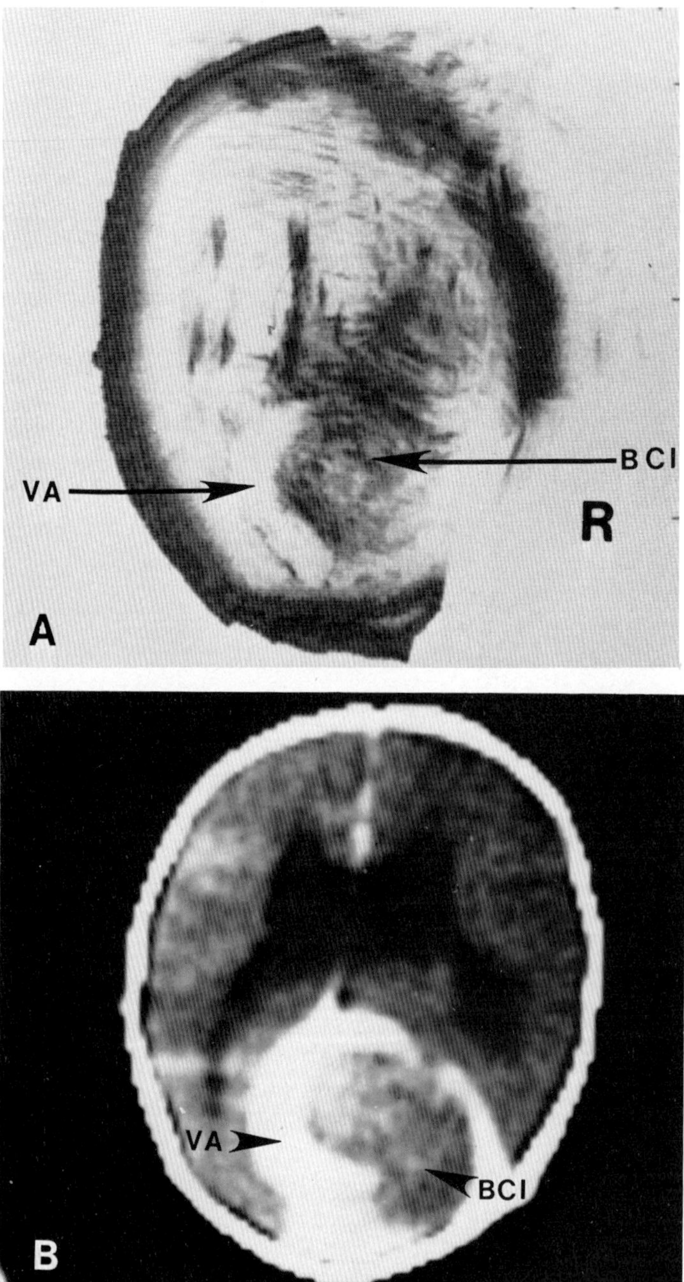

Figure 9.5 Arteriovenous malformation. Two-month-old infant with enlarging head, lethargy, and vomiting. (*A*) Axial and (*B*) corresponding CT scans show moderate enlargement of lateral ventricles and large echogenic mass (*BCI*) in occipital area with surrounding semicircular anechoic zone of venous aneurysm (*VA*). CT findings similar: semicircular structure enhanced after contrast material injection, indicating its vascular nature. (*C* and *D*) Angiogram shows large complex dural venous aneurysm containing blood clot in region of straight sinus and posterior falx cerebri. (Reproduced with permission from D. S. Babcock, B. K. Han, and G. W. LeQuesne: *American Journal of Roentgenology, 134:*457–468, 1980.[3])

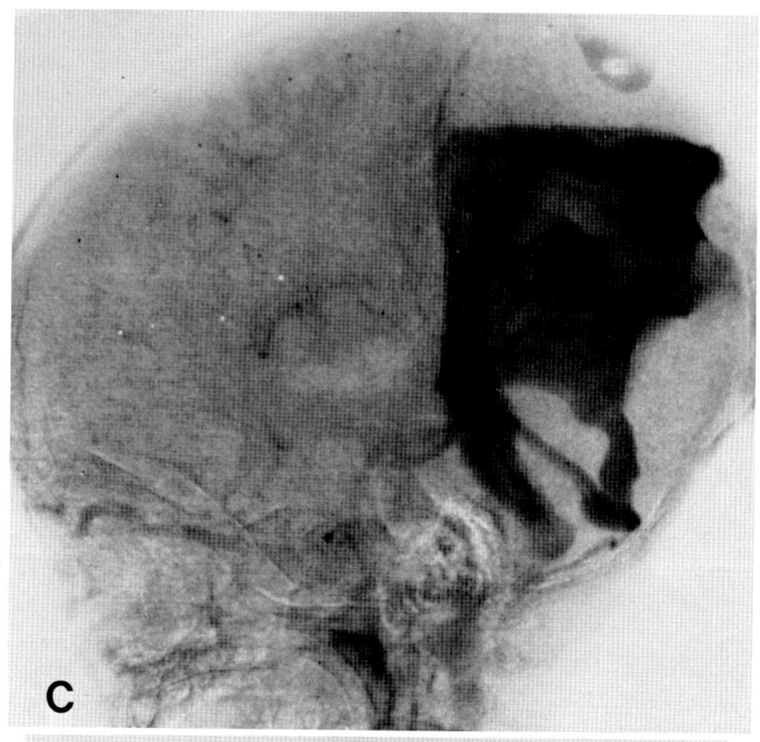
C

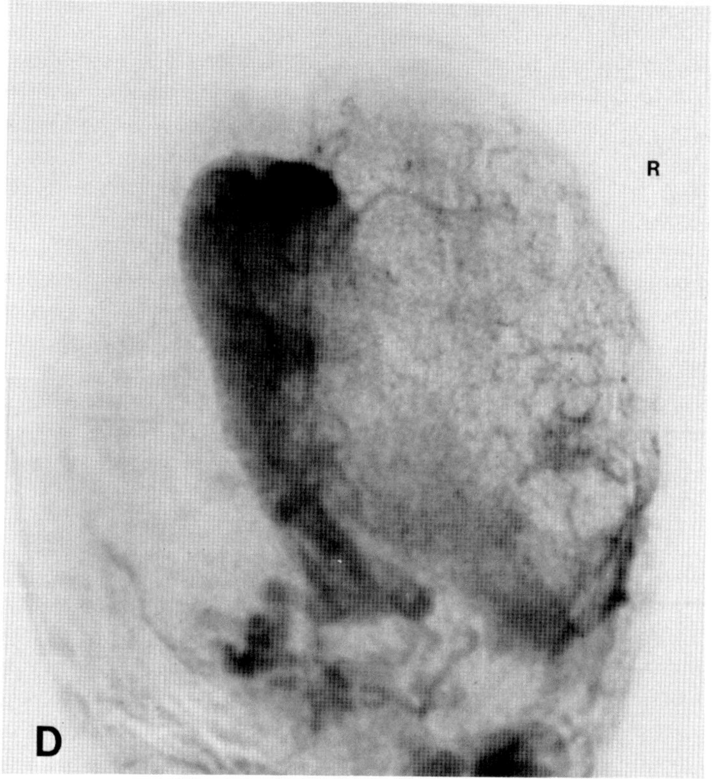
R
D

CHAPTER 10

Intracranial Infection

In our hospital, most infants and children with intracranial inflammatory processes are recognized and dignosed clinically, and are treated medically. Those patients with focal or progressive neurological signs, or prolonged or recurrent fevers, require neuroradiologic investigation to look for a surgically treatable collection of pus such as a subdural empyema or an intracerebral abscess.

Intracranial infections can be diffuse or focal and can involve either the brain or the dural covering. Meningitis or meningoencephalitis is a relatively common infectious disease of infancy. The incidence has been stated to be 2 in every 10,000 full-term births and 20 in every 10,000 premature births.[1] Meningitis and encephalitis often occur together and neuroradiology may show signs of both. The infection may be bacterial (most commonly *Haemophilus influenzae* or *Diplococcus pneumoniae*) or viral (most commonly mumps or herpes simplex). Meningitis or meningoencephalitis in the acute phase may be focal or diffuse and produce mass effect, vessel narrowing associated with cerebral edema, or local dilatation of vessels. These vascular changes are best seen on angiography.[2]

The organisms may reach the meningeal region from direct hematogenous spread, passage through the choroid plexus, rupture of superficial cortical abscesses, and contiguous spread of an adjacent infection such as otitis media, sinusitis, or osteomyelitis. Developmental anomalies such as a dermal sinus, or penetrating injuries of the skull which establish continuity between the central nervous system and the external environment, also may lead to meningitis. The inflammation of the leptomeninges is accompanied by subarachnoid exudate and vascular abnormalities. Communicating hydrocephalus (Fig. 10.1) may result from exudate in the subarachnoid space which interferes with the flow of cerebrospinal fluid from the basal cisterns over the cortical convexities to the arachnoid villi where it is absorbed. In the later stages of meningitis, noncommunicating hydrocephalus may also be produced by subarachnoid exudate extending into the foramina of Luschka and Magendie. The exudate may resorb with treatment with no sequelae, or chronic adhesive arachnoiditis may occur. In one-third of the patients, meningitis is associated with ventriculitis[3] with involvement of the ependyma, choroid plexus, and subependymal tissues. This may result in obliteration of the aqueduct of Sylvius or fourth ventricular foramina and noncommunicating hydrocephalus.

Subdural Effusions and Empyemas

Subdural effusions are a complication of meningitis and are most common over the parietal or frontoparietal region (Figs. 10.2 and 10.3). They are most commonly seen following inadequately treated Haemophilus influenza meningitis and contain proteinaceous yellow fluid.[2] The condition can be diagnosed by subdural taps, although the presence of the effusion may be suggested by transillumination of the skull or by a progressive enlargement of the head circumference.

Indications for suspecting a subdural effusion in infants with purulent meningitis include[4]:

1. Failure of temperature curve to show progressive decline after 72 hours of adequate antibiotic and supportive treatment.
2. Persistent positive spinal fluid cultures after 72 hours of appropriate antibiotic therapy.
3. Occurrence of focal or persistent convulsions.
4. Persistence of vomiting.
5. Development of focal neurologic signs.
6. An unsatisfactory clinical course, particularly evidence for increased intracranial pressure after 72 hours of antibiotic therapy.

This list also represents the indications for cranial ultrasonography in patients with meningitis. Patients with meningitis demonstrate mild dilatation of the ventricular system (Figs. 10.1, 10.2, and 10.4), usually involving all ventricles, and a prominent interhemispheric fissure (Fig. 10.4) and sulci. Subdural effusions over the brain convexities (Figs. 10.2 and 10.3) are not imaged unless they are relatively large, however fluid in the interhemispheric fissure (Fig. 10.4) is usually associated with small collections of fluid over the convexities.

Brain Abscesses

A brain abscess consists of localized free or encapsulated pus within the brain substance. They may be single or multiple; and they may occur by hematogenous spread from a distant infection or sepsis, by extension of a contiguous infection such as the middle ear or sinuses, as a complication of a penetrating wound, and in heart disease with right to left shunting. Clinical symptoms may initially be minimal, but later progress and become localized. Frontal lobe involvement is most common (33%), followed by temporal lobe, parietal lobe, occipital lobe, and, least frequently, posterior fossa.[2] A variety of organisms may be involved. Of 135 infants and children with intracranial abscesses reported by Harwood-Nash,[2] 23% were infants under 1 year of age. Other series have reported a somewhat lower figure for this age group; however, in our three year experience with cranial ultrasonography in the under-2-year age group, we have had no case of intracranial abscess. The reason for this is not known, but it may be due to earlier or more aggressive antibiotic therapy.

Ultrasound findings of intracranial abscess include mass effect with displacement of the ventricles and midline falx echoes, compression of the ventricles and adjacent tissue, and obliteration of the normal anatomy in the region. The pus-filled liquified portion of the abscess may be sonolucent with good through transmission or may have echoes of varying intensity caused by debris (Fig. 10.5).

Congenital Infections of the Nervous System

Infections of the fetal nervous system may cause significant damage to development and thus produce multiple defects. Etiologic agents include toxoplasmosis, rubella, cytomegalovirus, and syphilis. Ultrasound findings in these babies include generalized microcephalus with enlargement of the ventricles. The interhemispheric fissure may also be prominent, indicating diffuse brain atrophy. Calcifications in the brain parenchyma or ventricular wall may be demonstrated by ultrasound (Fig. 10.6).

Summary

Ultrasonography is useful in the investigation of patients with intracranial infection who are not responding satisfactorily to the usual therapy. Hydrocephalus and brain abscesses are readily identified. Subdural effusions and empyemas can be demonstrated when moderate in size.

References

1. Overall JC. Neonatal bacterial meningitis: analysis of predisposing factors and outcome compared with matched control subjects. J Pediatr 1970; 76:499.
2. Harwood-Nash DC, Fitz CR. *Neuroradiology in Infants and Children.* St. Louis: C. V. Mosby, 1976; 855–901.
3. Menke JH. *Textbook of Child Neurology.* Philadelphia: Lea & Febiger, 1974; 216.
4. Matsen DD. *Neurosurgery of Infancy and Childhood,* Ed. 2. Springfield, Ill.: Charles C Thomas, 1969; 734.
5. Babcock DS, Han BK. The accuracy of high resolution real-time ultrasonography of the head in infancy. Radiology 1981; 139:665–676.

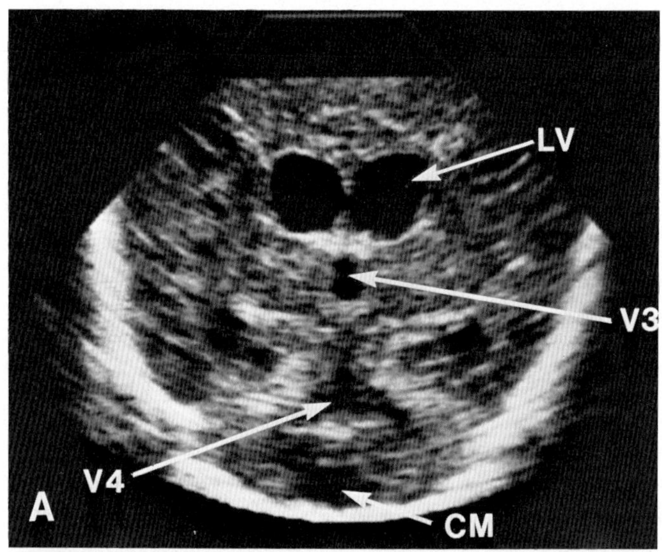

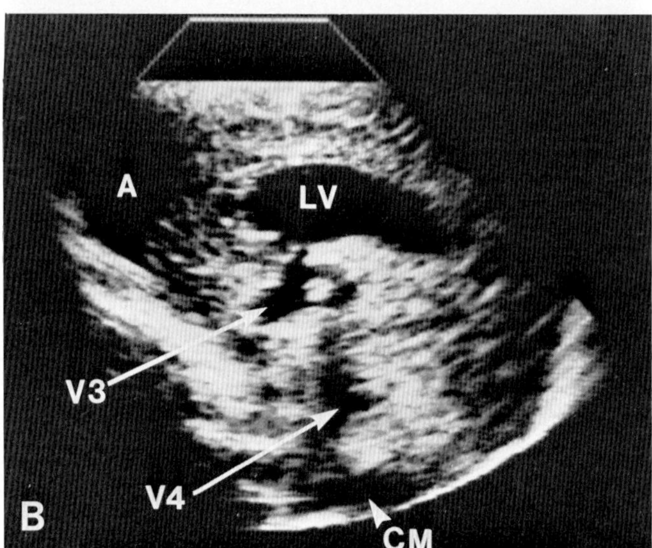

Figure 10.1 Communicating hydrocephalus. A 6 ½-month-old infant with *Haemophilus influenzae* meningitis. (*A*) Coronal and (*B*) sagittal scans. Mild dilatation of lateral (*LV*), third (*V3*), and fourth (*V4*) ventricles. Cisterna magna (*CM*) slightly prominent. Artifactual echolucent area (*A*) seen anteriorly on sagittal scan. (Reproduced by permission from D. S. Babcock and B. K. Han: *Radiology*, *139:* 665–676, 1981.[5])

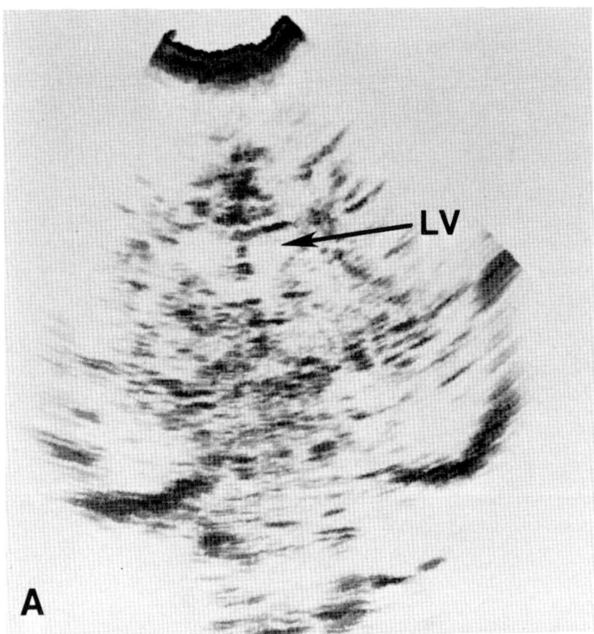

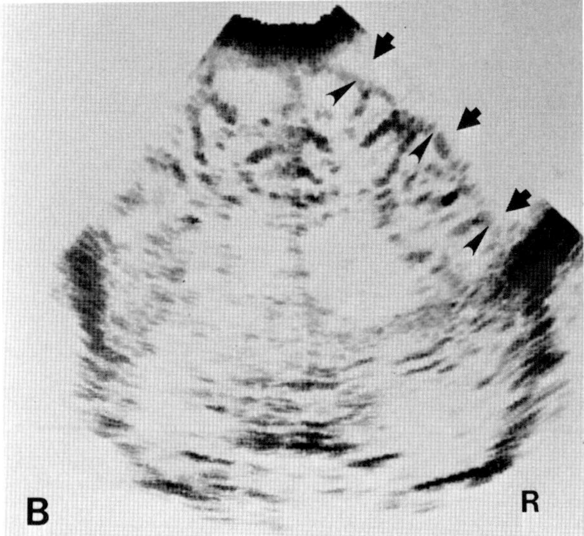

Figure 10.2 Subdural effusion and hydrocephalus. A 5 ½-month-old infant with *Haomophilus influenzae* meningitis and positive transillumination on right. (*A*) Modified coronal and (*B*) coronal scans. Mild enlargement of lateral ventricles (*LV*). Localized subdural effusion (*arrows*) demonstrated on right. Brain surface (*arrowheads*) including gyri and sulci, normally not seen, but well demonstrated when outlined by subdural effusion.

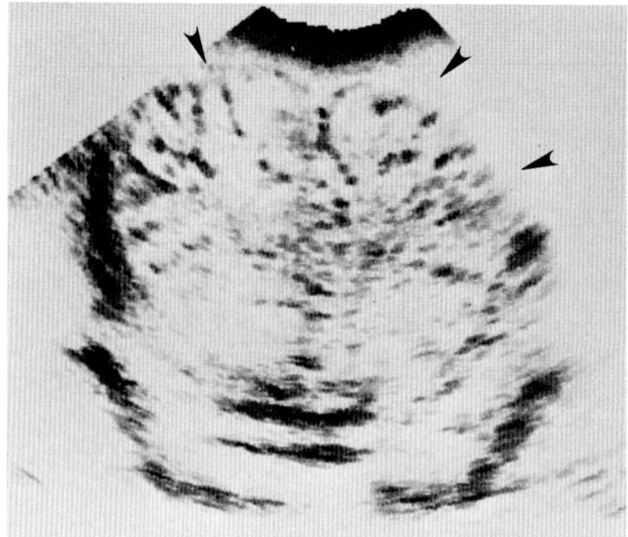

Figure 10.3 Subdural effusions. A 3-month-old infant with *Heamophilus influenzae* meningitis. Coronal scan shows bilateral subdural effusions (*arrowheads*) with prominent brain gyri and sulci.

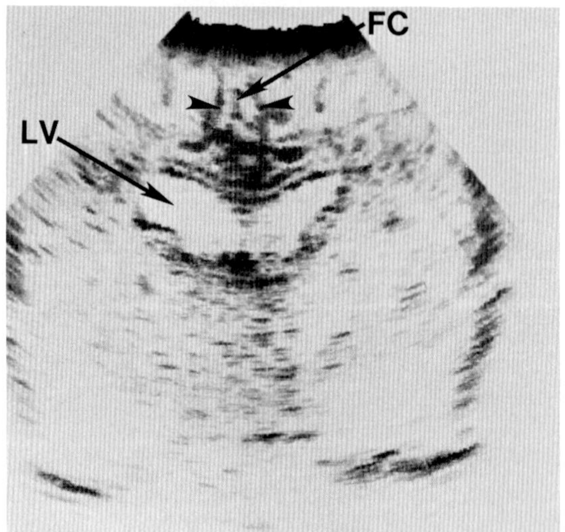

Figure 10.4 Prominent interhemispheric fissure. Coronal scan shows widening of interhemispheric fissure (*arrowheads*) and falx cerebri (*FC*) outlined by fluid. Mild enlargement of lateral ventricles (*LV*).

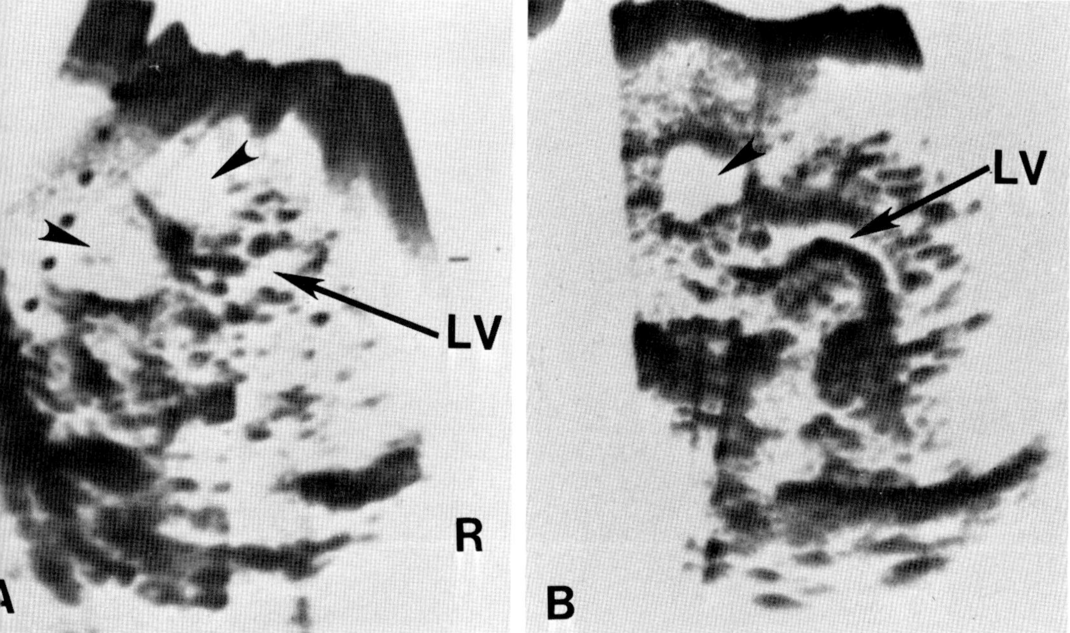

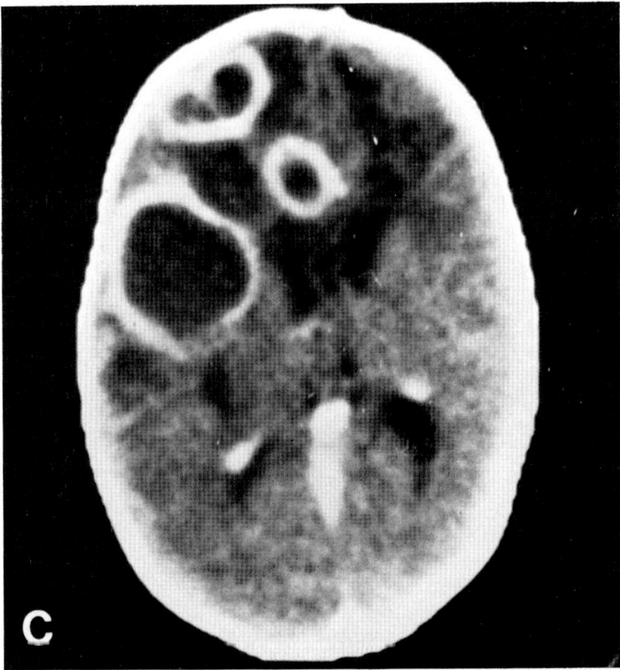

Figure 10.5 Brain abscess. A 2-month-old infant with increasing head size and irritability. Meningitis diagnosed at 7 days of life. (*A*) Coronal and (*B*) left parasagittal scans show echolucent masses in left frontoparietal area (*arrowheads*). Lateral ventricles (*LV*) slightly dilated. (*C*) Enhanced CT scan shows three ring lesions in left hemisphere. Abscesses surgically removed and shunt tube placed. Culture grew *Citrobacter diversis.* (This case courtesy of David Cavanaugh, M.D., Dayton, Ohio).

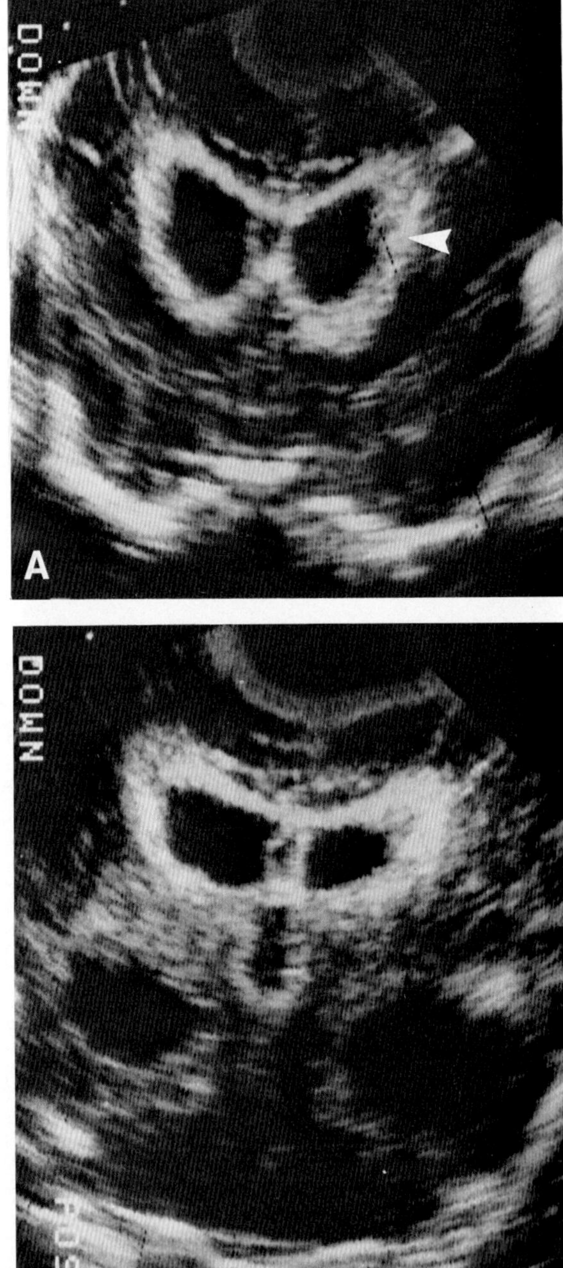

Figure 10.6 Newborn infant with intrauterine infection (cytomegalic inclusion disease). (*A* and *B*) Coronal and (*C*) sagittal scans show mild ventricular enlargement and periventricular echogenic areas of calcification (*arrowheads*). (*D*) CT scan with hydrocephalus and periventricular calcifications. (This case courtesy of David Martin, M.D., Toronto, Ontario.)

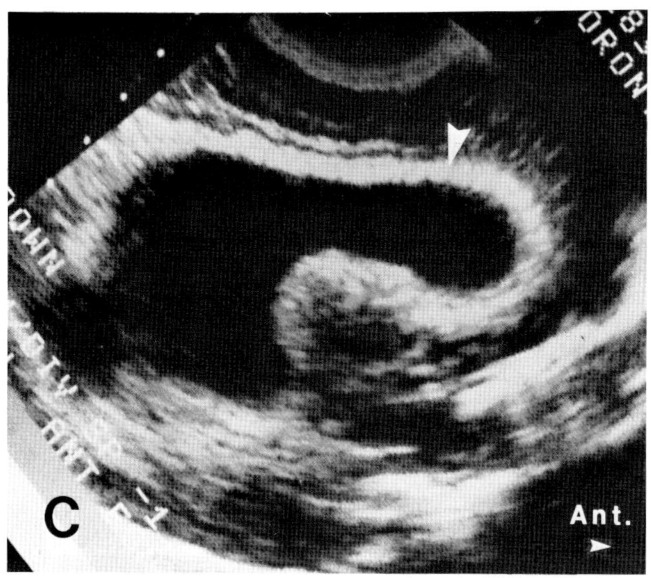
C
Ant.

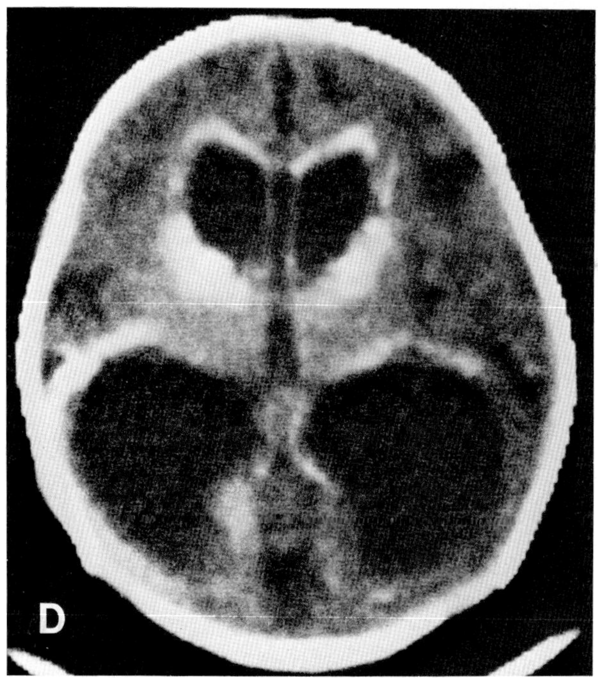
D

CHAPTER 11

Cranial Hemorrhage

Craniocerebral hemorrhage is a relatively common problem in infancy and accounts for a large percentage of cranial ultrasonograms at our institution. The hemorrhage and hematoma formation may occur as a result of trauma, may occur spontaneously in normal infants or infants with bleeding diathesis, or may occur in premature infants for as yet incompletely understood reasons. The hematoma may occur in relationship to the skull, the meninges, the brain, or the ventricles.

Cephalohematoma

A cephalohematoma or subperiosteal hematoma occurs frequently in the newborn as a result of a traumatic delivery. It most frequently occurs in the parietal region and because of the subperiosteal location the hematoma is limited by the adjacent sutures where the pericranium attaches to the edge. Fractures of the underlying bone are associated in approximately one-fourth of the cases.[1]

On ultrasonography the cephalohematoma is seen as a mildly echogenic mass separating the scalp from the bony skull (Fig. 11.1). Reverberation lines paralleling the skull can frequently be seen within the calvarium when scanning over the side of the hematoma and should not be mistaken for a subdural hematoma. With reverberations there is no shift of the midline echoes and the reverberation lines are seen outside of the head when the patient is scanned from the side opposite the hematoma (Fig. 11.1*C*).

Epidural and Subdural Hematoma and Hygroma

Hemorrhage can occur in the spaces between the bony calvarium and the brain, most commonly as a result of trauma. An epidural hematoma occurs between the inner table of the skull and the dura mater and is most common in the temporal, frontal and occipital areas.[1] A subdural hematoma results from hemorrhage between the dura mater and the arachnoid membrane and is more common. It can also occur with hypervitaminosis A, blood dyscrasia, or as a sequela of meningitis. A subdural hematoma is most often venous in origin and usually results from tearing of the cerebral veins as they pass through the meninges, whereas an epidural hematoma usually results from laceration of an arterial channel. An epidural hematoma tends to be localized and join the inner table at well defined angles whereas an acute subdural hematoma tends to be more diffuse and has tapering edges.

On ultrasonography, epidural and subdural fluid collections are seen as relatively sonolucent spaces separating the very echogenic bony calvarium from the moderately echogenic brain parenchyma (Figs. 11.2 and 11.3). The gyri and sulci of the brain are more easily demonstrated because they are outlined by fluid (Fig. 11.3). Fluid collections, whether epidural or subdural, are difficult to demonstrate by B-mode ultrasonography when localized over the convexity on the side of the head near the transducer because of near-field artifacts caused by the bony calvaria. We have demonstrated extra-axial fluid collections over the convexities only when they are relatively large, i.e. greater than 5 mm. Subdural fluid collections can extend into the interhemispheric fissure and are seen as widening of the interhemispheric fissure on coronal scans. The falx cerebri in such cases may be demonstrated outlined by the fluid (Fig. 11.3). We have noted that in several cases of small subdural fluid collections the prominent interhemispheric fissure was the only ultrasound finding. Another secondary sign is shift of the midline structures, and this can be demonstrated when the epidural or subdural hematoma is unilateral.

A subdural hygroma consists of clear fluid, resembling cerebrospinal fluid, in the subdural space and frequently is a residual finding after resolution of a subdural hematoma. On ultrasonography both subdural hematomas and hygromas are sonolucent and cannot be differentiated.

At the present time we consider cranial ultrasonography somewhat limited in its ability to identify eidural and subdural fluid collections, unless they are large, because of technical problems in imaging the area adjacent to the bony calvarium. In clinical situations where these abnormalities are suspected, cranial computerized tomography (CT) is recommended as the preferable diagnostic modality when available.

We have not identified an epidural hematoma to date, and it is said to be uncommon in young children compared to the subdural hematoma.[2]

Intracerebral Hematoma

Intracerebral hemorrhage in children is most often due to trauma, and there may be associated subdural or extradural hemorrhage as well. It is most often found in the cerebral hemispheres but can occur in the cerebellum or brainstem.[2] In neonates, intracerebral hemorrhage is due to distortion of the head in the birth canal or by forceps delivery, usually in full-term infants. Frontal and parietal lobe involvement is most common, with temporal lobe involvement less common, and occipital lobe rare. The hematoma may be small, or rarely, massive. Spontaneous intracerebral hemorrhage may occur with blood dyscrasias, and in patients with leukemia, thrombocytopenia, hemophilia and thrombocytopenic purpura can occur with minor trauma. The infant may present with convulsions and bloody spinal fluid.

On cranial ultrasonography an intracerebral mass is seen with displacement of the midline structures and ventricles away from their normal position (Fig. 11.4). Initially, the hemorrhage is echogenic. As in hematomas elsewhere in the body,[3] the blood will, over a period of time, liquefy with retraction of the blood clot.

The hemorrhage may communicate with or involve the ventricles as well, with dilatation of the ventricular system of varying degree. Chronic hydrocephalus may develop due to occlusion of one or both foramina of Monro, the aqueduct of Sylvius, or the fourth ventricle foramina. Bleeding into the subarachnoid space with arachnoid adhesions or plugging of arachnoid villi can produce extraventricular obstructive hydrocephalus.

Large areas of cerebral or cerebellar destruction may develop as well as ventricular dilatation due to more diffuse brain atrophy. Post-traumatic porencephalic cysts filled with cerebrospinal fluid (CSF) may result. Ultrasonography can identify the acute hemorrhage as well as follow its resolution or the development of a porencephalic cyst and hydrocephalus (Fig. 11.4).

Subependymal and Intraventricular Hemorrhage in Premature Infants

Spontaneous intracranial hemorrhage is a phenomenon that occurs in premature infants and, according to Leech and Kohnen,[4] is the most common central nervous system abnormality in neonatal autopsies. The incidence at autopsy in premature infants is found to be 56–71%.[4–6] The hemorrhage usually originates in the germinal matrix which is a tissue located beneath the ependymal lining of the lateral ventricles. The germinal matrix is largest lateral to the groove between the head of the caudate nucleus and the thalamus and is a highly vascular structure with little supporting tissue. It is a source of neuroblasts which migrate peripherally during development of the fetal brain. The germinal matrix is largest at 24–32 weeks gestation and then involutes so that it is virtually absent in the full-term infant.[7]

There are numerous theories of pathogenesis of subependymal hemorrhage including infarction due to thrombosis of the deep cerebral vessels, increased venous pressure, increased arterial pressure, and increased subependymal capillary pressure.[8–10] Hypoxia, pulmonary disease, pneumothorax, acidosis, administration of excess $NaHCO_3$, and maternal aspirin ingestion have been associated with intracranial hemorrhage. The exact mechanisms are not yet known but are the subject of much current investigation.

The hemorrhage can remain isolated in the germinal matrix or may extend into the brain parenchyma adjacent to the germinal matrix. The hemorrhage may also rupture through the ependymal lining into the ventricular system. Hydrocephalus may result from obstruction of the CSF pathways by clot, organizing ependymitis, or basilar arachnoiditis.

The clinical diagnosis of intracranial hemorrhage in premature infants is based on changes in muscular tone and activity, the presence of seizures, increasing head circumference, a bulging anterior fontanelle, vascular hypotension, greater than 10% drop in hematocrit, and the presence of blood and/or elevated protein content in the CSF. Hydrocephalus is diagnosed by a bulging anterior fontanelle, abnormally increasing head circumference, and transillumination of the head. Prospective studies of intracranial hemorrhage using CT have shown that clinical methods are inaccurate and underestimate the incidence.[11-14] Cranial CT has been shown to be accurate in diagnosing intracranial hemorrhage in premature infants[12-18] but has practical limitations for this purpose: the patient must be transported to the radiology department for the scan, sedation is often required, CT uses ionizing radiation which has a potential long term deleterious effect on the infant, and CT is relatively expensive.

In the last several years, B-mode ultrasonography has proven to be an accurate method for diagnosing intracranial hemorrhage.[19-28] Ultrasound has advantages over CT: it uses nonionizing radiation, can be performed portably in the isolette in the intensive care unit with the newer real-time ultrasound equipment, no sedation is necessary, and the examination is less expensive.

On normal cranial ultrasonograms, the caudate nucleus is a moderately echogenic area in the inferolateral wall of the lateral ventricles from the frontal horn to the base of the temporal horn and is indistinguishable from the adjacent brain parenchyma (Fig. 11.5). The head of the caudate nucleus lies anterior to the foramen of Monro. In patients with hemorrhage limited to the subependymal germinal matrix, ultrasonography demonstrates areas of increased echogenicity in the wall of the lateral ventricle, most frequently in the region of the head of the caudate nucleus (Fig. 11.6). A normal highly echogenic structure, the choroid plexus, is also seen in the floor of the lateral ventricle and should not be confused with a subependymal hemorrhage. The choroid plexus is a sharply marginated structure and extends posteriorly from the foramen of Monro into the atrium and temporal horn (Fig. 11.5). The choroid plexus has also been implicated as a source of intraventricular hemorrhage and in such cases it appears enlarged and more echogenic than normal.

The diagnosis of intraventricular extension of the hemorrhage can be made when echogenic clot is seen within the ventricles forming a clot fluid level, or cast of the ventricles. Since the thin ependymal lining of the ventricles is not identifiable by ultrasound, it is sometimes impossible to differentiate an intraventricular clot attached to the wall of the ventricle from a large subependymal clot (Figs. 11.7 and 11.8). With intraventricular extension of the hemorrhage the ventricles enlarge and, rather than being slitlike, as in the normal infant, are seen as fluid-filled or echogenic clot-filled, rounded structures (Figs. 11.7–11.9). The ventricular dilatation may be mild, moderate or marked (Fig. 11.9) and may remain stable, regress, or progress with time and require permanent ventricular shunting. In our experience, enlargement of the ventricles with sonolucent fluid in a patient with visible subependymal hemorrhage indicates intraventricular hemorrhage with CSF-diluted blood.

With intraparenchymal extension of the hemorrhage, an area of increased echoes is seen not only in the immediate periventricular germinal matrix region, but extending diffusely into the brain parenchyma—the cerebral hemispheres or basal ganglia (Figs. 11.10 and 11.11). Over a several week period, the echogenic intraparenchymal hemorrhage becomes partially anechoic with liquefaction and retraction of the clot and eventual cavitation of that portion of the brain (Figs. 11.10, *E* and *F*, and 11.11, *C–E*). Small cystic areas of porencephaly can be identified in the subependymal region on follow-up examination (Fig. 11.12) and large intraparenchymal hemorrhages can result in large areas of porencephaly (Fig. 11.11). We have also noted areas of porencephaly secondary to multiple ventricular taps and dilatation of the needle tract (Fig. 11.13).

A prominent extra-axial or subarachnoid space can occasionally be seen on ultrasound examinations of premature infants. This appears as separation of the brain from the bony calvaria over the parietal and temporal region and a prominent Sylvian fissure (Fig. 11.14). On subsequent examinations this gradually resolves, usually with no demonstrable consequence, and may be a normal variant in premature infants similar to that described on CT[29] or may be evidence of subarachnoid hemorrhage.

Ischemic brain damage, which consists of periventricular and cortical areas of necrosis and/or infarction is seen at autopsy, but is not usually diagnosable by ultrasound, probably because of the small size of the lesions and the echogenicity is similar to that of the adjacent brain. Occasionally with severe asphyxia the brain appears diffusely abnormal in its echogenicity. The late manifestation of ischemic brain damage, diffuse brain atrophy with hydrocephalus ex vacuo, is diagnosible by ultrasound.[28] The ultrasound findings consist of enlarged ventricles with normal ventricular angles and sometimes a prominent interhemispheric fissure and extra-axial spaces (Fig. 13.3, Chapter 13). The clinical information of decreasing or stationary head size confirms the diagnosis.

Conclusion

Ultrasonography is useful for the diagnosis and follow-up of hemorrhage in relationship to the skull, meninges, brain, and the ventricles. It is particularly useful for evaluating intracerebral and intraventricular hemorrhage and their sequelae in premature infants and with the advent of portable real-time equipment has become a routine part of patient care in these infants.

Extra-axial hematomas in the epidural, subdural, and subarachnoid spaces can be demonstrated by ultrasonography but, because of technical problems in imaging the region immediately adjacent to the bone, small hematomas may be missed by this technique. If the primary consideration is a hemorrhage in this area, then CT is suggested as a more accurate method of evaluating these patients.

References

1. Taveras JM, Wood EH. *Diagnostic Neuroradiology*, Vol. II. Baltimore: Williams & Wilkins, 1977; 1062–1090.
2. Harwood-Nash DC, Fitz CR. *Neuroradiology in Infants and Children*. St. Louis: C. V. Mosby, 1976; 827.
3. Wicks JD, Silver TM, Bree RL. Gray scale features of hematomas; an ultrasonic spectrum. AJR 1978; 131:977–980.
4. Leech RW, Kohnen P. Subependymal and intraventricular hemorrhages in the newborn. Am J Pathol 1974:77:465–476.
5. Coen RW, Sutherland JM, Bove K, McAdams AJ. Anatomic and epidemiologic features of the stroke lesion of newborn infants. Trans Am Neurol Assoc 1970; 95:36–40.
6. Tsiantos A, Victorin L, Reiler JP, Dyer N, Sundell H, Brill AB, Stahlman M. Intracranial hemorrhage in the prematurely born infant: timing of clots and evaluation of clinical signs and symptoms. J Pediatr 1971; 85:854–859.
7. Friede RL. *Developmental Neuropathology*. New York: Springer, 1976; 1–37.
8. Volpe J. Intracranial hemorrhage in the newborn. Current understandings and dilemmas.

Neurology 1979; 29:632–635.

9. Hambleton G, Wigglesworth J. Origin of intraventricular hemorrhages in the pre-term infant. Arch Dis Child 1976; 51:651–659.
10. Wigglesworth J, Pape K. An integrated model for haemorrhagic and ischaemic lesion in the newborn brain. Early Hum Dev 1978; 2:179–199.
11. Papile LA, Burstein J, Burstein R, Koffler H. Incidence and evolution of subependymal and intraventricular hemorrhage: a study of infants with birth weights less than 1,500 gm. J Pediatr 1978; 92:529–534.
12. Burstein J, Papile LA, Burstein R. Intraventricular hemorrhage and hydrocephalus in premature newborns: a prospective study with CT. AJR 1979; 132:631–635.
13. Lee BCP, Grassi AE, Schechner S, Auld PAM. Neonatal intraventricular hemorrhage: a serial computed tomography study. J Comput Assist Tomogr 1979; 3:483–490.
14. Lazzara A, Ahmann P, Dykes F, Brann AW, Schwartz J. Clinical predictability of intraventricular hemorrhage in preterm infants. Pediatrics 1980; 65:30–34.
15. Pevsner PH, Garcia-Bunuel R, Leeds N, Finkelstein M. Subependymal and intraventricular hemorrhage in neonates. Early diagnosis by computed tomography. Radiology 1976; 119: 111–114.
16. Krishnamoorthy KS, Fernandez RA, Momose KJ et al. Evaluation of neonatal intracranial hemorrhage by computerized tomography. Pediatrics 1977; 59:165–172.
17. Burstein J, Papile L, Burstein R. Subependymal germinal matrix and intraventricular hemorrhage in premature infants: diagnosis by CT. AJR 1977; 128:971–976.
18. Rumack CM, McDonald MM, O'Meara OP, Sanders BB, Rudikoff JC. CT detection and course of intracranial hemorrhage in premature infants. AJR 1978; 131:493–497.
19. Pape KE, Blackwell RJ, Cusick G et al. Ultrasound detection of brain damage in preterm infants. Lancet 1979; 1:1261–1264.
20. London DA, Carroll BA, Enzmann DR. Sonography of ventricular size and germinal matrix hemorrhage in premature infants. AJR 1980; 135:559–564.
21. Grant EG, Schellinger D, Borts FT et al. Real-time sonography of the neonatal and infant head. AJNR 1980; 1:487–492.
22. Sauerbrei EE, Harrison PB, Ling E, Cooperberg PL. Neonatal intracranial pathology demonstrated by high-frequency linear array ultrasound. J Clin Ultrasound 1981; 9:33–36.
23. Johnson ML, Rumack CM, Mannes EJ, Appareti KE. Detection of neonatal intracranial hemorrhage utilizing real-time and static ultrasound. Presented at the 25th Annual Convention of the American Institute of Ultrasound in Medicine, New Orleans, September 1980.
24. Pape KE, Szymonowicz W, Bennett Britton S, Murphy W, Martin DJ. Ultrasound diagnosis of neonatal intracranial bleeding. Presented at the Perinatal Intracranial Hemorrhage Conference, Washington DC, December 11–13, 1980.
25. Slovis TL, Shankaran S, Bedard MP, Poland RL. Assessment of intracranial hemorrhage utilizing real time ultrasonic sector scanning as the primary modality: a one-year experience. Presented at the Perinatal Intracranial Hemorrhage Conference, Washington DC, December 11–13, 1980.
26. Bejar R, Curbelo V, Coen RW, Leopold G, James H, Gluck L. Technique for diagnosis and follow-up of intraventricular and intracerebral hemorrhages by ultrasound studies of the infant's brain through the fontanelles and the sutures. Presented at the Perinatal Intracranial Hemorrhage Conference, Washington DC, December 11–13, 1980.
27. Silverboard G, Horder MH, Ahmann PA, Lazzara A, Schwartz JF. Reliability of ultrasound in the diagnosis of intracerebral hemorrhage and posthemorrhagic hydrocephalus: comparison with computed tomographic scan. Presented at the Perinatal Intracranial Hemorrhage Conference, Washington DC, December 11–13, 1980.
28. Babcock DS, Bove K, Han BK. Ultrasound and pathologic correlation in premature infants with intracranial hemorrhage. Presented at the 81st Annual Meeting of the American Roentgen Ray Society, San Francisco, March 1981.
29. Picard L, Claudon M, Roland J, Jeanjean E, Andre M, Plenat P, Vert P. Cerebral computed tomography in premature infants, with an attempt at staging developmental features. J Comput Assist Tomogr 1980; 4:435–444.
30. Babcock DS, Han BK, LeQuesne GW. B-Mode gray scale ultrasound of the head in the newborn and young infant. AJR 1980; 134:457–468.
31. Babcock DS, Han BK. The accuracy of high resolution real-time ultrasonography of the head in infancy. Radiology 1981; 139:665–676.

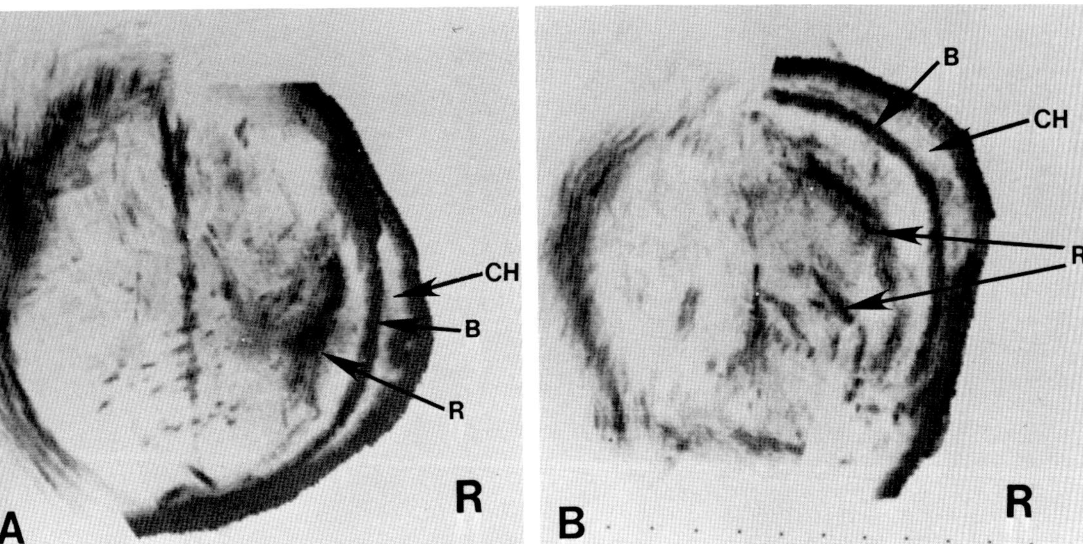

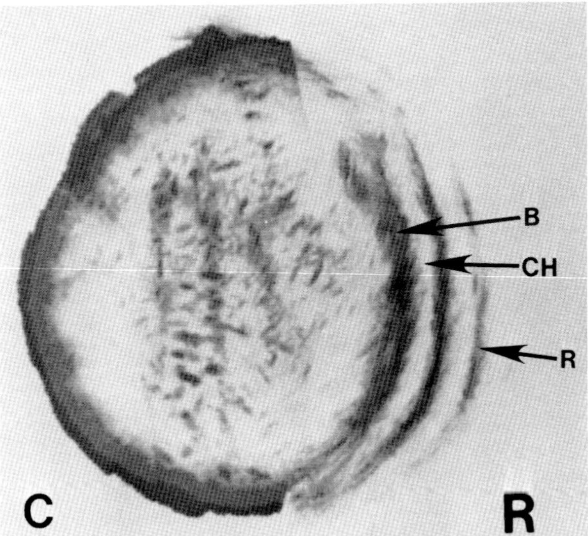

Figure 11.1 Cephalohematoma. Three-day-old infant with swelling over right parietal region noted at birth. (*A*) Axial and (*B*) coronal scans show cephalohematoma (*CH*) in right posterior parietal region with separation of scalp from bony skull (*B*) by hematoma. Reverberation lines (*R*) paralleling skull, apparently within calvarium are thought to be artifactual, but are suspicious for subdural hematoma although there is no shift of midline echoes. (*C*) Axial scan from opposite side shows reverberation lines outside of head. (Reproduced with permission from D. S. Babcock, B. K. Han, and G. W. LeQuesne: *American Journal of Roentgenology, 134:*457–468, 1980.[30])

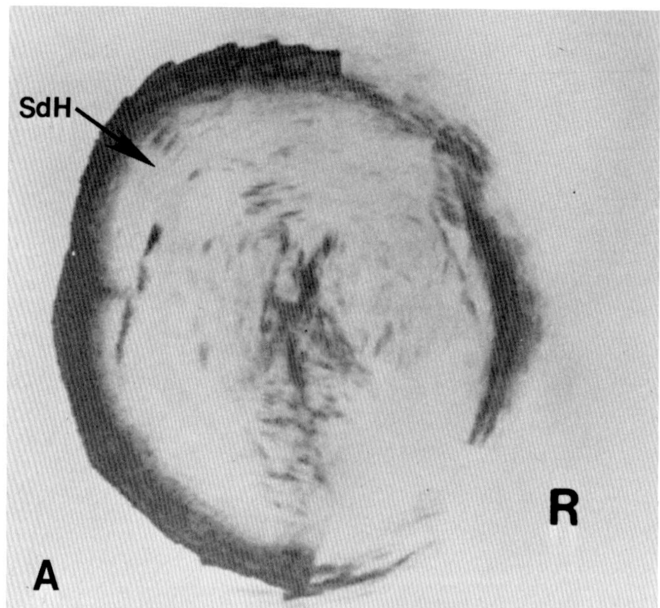

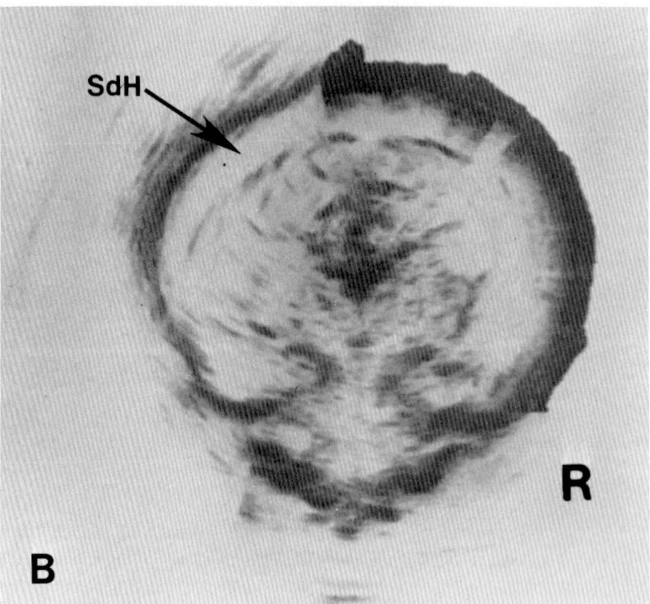

Figure 11.2 Subdural hematoma. Three-week-old infant with birth history of difficult, traumatic forceps delivery and right parietal cephalohematoma. She did well at home until seizures developed at age 3 weeks. (*A*) Axial and (*B*) coronal scans show large bilateral subdural fluid collections (*SdH*) and subdural taps yielded bloody fluid. Subdural hematomas repeatedly tapped but reaccumulated.

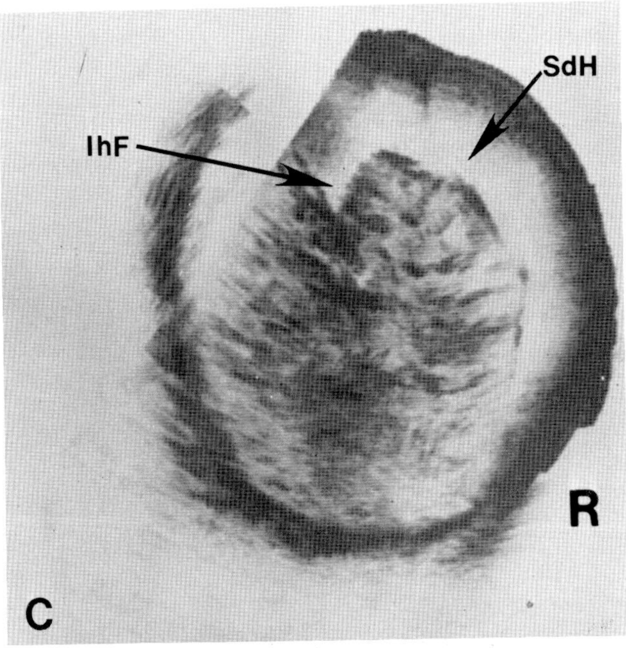

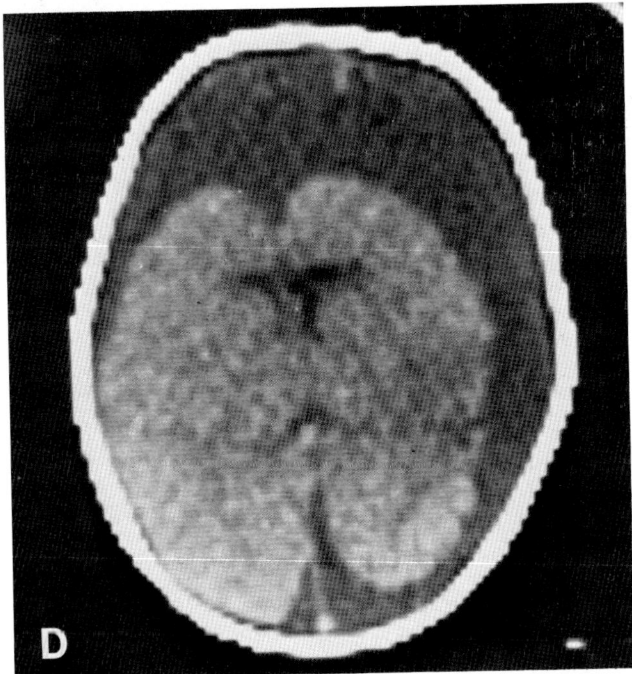

(*C*) Follow-up axial ultrasound scan and (*D*) CT scan show enlargement of subdural hematoma extending into interhemispheric fissure (*IhF*). (Reproduced with permission from D. S. Babcock, B. K. Han, and G. W. LeQuesne: *American Journal of Roentgenology, 134:*457–468, 1980.[30])

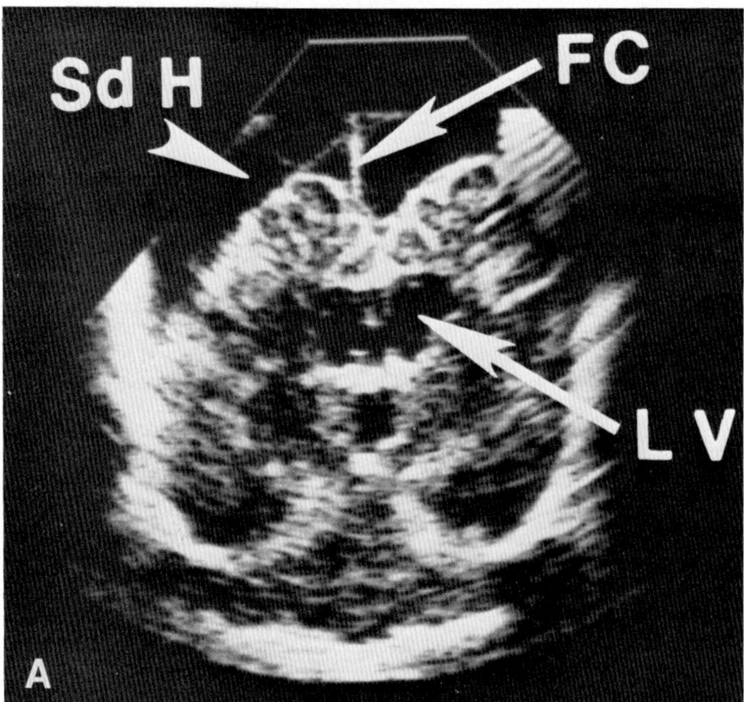

Figure 11.3 Subdural hematoma. Three-month-old premature infant with apneic episodes and recent history of mild trauma. (*A*) Coronal and (*B* and *C*) parasagittal scans show large bilateral subdural hematomas (*SdH*). Falx cerebri (*FC*) seen as linear midline structure outlined by fluid. Gyri (*G*) and sulci of brain are more easily demonstrated. (Reproduced with permission from D. S. Babcock and B. K. Han: *Radiology, 139:*665–676, 1981.[31])

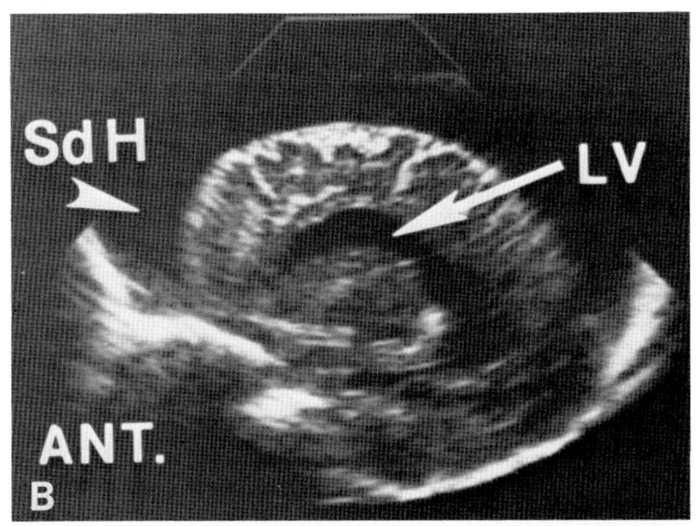
SdH
LV
ANT.
B

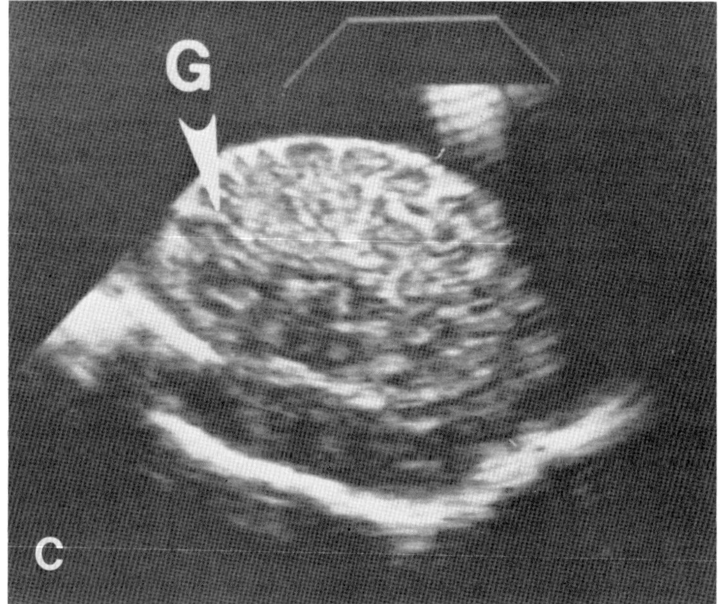
G
C

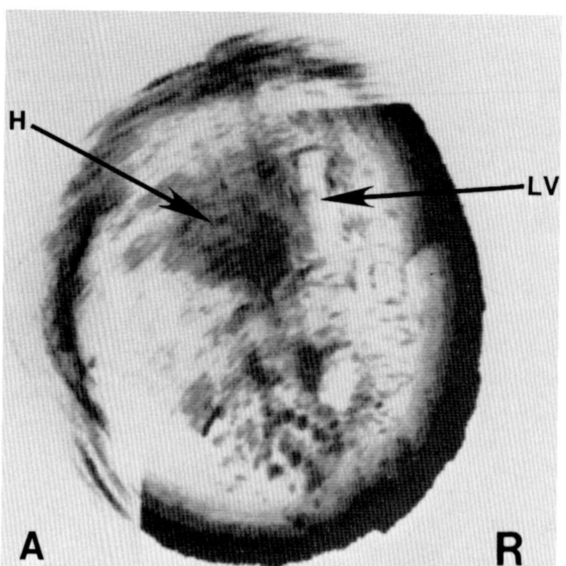

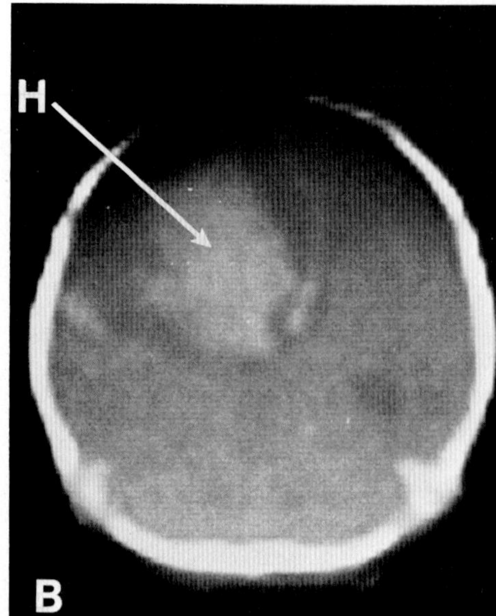

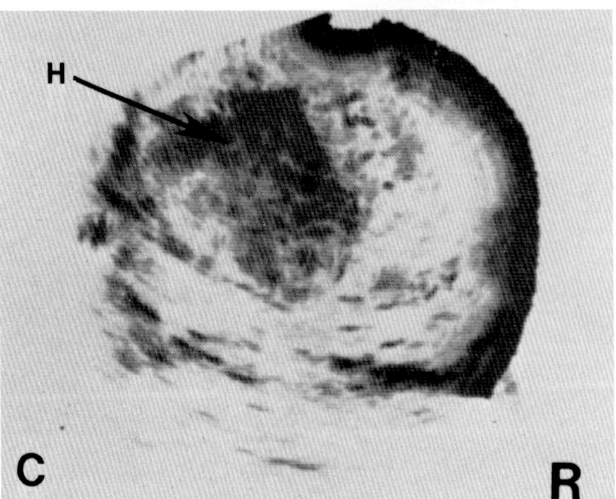

Figure 11.4 Intracerebral hemorrhage. Full-term infant who had right-sided seizure at age 2 days. (*A*) Axial and (*C*) coronal scans show large, highly echogenic mass in left frontal lobe representing intracerebral hematoma (*H*). Right lateral ventricle (*LV*) mildly dilated and mild shift of midline structures from left to right. (*B*) Axial CT scan without contrast shows large frontal lobe mass with area of increased density compatible with intracerebral hematoma (*H*). Patient did well clinically. (*D*) Follow-up coronal scan 6 weeks later shows large left frontal lobe mass has partially liquefied and become anechoic, blood clot retracting. (*E*) Axial scan 2 months later for increasing head size shows large porencephalic cyst (*Po*) in area of previous hematoma. Lateral ventricles now moderately dilated. (Reproduced with permission from D. S. Babcock, B. K. Han, and G. W. Lequesne: *American Journal of Roentgenology, 134:*457–468, 1980.[30])

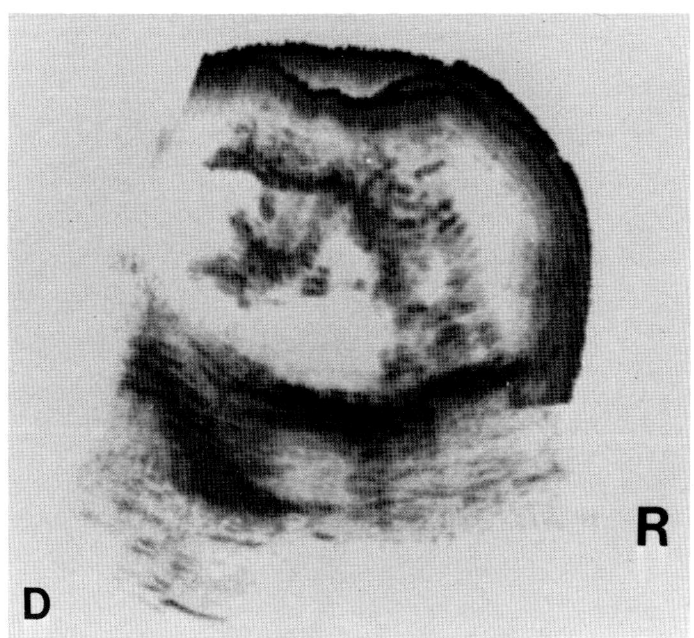
R
D

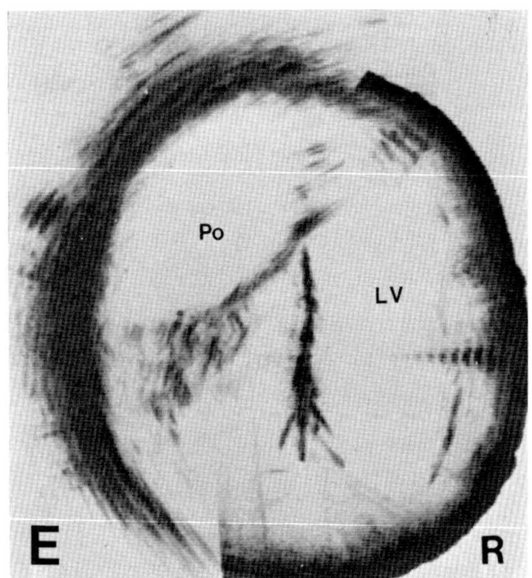
Po
LV
E
R

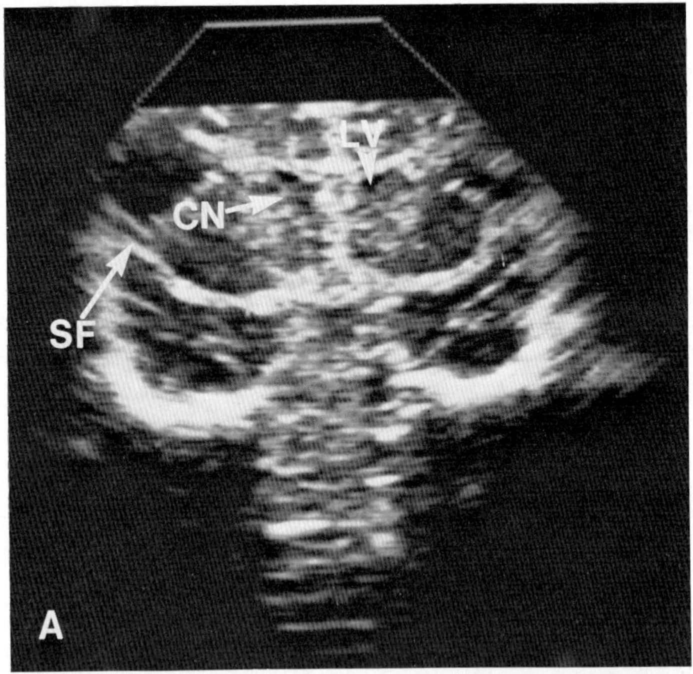

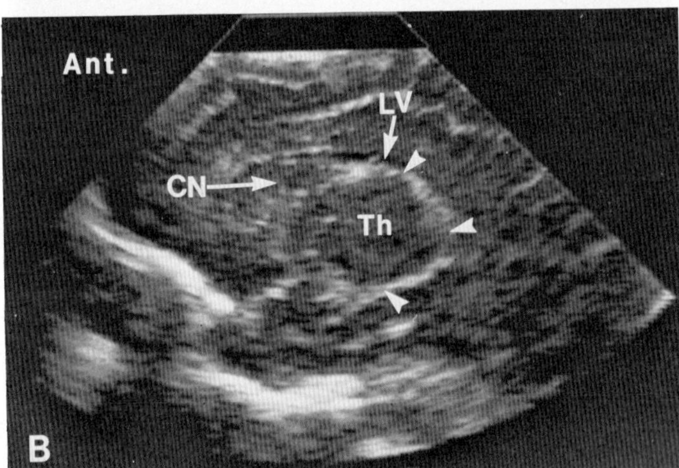

Figure 11.5 Normal (*A*) Coronal and (*B*) sagittal scans. Moderately echogenic head of caudate nucleus (*CN*) lies inferior to frontal horn of lateral ventricle (*LV*), and anterosuperior to thalamus (*Th*), which is inferior to body of lateral ventricle (*LV*). Densely echogenic choroid plexus (*arrowheads*) begins at foramen of Monro and lies posterior to head of caudate nucleus coursing along floor of LV into atrium and temporal horn of LV. *SF*, Sylvian fissure.

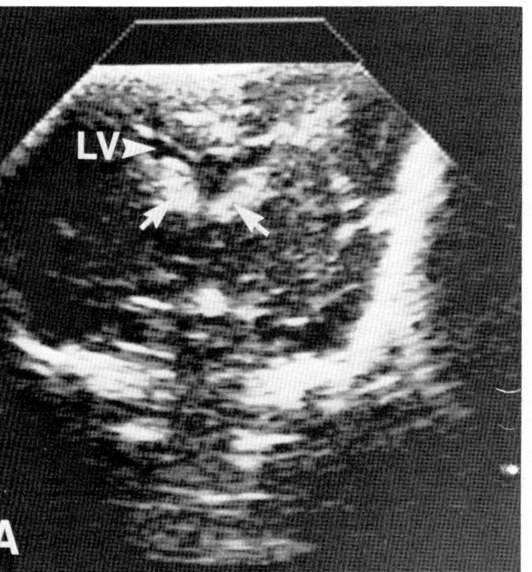

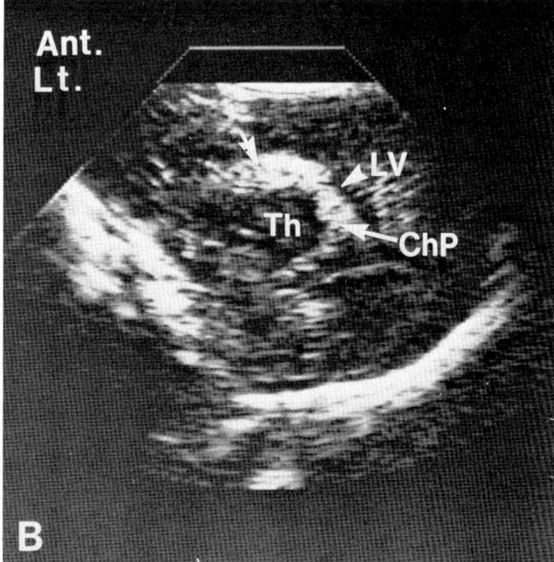

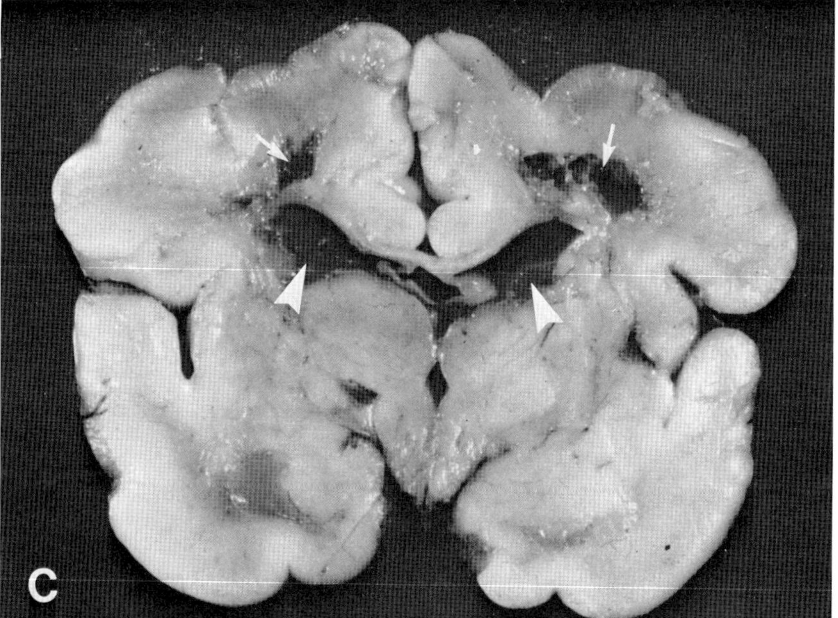

Figure 11.6 Subependymal hemorrhage. Infant 1320 g, 31-week gestation, with respiratory distress syndrome, severe pulmonary interstitial emphysema, and patent ductus arteriosus. (*A*) Coronal and (*B*) sagittal scans on 4th day of life show bilateral small echogenic areas in region of heads of caudate nuclei representing subependymal hemorrhages (*arrows*). Ventricles normal size. (*C*) Brain section shows bilateral subependymal hemorrhages (*arrowheads*). Periventricular necrosis found at autopsy (*arrows*) not detected by ultrasound 10 days prior to death. *Th*, thalamus, *ChP*, choroid plexus; *LV*, lateral ventricle.

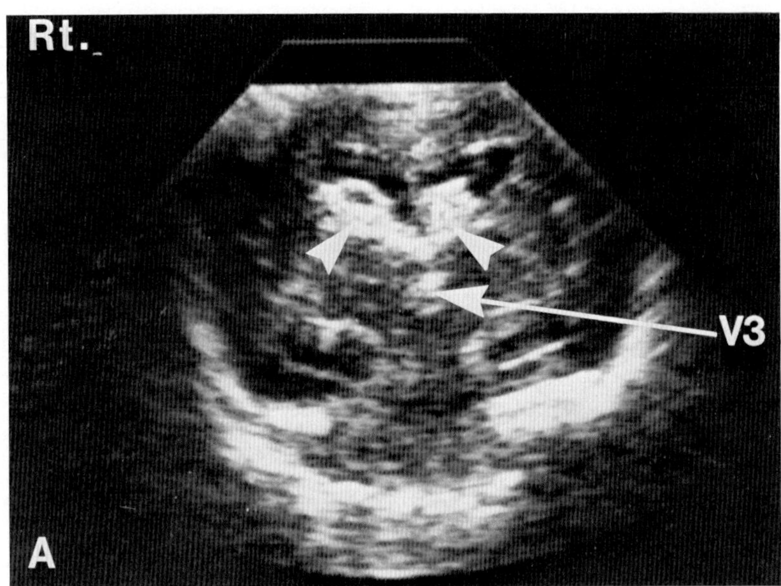

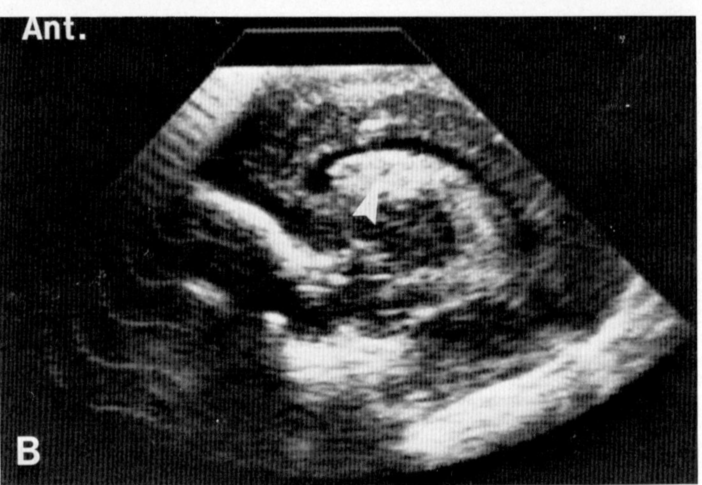

Figure 11.7 Subependymal hemorrhage with slight intraventricular extension. Infant, 1500 g, 30-week gestation, with VATER syndrome (vertebral and vascular abnormalities, anorectal malformation, tracheoesophageal fistula, esophageal atresia, radial limb hypoplasia, and renal abnormalities); respiratory distress syndrome; and seizures. (*A*) Coronal and (*B*) sagittal scans show bilateral small subependymal hemorrhages (*arrowheads*) in region of heads of caudate nuclei. Mild ventricular dilatation and echogenic cast clots within lateral and third ventricles (*V3*) represent intraventricular extension. (*C*) Brain section shows intraventricular hemorrhage with bilateral asymmetrical subependymal hemorrhage (*arrowheads*) and subarachnoid hemorrhage (*open arrows*).

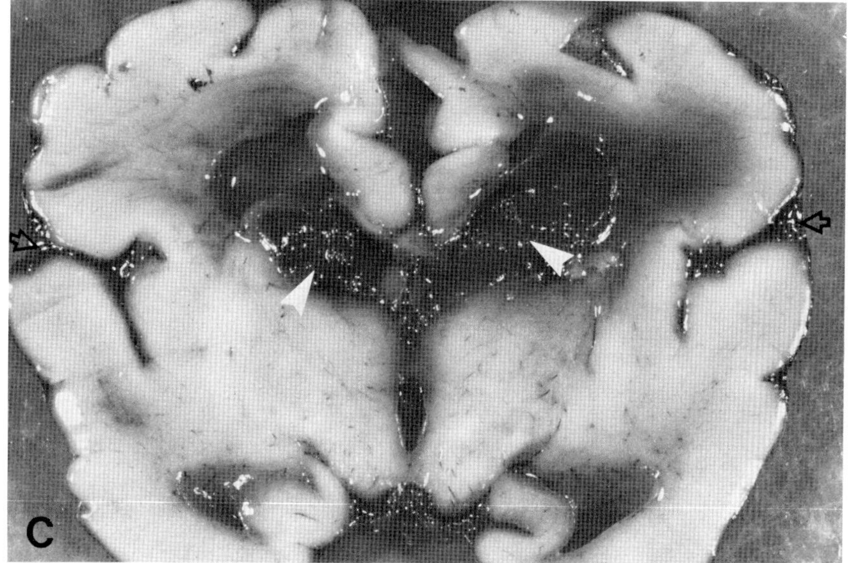
C

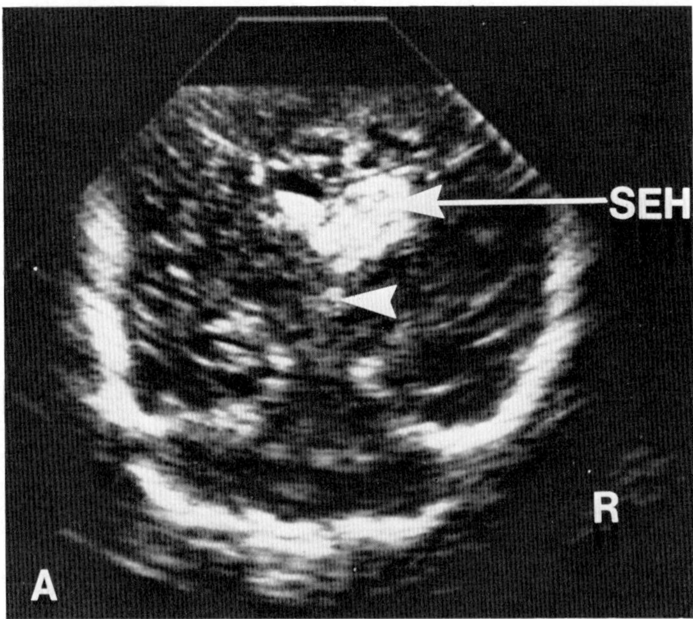

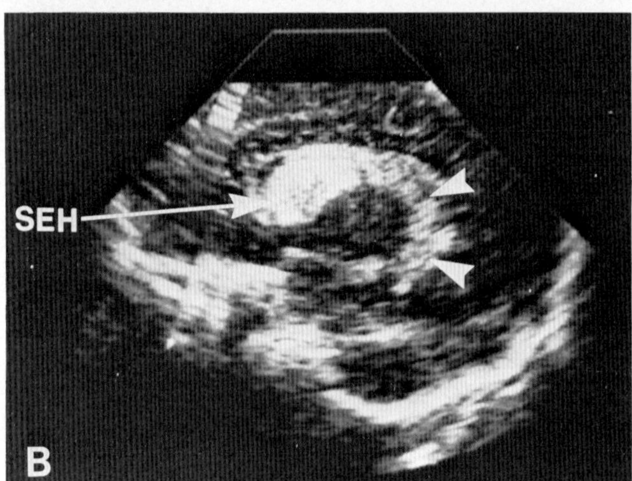

Figure 11.8 Subependymal and intraventricular hemorrhage. A 10-week-old, full-term infant with seizures and full fontanelle. Spinal tap grossly bloody. (*A*) Coronal and (*B*) sagittal scans show bilateral subependymal hemorrhages (*SEH*) larger on right and echogenic blood within mildly dilated lateral and third ventricles (*arrowheads*). (*C*) CT scan shows hematoma in same area with blood in lateral and third ventricles. (*D*) Six-week follow-up coronal ultrasound scan shows persistent mild hydrocephalus with resolution of hematoma. (Reproduced with permission from D. S. Babcock and B. K. Han: *Radiology*, *139:*665–676, 1981.[31])

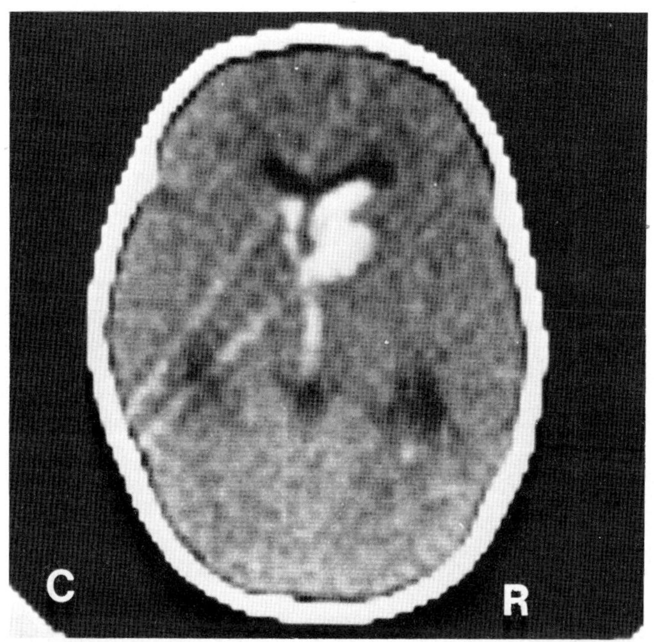
C
R

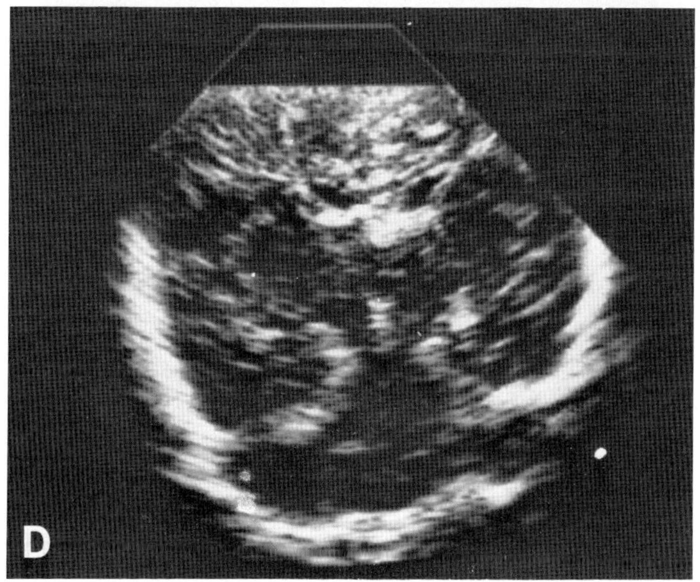
D

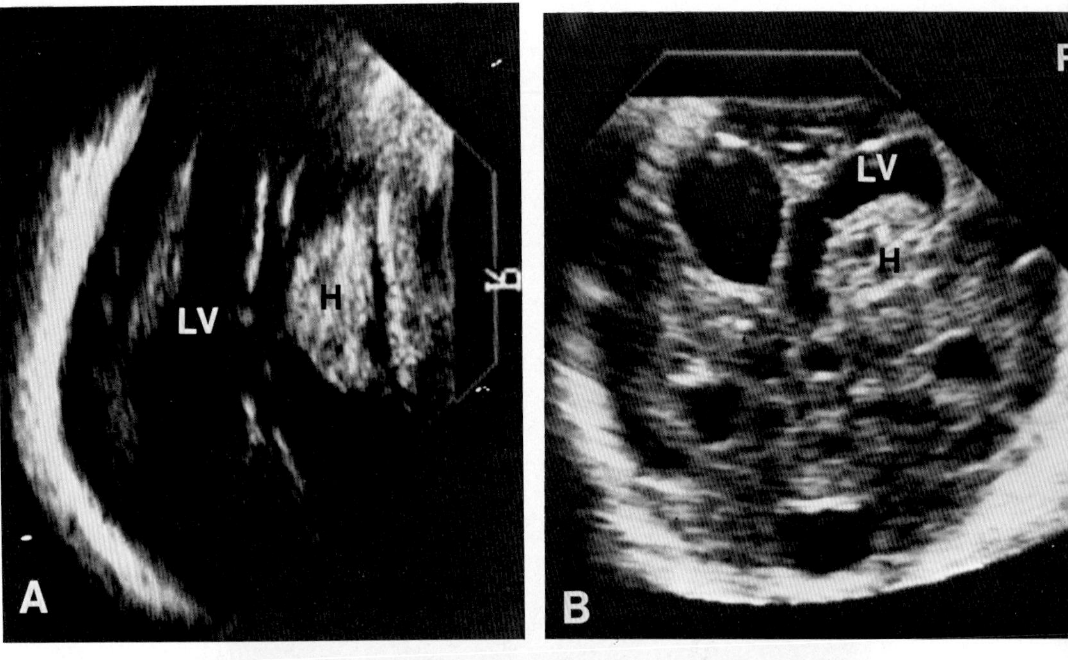

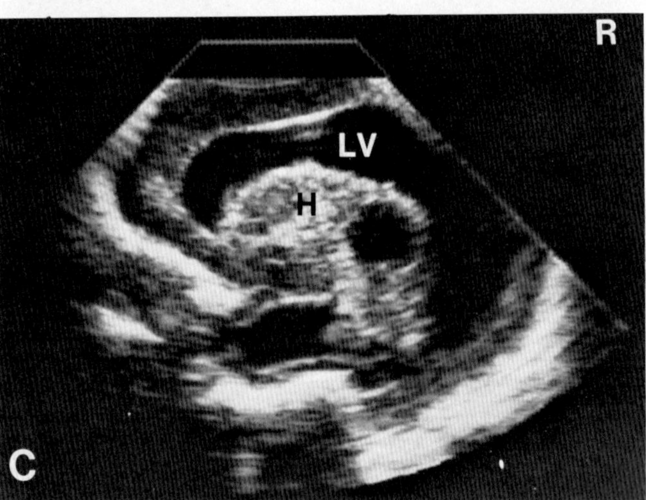

Figure 11.9 Subependymal and intraventricular hemorrhage with massive hydrocephalus. A 1400-g, 30-week gestation infant with history of birth asphyxia. Increasing head size and drop in hematocrit noted at 10 days of age. (*A*) Axial, (*B*) coronal, and (*C*) sagittal scans show large hematoma (*H*) on right with marked panhydrocephalus. Follow-up a week later: (*D*) Coronal and (*E*) sagittal scans show partial liquification (*arrowheads*) of hematoma. (*F*) Baby died 2 months later of ventriculitis and brain section shows massive panhydrocephalus, inflammatory exudate, and residual hematoma (*arrow*) in right caudate nucleus and thalamus. (Reproduced with permission from D. S. Babcock and B. K. Han: *Radiology*, *139*:665–676, 1981.[31])

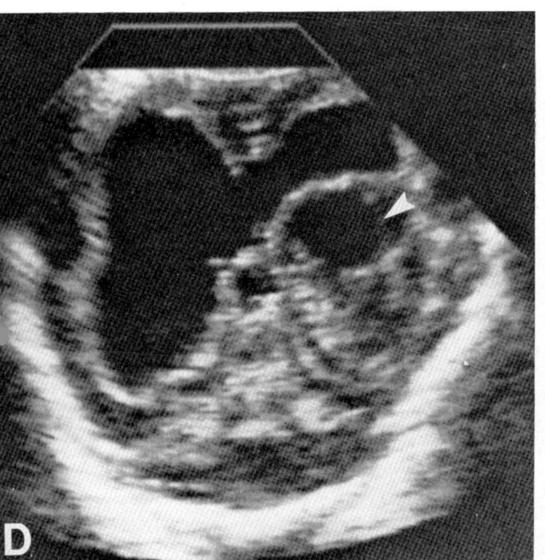
D

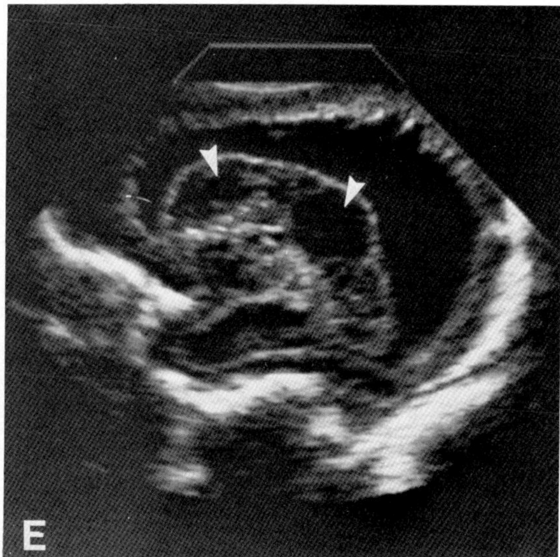
E

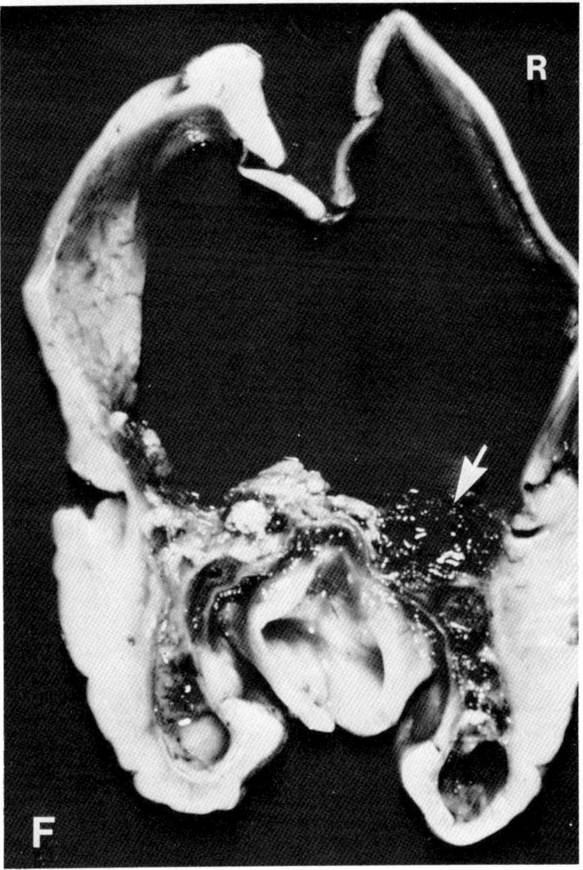
R
F

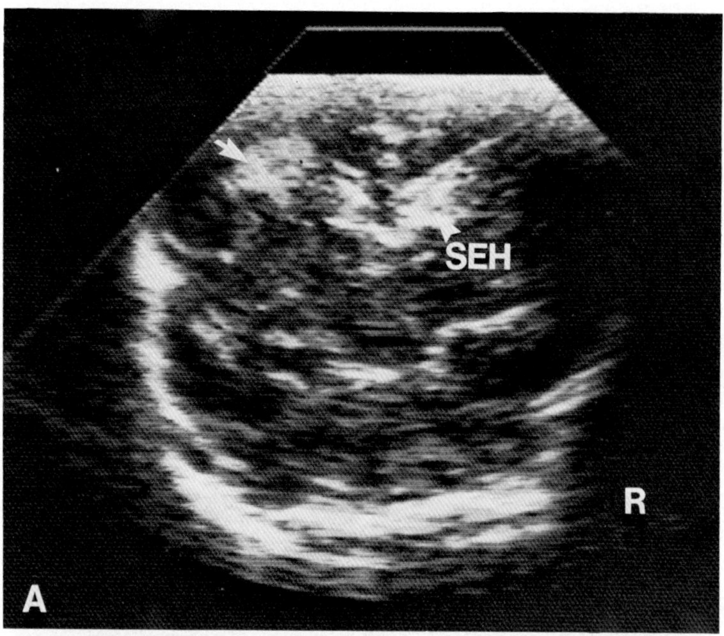

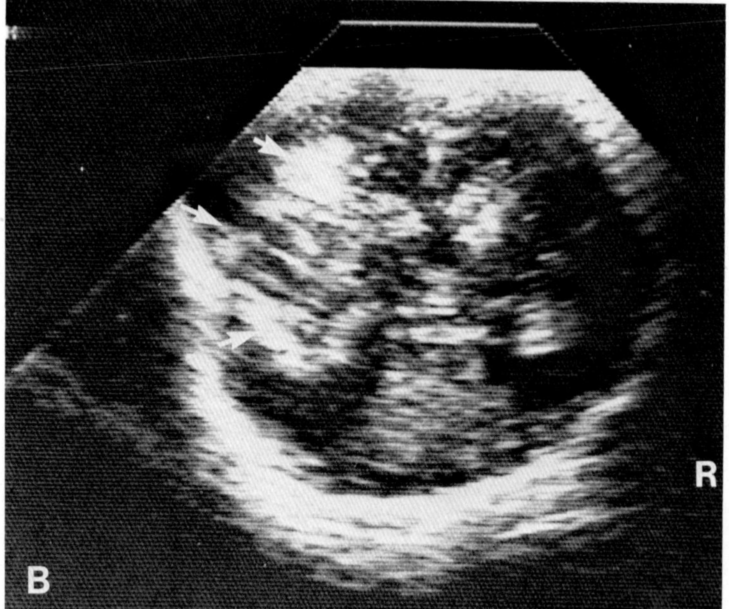

Figure 11.10 Subependymal and intraventricular hemorrhage with intraparenchymal extension. A 32-week gestation infant with sepsis and bloody spinal fluid tap. (*A*) Anterior coronal and (*B*) posterior coronal scans show bilateral subependymal hemorrhages (*SEH*) and periventricular parenchymal hemorrhage (*arrows*) on left. Ventricles normal in size. (*C*) One week follow-up coronal and (*D*) left parasagittal scans show moderately increased parenchymal hematoma (*arrows*). Ventricles moderately enlarged with blood clot within right lateral ventricle (*arrowhead*). (*E*) One week later coronal scan shows partial liquefication of parenchymal hematoma (*open arrows*). (*F*) Three weeks later, coronal scan shows moderate retraction of hematoma (*arrow*).

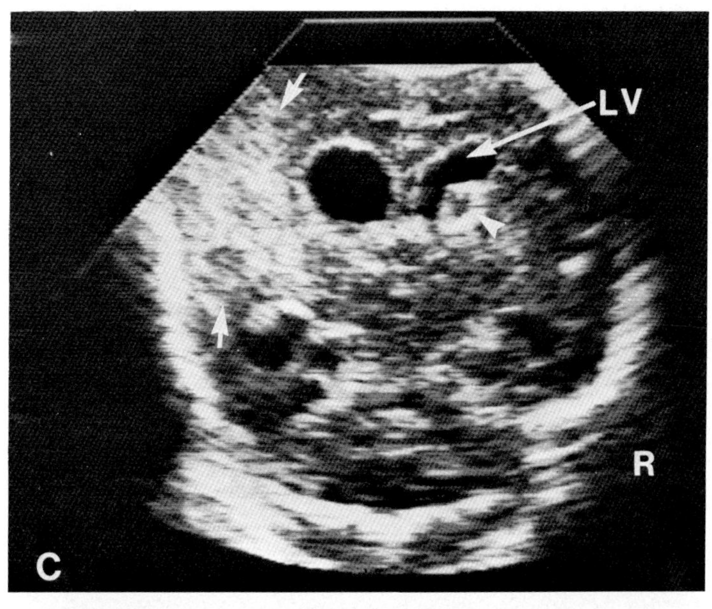
LV
R
C

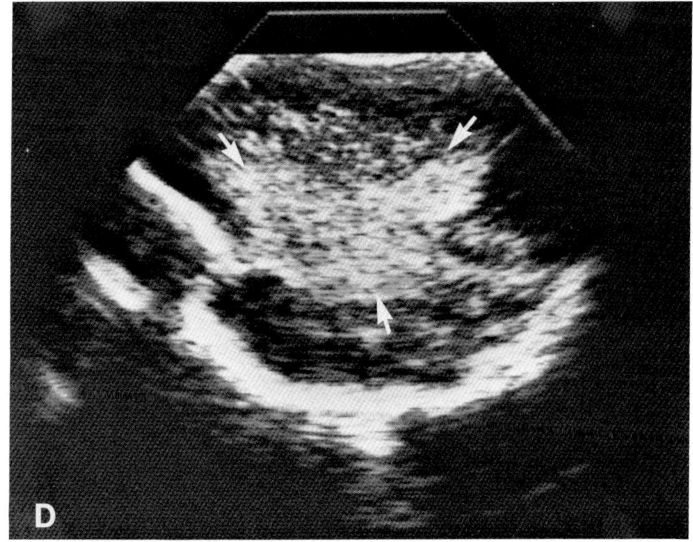
D

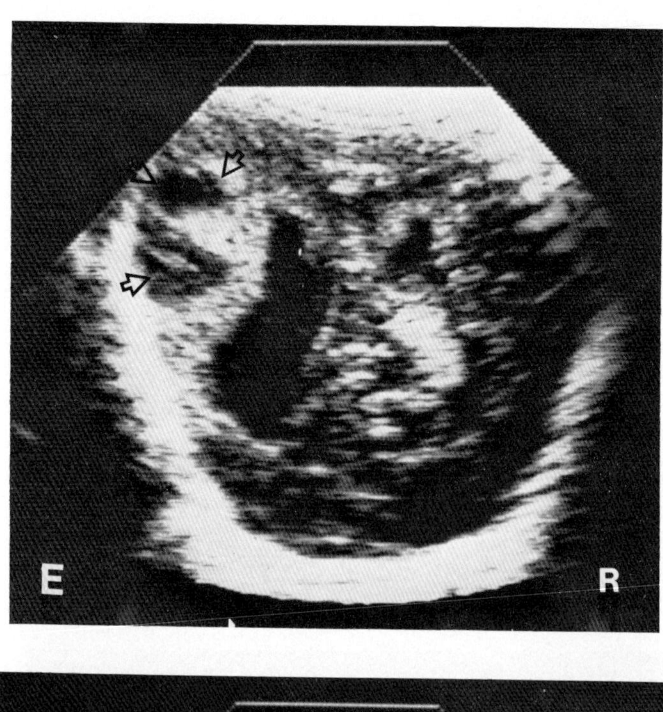

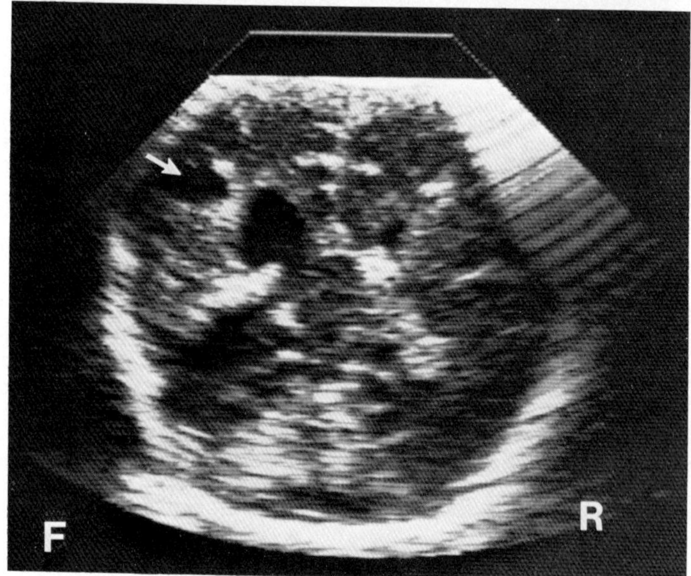

Figure 11.10 E and F

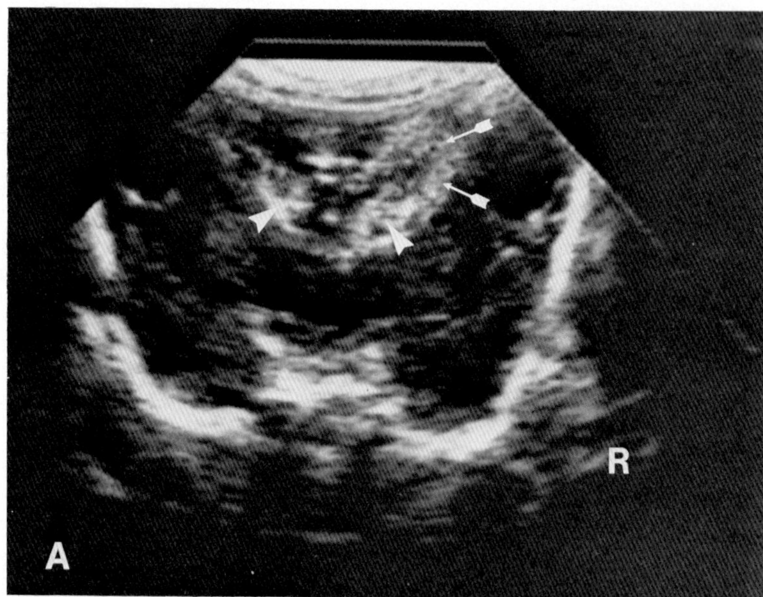

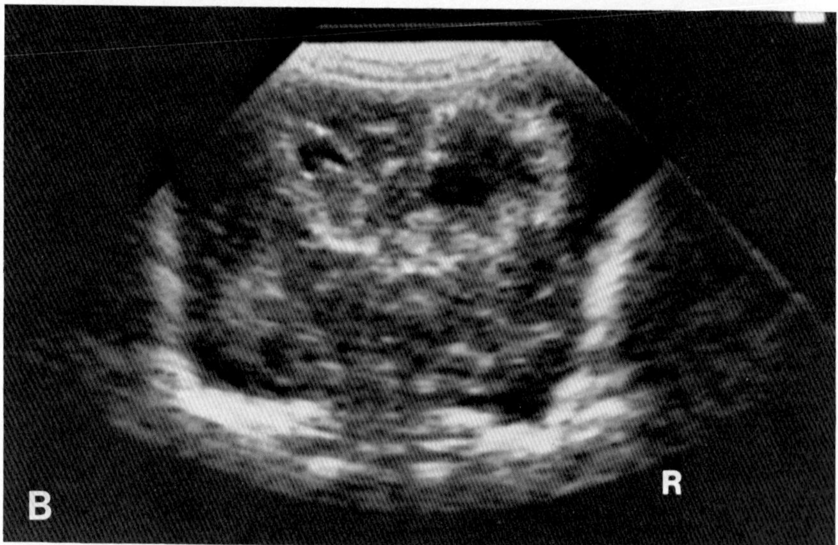

Figure 11.11 Subependymal, intraventricular and intraparenchymal hemorrhage with secondary porencephaly. A 1020-g, 27-week gestation infant with full fontanelle and metabolic acidosis. (*A*) Coronal scan on first day of life shows bilateral small subependymal hemorrhages (*arrowheads*) with slight parenchymal extension (*arrows*) on right. (*B*) Coronal scan, 10 days later. Subependymal hemorrhage increased with further parenchymal extension. (*C*) Two weeks later, coronal scan. Periventricular parenchymal hematoma (*H*) sloughed-off into ventricle which results in porencephalic dilatation of right lateral ventricle (*LV*). Ventricles moderately enlarged. (*D*) Coronal scan, 2 months later. Ventricles slightly decreased in size. Hematoma (*H*) in right lateral ventricle retracted. (*E*) Two months later, coronal scan. Hematoma liquefied and absorbed resulting in porencephaly.

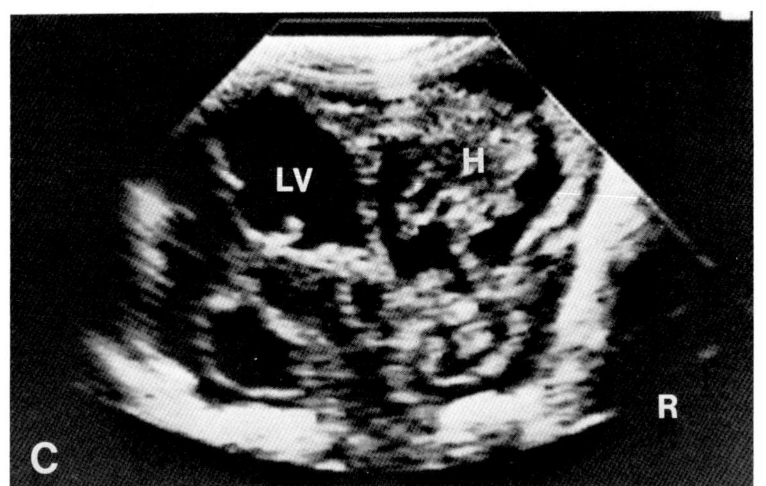
LV
H
R
C

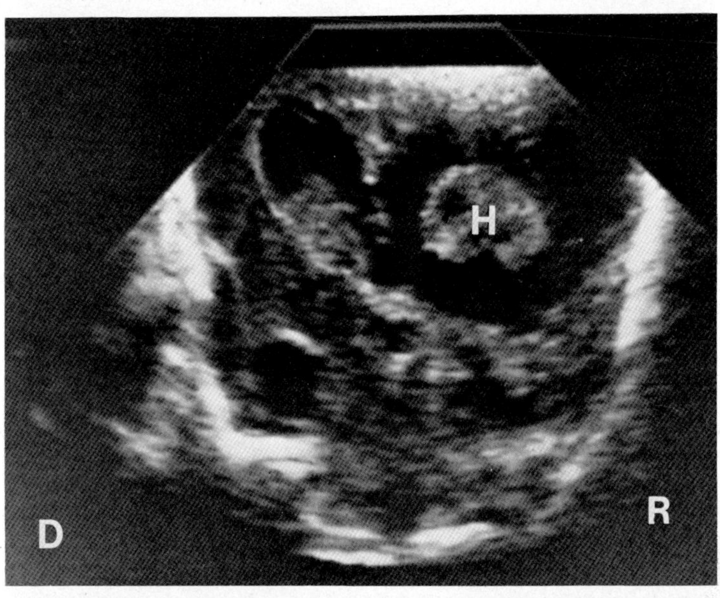
H
R
D

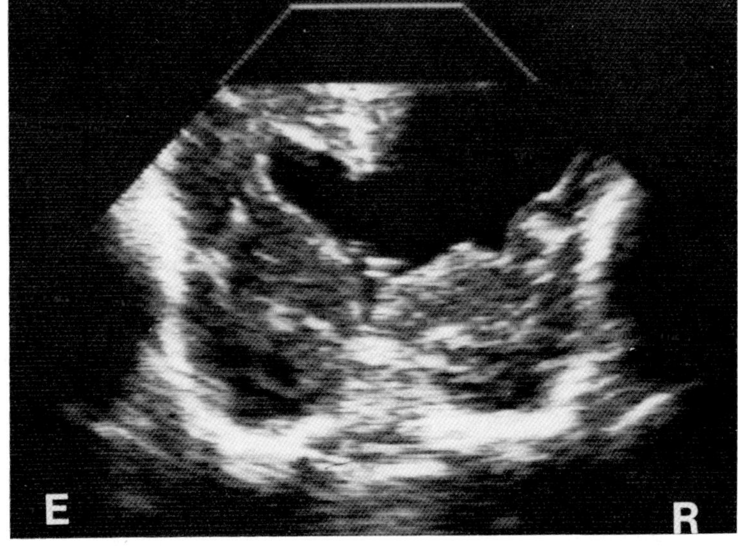
E
R

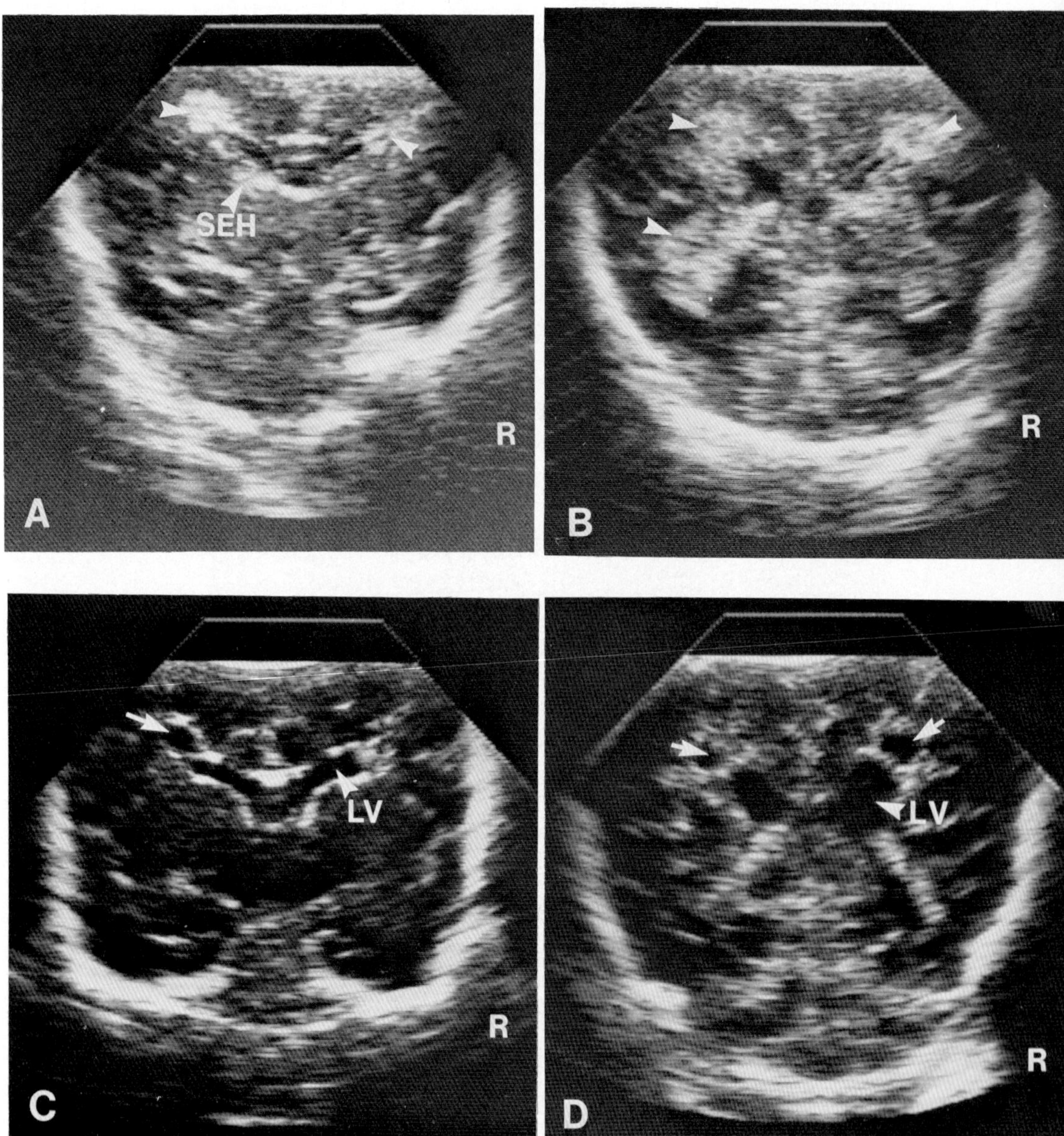

Figure 11.12 Periventricular cysts secondary to subependymal and intraparenchymal hemorrhage. A 1320-g, 30-week gestation infant. (*A*) Midcoronal and (*B*) posterior coronal scans on 3rd day of life show bilateral subependymal hemorrhages (*SEH*) with periventricular parenchymal extension (*arrowheads*). (*C*) One month later, midcoronal and (*D*) posterior coronal scans show several small periventricular cysts (*arrows*) in region of previous hemorrhage. Lateral ventricles (*LV*) slightly enlarged. (*E*) Two months later, anterior coronal and (*F*) posterior coronal scans. Previously noted small periventricular cysts have disappeared.

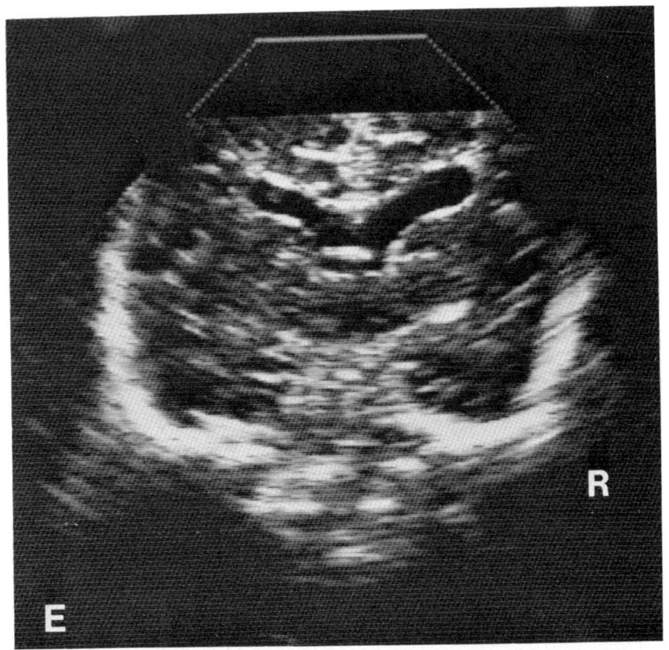
R
E

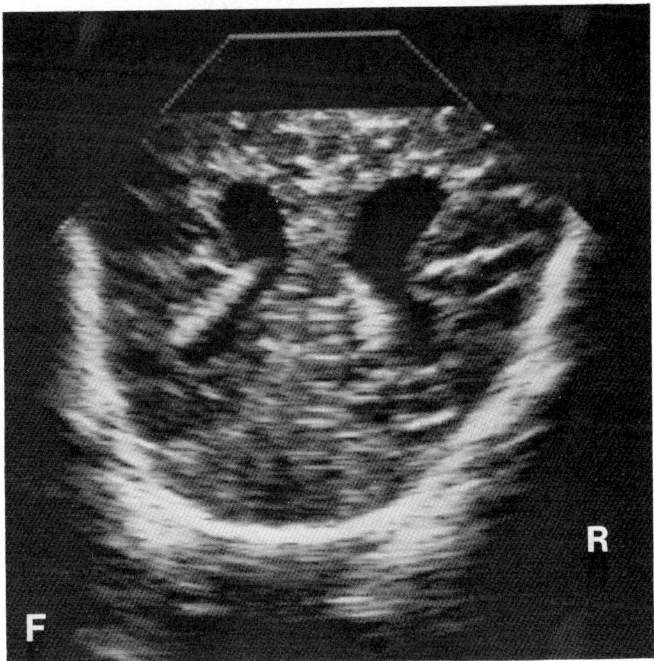
R
F

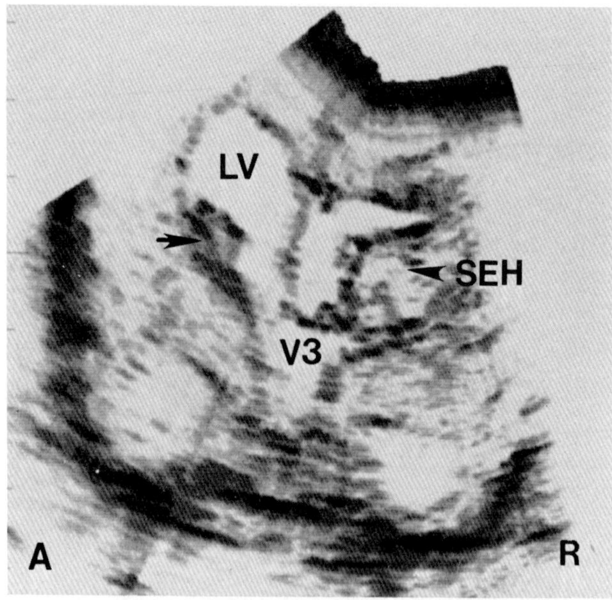

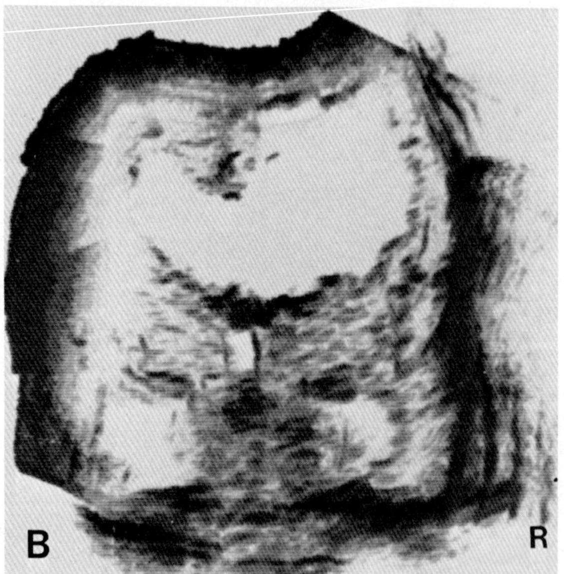

Figure 11.13 Porencephaly secondary to multiple ventricular taps. (*A*) Coronal scan shows moderate dilatation of lateral (*LV*) and third ventricles (*V3*). Large subependymal hematoma (*SEH*) seen on right. Small blood clot also seen in left lateral ventricle (*arrow*). Patient had multiple ventricular taps on right. (*B*) Two month follow-up coronal scan shows large porencephalic dilatation of right lateral ventricle secondary to multiple ventricular taps.

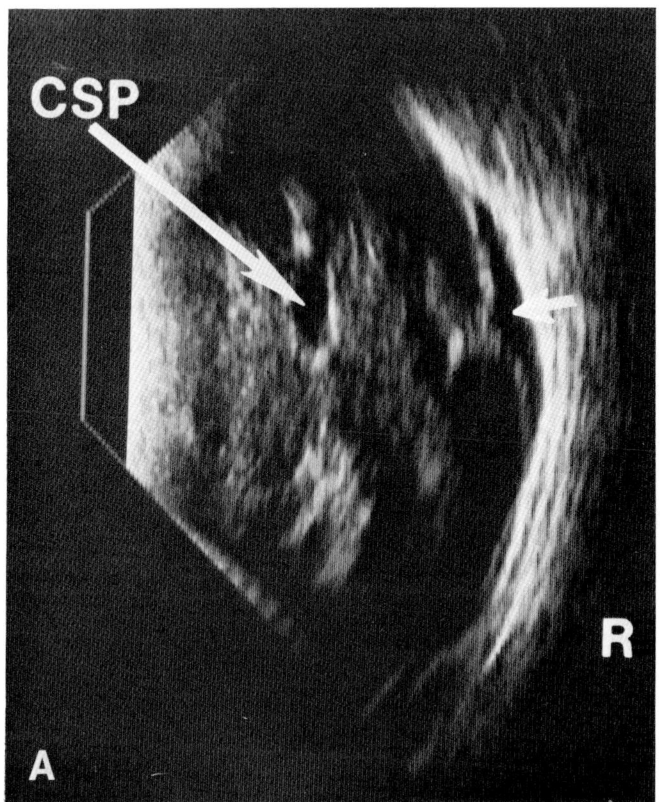

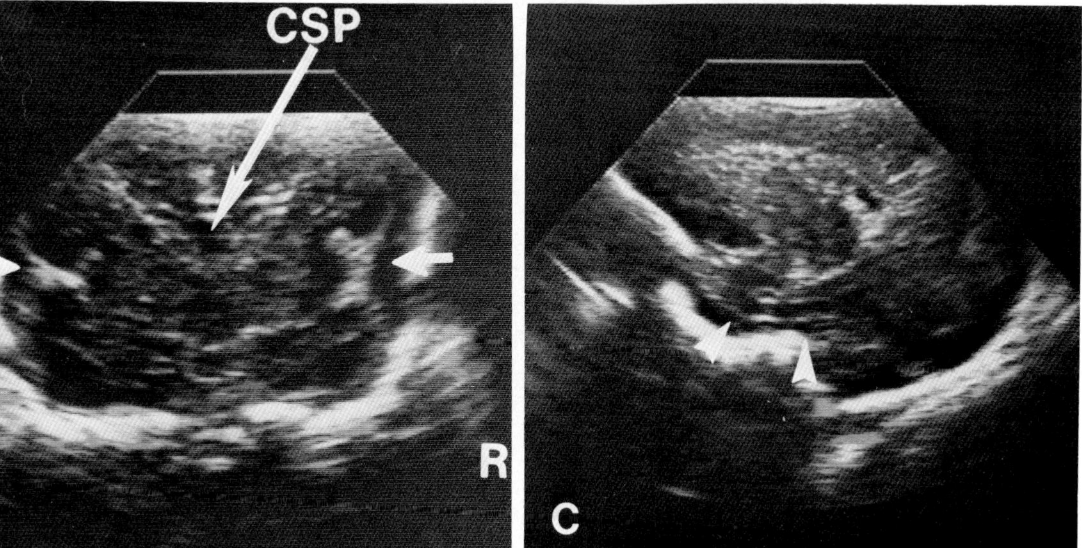

Figure 11.14 Subarachnoid hemorrhage. A 1400-g, 32-week gestation infant with respiratory distress syndrome, diffuse intravascular coagulation, and metabolic acidosis. (*A*) Axial, (*B*) coronal, and (*C*) sagittal scans show prominent subarachnoid space between brain surface and bony calvarium (*arrows*). Patient subsequently developed intraventricular hemorrhage with hydrocephalus. Brain section showed intraventricular and old subarachnoid hemorrhage. *CSP*, cavum septi pellucidi.

CHAPTER 12

Intracranial Tumors

Of all the neoplastic diseases seen in infants and children, intracranial neoplasms are second in frequency and are exceeded in occurrence only by leukemia. Intracranial neoplasms constitute 12% to 15% of the tumors encountered in infants and children.[1] While brain neoplasms are less frequent in infants under 2 years of age (the group of patients who can be examined by ultrasound) they do occur and can be identified by ultrasound. Both supratentorial and infratentorial neoplasms occur in this age group, with a variety of cell types including astrocytoma, ependymoma, choroid plexus papilloma, medulloblastoma, optic nerve glioma, and dermoid. The location of the tumor as well as its character, solid or cystic, can be evaluated with ultrasonography. Further evaluation, such as computerized tomography (CT) and angiography, are then performed.

Ultrasound Findings

A tumor can be identified by its mass effect on normal structures (Figs. 12.1–12.3). Cerebrospinal fluid (CSF)-containing ventricles and cisterns, the falx, and other normal structures may be displaced by the tumor mass. The tumor, particularly a posterior fossa mass, may compress and obstruct the CSF pathway resulting in hydrocephalus.

The echogenicity of the tumor is frequently different than that of normal brain tissue. A patient with a glioma in the region of the thalamus had increased echoes in the tumor compared to the normal thalamus on the opposite side (Fig. 12.2). This was appreciable even though the mass was not large. One patient with an intracranial teratoma (Fig. 12.1) was remarkable in that it was difficult to find any normal appearing brain tissue within the cranium. Areas of solid tissue as well as sonulucent fluid-filled spaces were visualized. Calcified areas were seen as echogenic with acoustic shadowing.

The location of the tumor as well as its character, as determined by its echogenicity, can be used to predict the neoplasm cell type; however, an exact diagnosis is not usually possible by ultrasonography and other non-neoplastic lesions such as intraparenchymal hemorrhage may have similar ultrasound findings.

Summary

While we do not advocate ultrasonography as the primary modality in the investigation of intracranial neoplasms, it can be of help as a screening procedure in infants with neurologic abnormalities, leading to further investigation with CT and angiography for a more specific diagnosis. One should be familiar with the appearance of neoplasms since they can be encountered when examining infants for other reasons.

References

1. Harwood-Nash DC, Fitz CR. *Neuroradiology in Infants and Children.* St. Louis: C. V. Mosby, 1976; 668.
2. Babcock DS, Han BK. The accuracy of high resolution real-time ultrasonography of the head in infancy. Radiology 1981; 139:665–676.

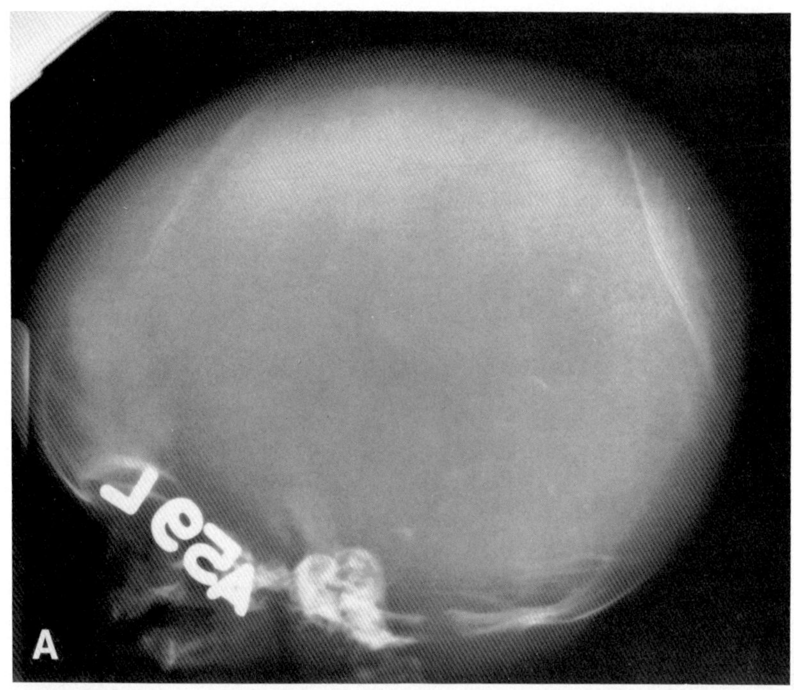

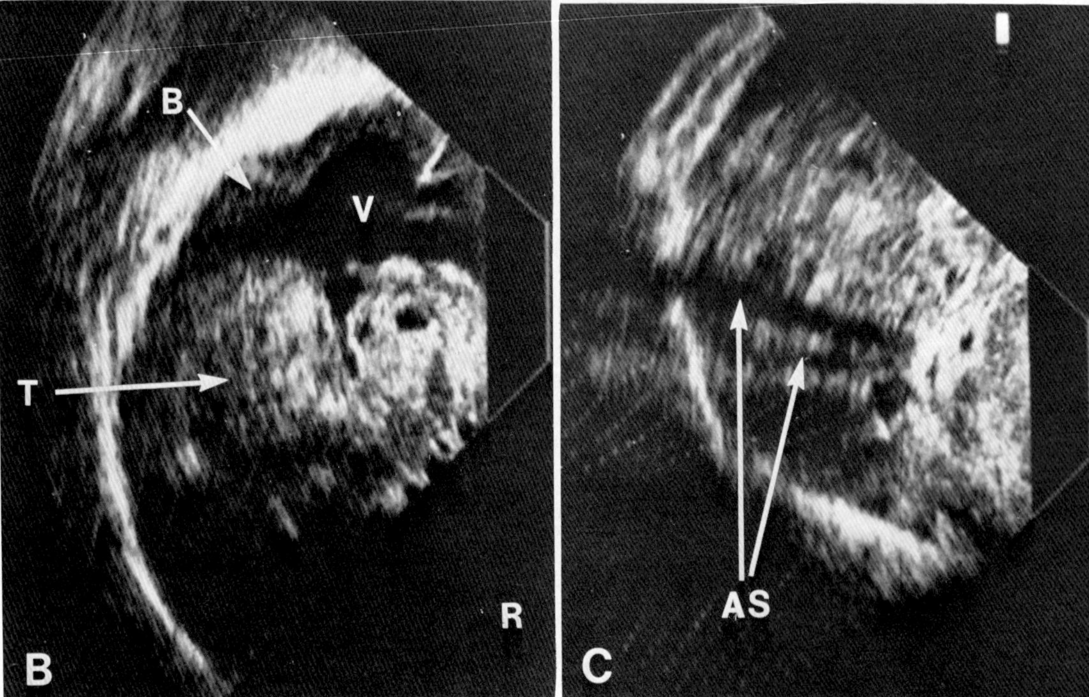

Figure 12.1 Large intracranial teratoma. Newborn infant with enlarged head. (*A*) plain film of skull shows markedly enlarged head with multiple irregular intracranial calcifications. (*B*) Axial, (*C*) more posterior axial, and (*D*) CT scan. Large tumor mass (*T*) with echolucent areas as well as echogenic areas with

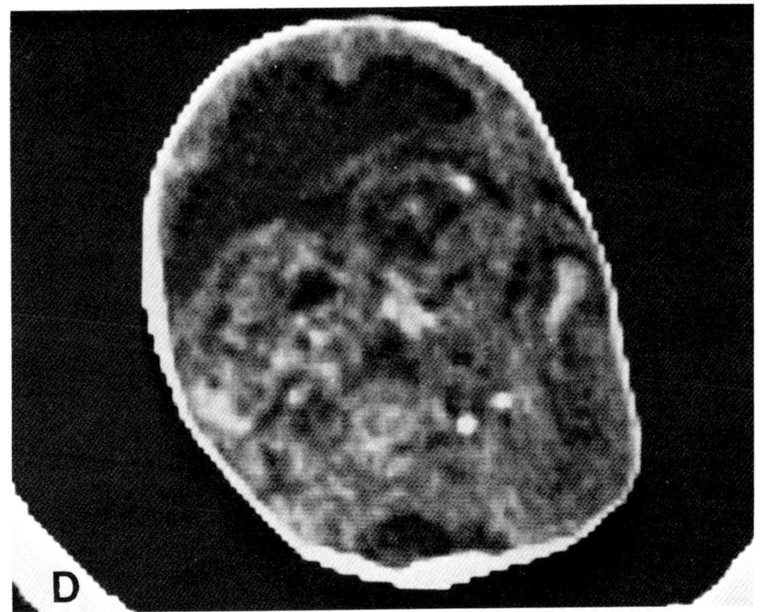

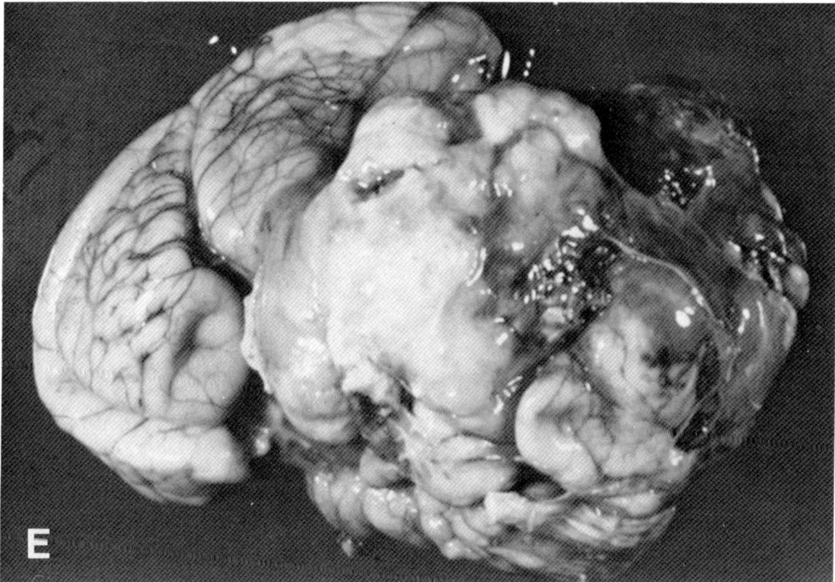

acoustic shadowing (*AS*) representing calcifications occupies posterior two-thirds of head. Brain (*B*) and dilated ventricles (*V*) are displaced and compressed anteriorly by tumor mass. Baby died. (*E*) brain specimen shows large teratoma posteriorly and brain anteriorly.

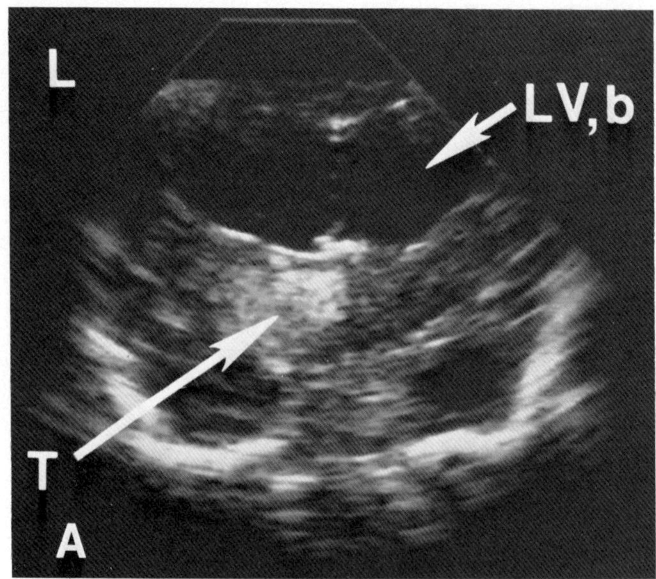

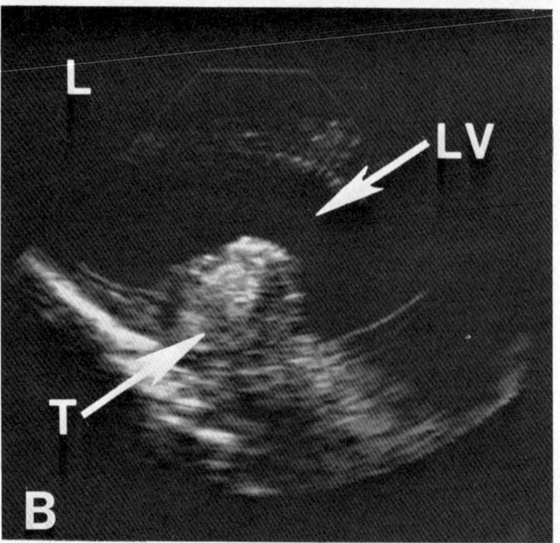

Figure 12.2 Astrocytoma. Four-month-old infant with seizures and macrocrania. (*A*) Coronal scan, (*B*) sagittal scan through left lateral ventricle (*LV*), and (*C*) sagittal scan through right lateral ventricle (*LV*). Echogenic tumor (*T*) in region of left thalamus. Compare to normal right thalamus. Moderate dilatation of lateral ventricles without enlargement of third and fourth ventricles suggests obstruction at foramina of Monro. (*D*) CT scan shows enhancing tumor in region of left thalamus and moderate dilatation of lateral ventricles. Cerebral angiography (not shown) showed possible tumor blush without evidence of arteriovenous malformation. Ventriculoperitoneal shunt placed. CSF cytology showed cells consistent with malignant glioma, probably astrocytoma. (Reproduced with permission from D. S. Babcock and B. K. Han: *Radiology*, *139:*665–676, 1981.[2])

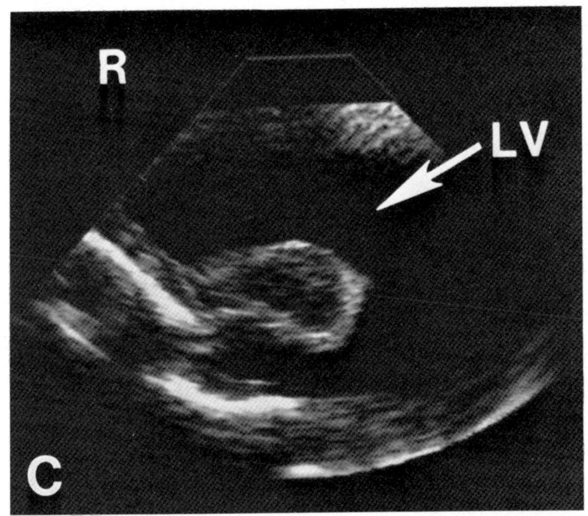
R
LV
C

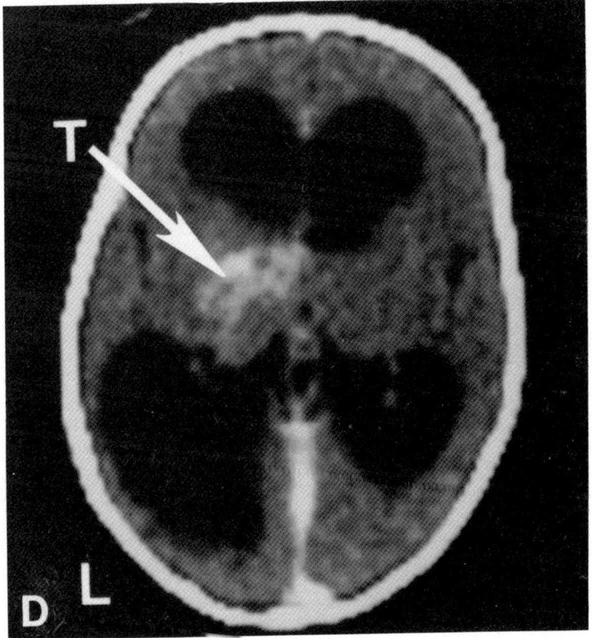
T
D
L

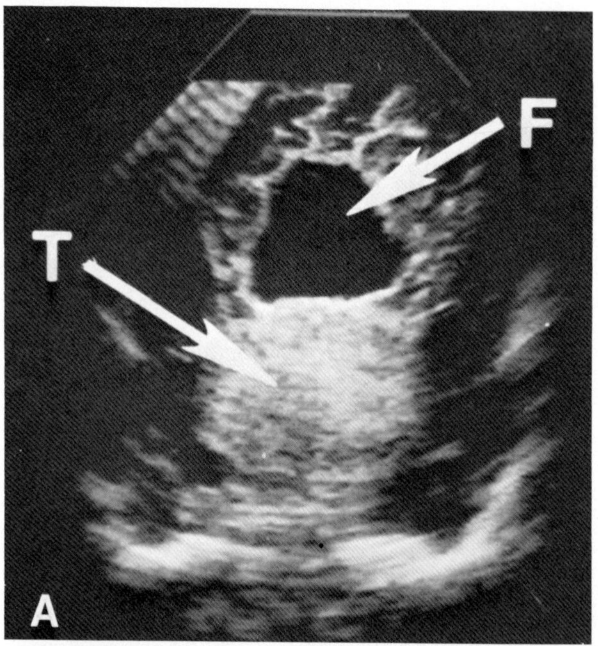

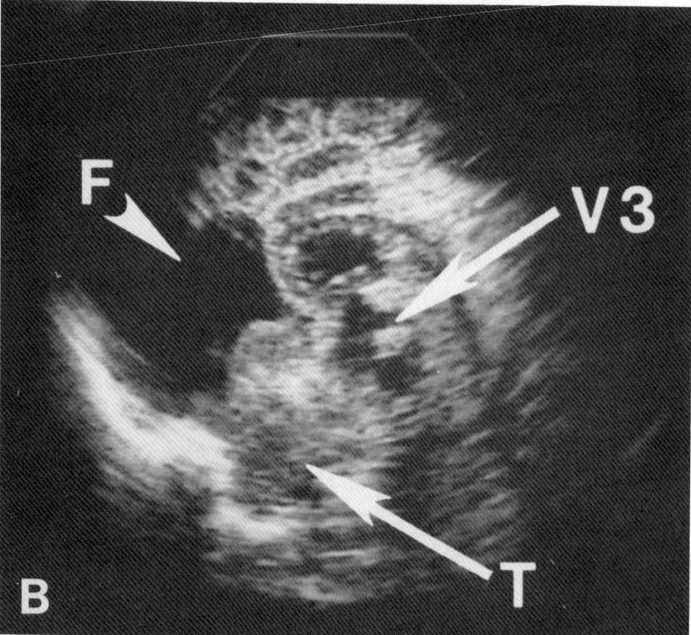

Figure 12.3 Chiasmatic astrocytoma. Six-month-old infant with macrocrania and searching nystagmus. (*A*) Coronal and (*B*) sagittal scans. Third ventricle (*V3*) is displaced superiorly and posteriorly by suprasellar tumor (*T*) and loculated fluid collection (*F*) between frontal lobes. (*C*) CT scan shows enhancing tumor in chiasmatic hypothalamic/thalamic region with fluid (*F*) in interhemispheric fissure between frontal lobes and under tips of both temporal lobes. (*D*) Brain angiography shows slightly vascular mass with vessel displacement. Biopsy proven pilocytic astrocytoma with secondary pseudocyst. (Reproduced with permission from D. S. Babcock and B. K. Han: *Radiology*, *139*:665–676, 1981.[2])

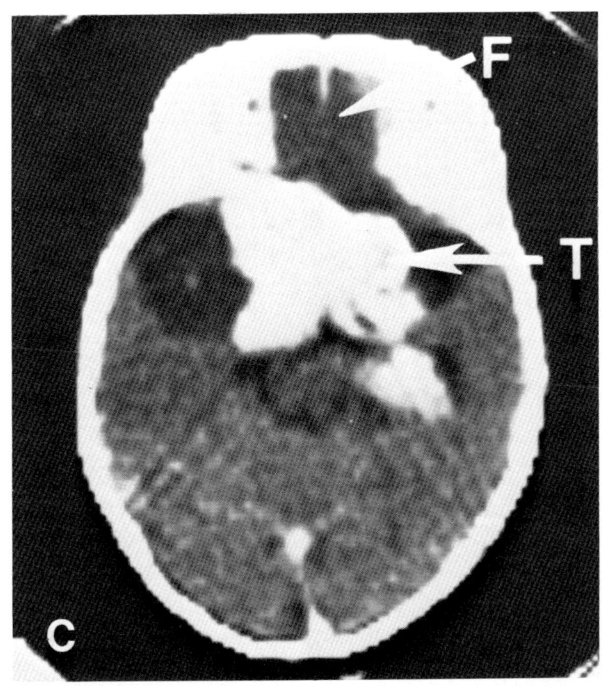
F
T
C

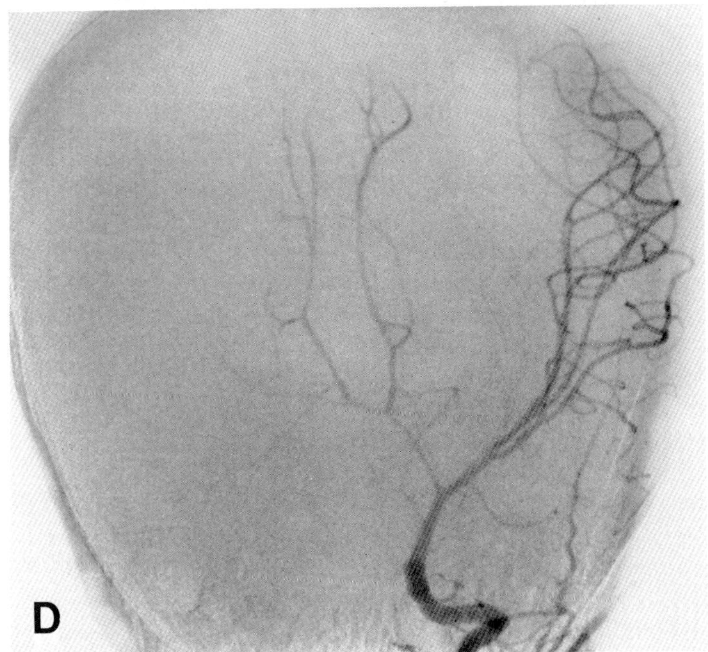
D

CHAPTER 13

Evaluation of Ventricular Shunt Function

The treatment of hydrocephalus with increased intraventricular pressure is insertion of a shunting system which shunts the cerebrospinal fluid (CSF) from the ventricles to another body compartment such as the peritoneum, right atrium, et cetera. The decrease in intraventricular pressure usually results in diminished intraventricular volume. The hemispheres sometimes fall away from the inner table of the skull, the cisterns increase minimally in volume, and the sulci occasionally become more prominent. In the young infant, the skull bones overlap where previously the sutures had been split, and the anterior fontanelle sinks. In older children whose sutures are already closed, the hemispheres fall away from the inner table of the skull and bridging veins may tear with the resultant accumulation of a subdural hematoma.[1]

With hydrocephalus and increased pressure the ventricles are dilated and there is rounding of the ventricular angles, most easily identified as rounding of the lateral angles of the lateral ventricles (Figs. 13.1, *B* and *F*, and 13.2, *B* and *D*).[2] With enlargement of the ventricles due to hydrocephalus ex vacuo or brain atrophy, the ventricles may be enlarged, but the intraventricular pressure is not increased and the angles are usually preserved (Fig. 13.3). Ultrasonography has proven accurate for evaluating the presence and severity of dilatation of the ventricles.[3] The atria and occipital horns of the lateral ventricles dilate more and earlier than the frontal horns (Fig. 13.1*A*). The anterior third ventricle and suprapineal recess dilate early and significantly in obstructions distal to these structures.

After ventricular shunting, the ventricles decrease in size and the angles become less rounded (Fig. 13.1), although they may not return to normal size. The cortical thickness sometimes increases. Ultrasonography has proven useful in evaluating for possible shunt malfunction, particularly when a shunted infant presents with nonspecific symptoms, such as irritability, and the clinician cannot readily differentiate between shunt malfunction and other diseases of childhood. The ultrasound examination in the case of shunt malfunction will demonstrate increasing ventricular size and aid in making a proper diagnosis.

The cause of the shunt malfunction is usually not identified on cranial ultrasonography; however, occasionally, occlusion of the pathway such as at the foramen of Monro may be suspected when there is unilateral dilatation of a lateral ventricle (Fig. 13.2). This patient required bilateral ventricular shunting before the symptoms were relieved.

Intra-abdominal Complications

With ventriculoperitoneal shunts, peritoneal adhesions may cause encysted collections of CSF, creating a large abdominal mass and poor absorption of the CSF by the peritoneal lining. Such CSF pseudocysts are readily demonstrable by abdominal ultrasonography (Fig. 13.4).[4–7]

Summary

Ultrasonography is an accurate and easy method for diagnosing the presence and severity of hydrocephalus and for evaluating ventricular shunt function. Since repeated examinations can be performed with no known hazard to the patient, it provides a method for studying the changes in ventricular size and configuration in the immediate postventricular shunt placement period. An additional discussion of the evaluation of ventricular size and shunt function is given in Chapter 6.

References

1. Harwood-Nash DC, Fitz CR. *Neuroradiology in Infants and Children.* St. Louis: C. V. Mosby, 1976; 609–667.
2. Naidick TP, Gado M. Hydrocephalus. In: *Radiology of the Skull and Brain*, Newton TH, Potts DG, (eds). St. Louis: C. V. Mosby, 1978; 3764–3834.
3. Skolnick ML, Rosenbaum AE, Matzuk T, Guthkelch AN, Heinz ER. Detection of dilated cerebral ventricles in infants: a correlative study between ultrasound and computed tomography. Radiology 1979; 131:447–451.
4. Cunningham JJ. Evaluation of malfunctioning ventriculoperitoneal shunts with gray scale echography. JCU 1976; 4:369–370.
5. Lee TG, Parsons PM. Ultrasound diagnosis of cerebrospinal fluid abdominal cyst. Radiology 1978; 127–220.
6. Goldfine SL, Turetz F, Beck AR, Eiger M. Cerebrospinal fluid intraperitoneal cyst: an unusual abdominal mass. AJR 1978; 130:568–569.
7. Fried AM, Adams WE, Ellis GT, Hatfield DR, Walsh JW. Ventriculoperitoneal shunt function: evaluation by sonography. AJR 1980; 134:967–970.
8. Babcock DS, Han BK, LeQuesne GW. B-Mode gray scale ultrasound of the head in the newborn and young infant. AJR 1980; 134:457–468.
9. Babcock DS, Han BK. Cranial sonographic findings in meningomyelocele. AJNR 1980; 1: 493–499.

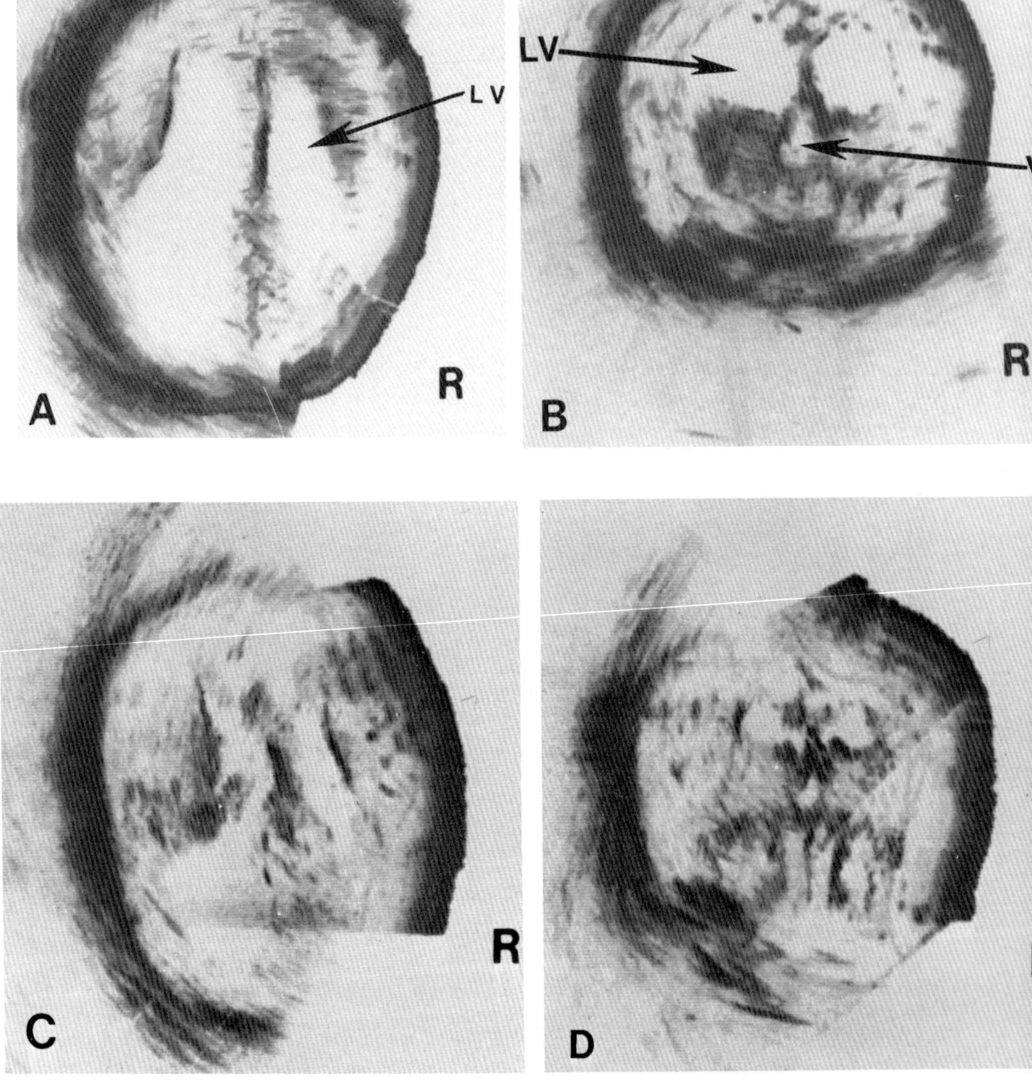

Figure 13.1 Ventricular shunt function. A 37-week gestation newborn with meningomyelocele and mild head enlargement. (*A*) Axial and (*B*) coronal scans at age 2 days. Moderate to severe dilatation of lateral (*LV*) and third (*V3*) ventricles shown with rounding of ventricular angles. Atria and occipital horns dilated more than frontal horns. (*C* and *D*) Follow-up examination 9 days later after temporary ventricular shunt. Lateral and third ventricles diminished, although still mildly enlarged. Ventricular angles less rounded. (*E* and *F*) Two week follow-up for increasing head size. Increased ventricular size and rounded ventricular angles shown indicating shunt (*S*) malfunction. Malfunctioning shunt was replaced. (*G* and *H*) Postoperative examination 1 month later. Ventricles collapsed and slitlike. (Reproduced with permission from D. S. Babcock, B. K. Han, and G. W. LeQuesne: *American Journal of Roentgenology*, *134*:457–468, 1980.[8])

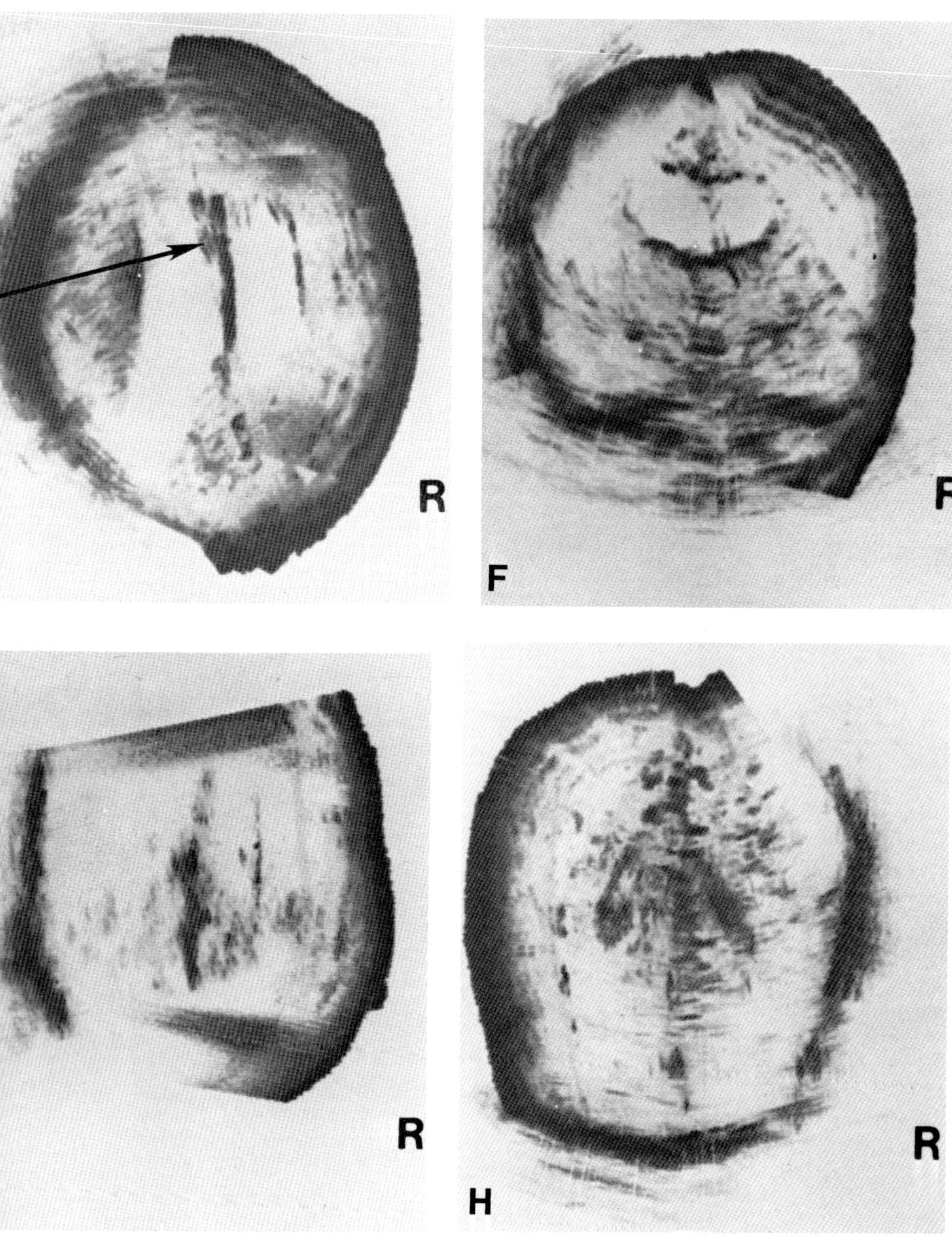
R
R
F
R
R
H

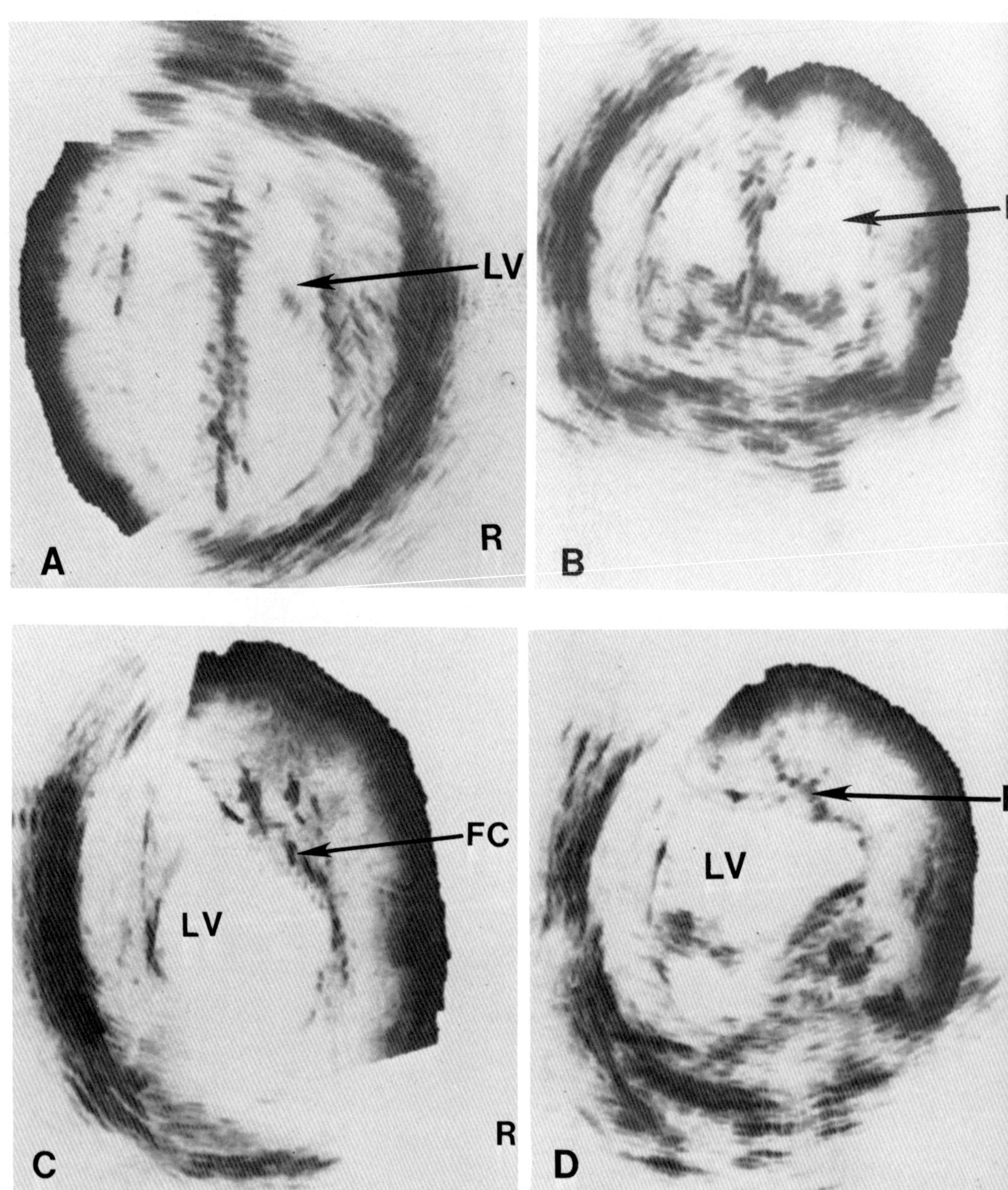
LV
R
A
B
FC
LV
R
C
LV
D

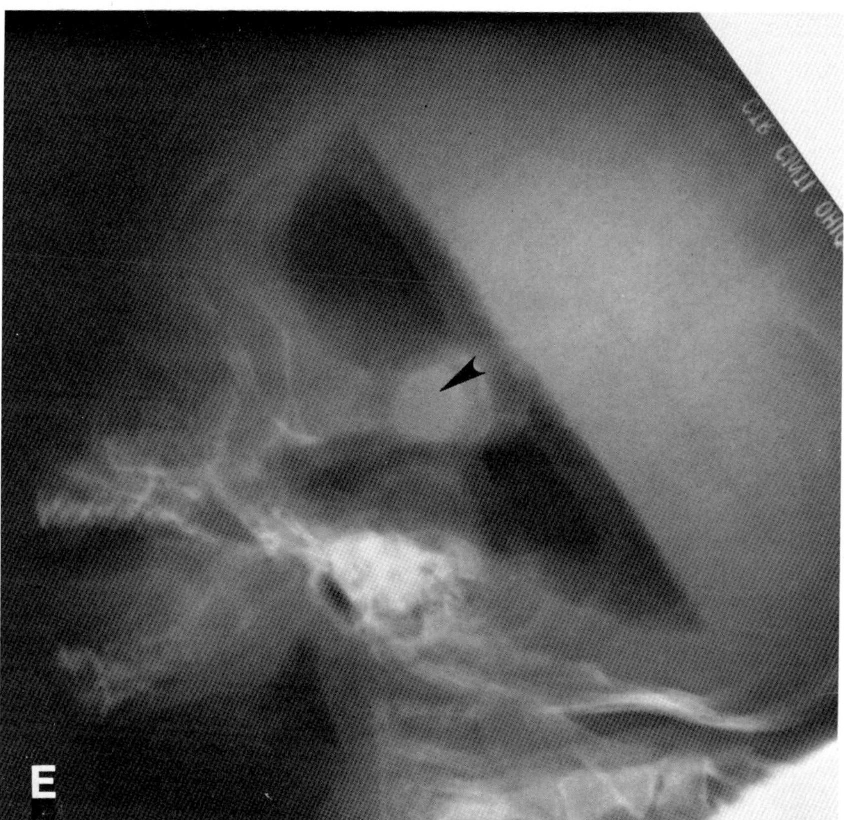

Figure 13.2 Obstruction of foramen of Monro. Two-day old infant with meningomyelocele. (*A*) axial and (*B*) coronal scans prior to shunting. Moderate dilatation of lateral ventricles (*LV*) seen. Third ventricle obliterated by enlarged massa intermedia. (*C*) Axial and (*D*) coronal scans after unilateral ventricular shunting show collapse of ipsilateral ventricle and further enlargement of contralateral ventricle. Displaced falx cerebri (*FC*). (*E*) ventriculography shows enlarged massa intermedia (*arrowhead*) which may be obstructing foramen of Monro. (Reproduced with permission from D. S. Babcock, B. K. Han: *American Journal of Neuroradiology*, *1*:493–499, 1980.[9])

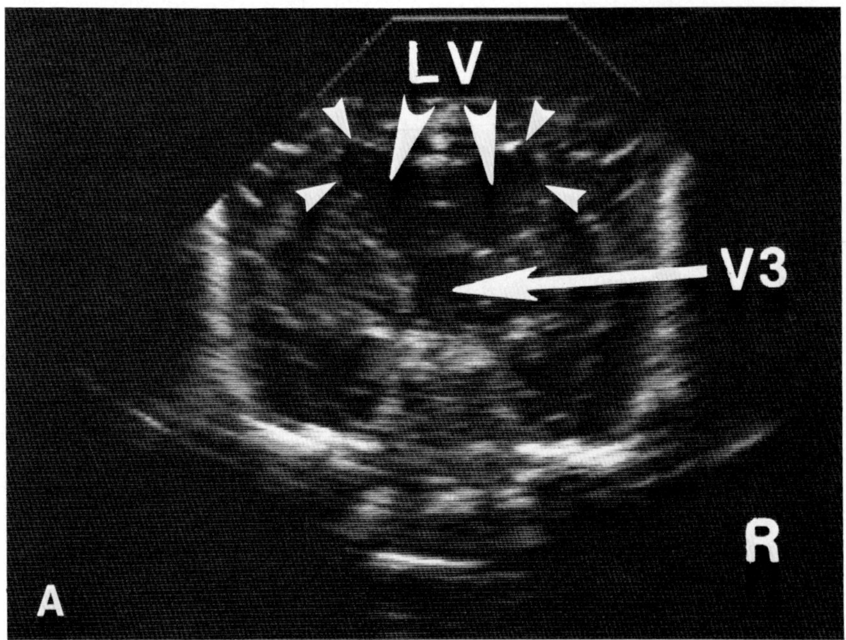

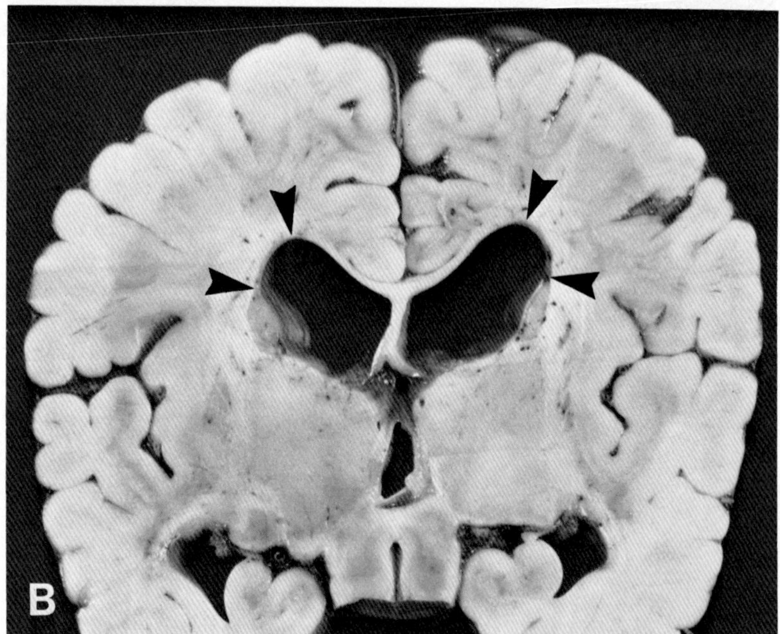

Figure 13.3 Hydrocephalus ex vacuo. Eight-month-old former premature infant with respiratory distress syndrome, bronchopulmonary dysplasia, and patent ductus arteriosus. Mild enlargement of lateral (*LV*) and third (*V3*) ventricles which retain relatively sharp angles (*arrowheads*) suggesting enlargement due to brain atrophy, rather than increased pressure. (*B*) Brain section shows hydrocephalus ex vacuo.

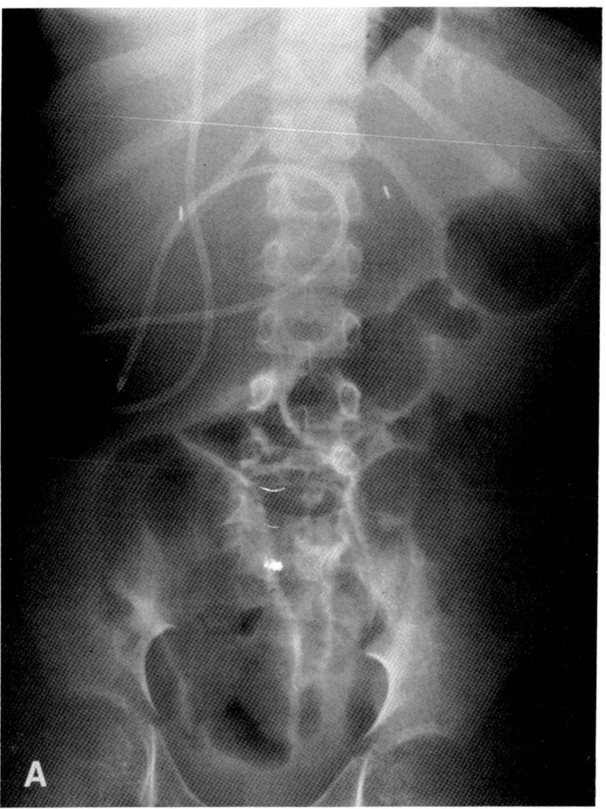

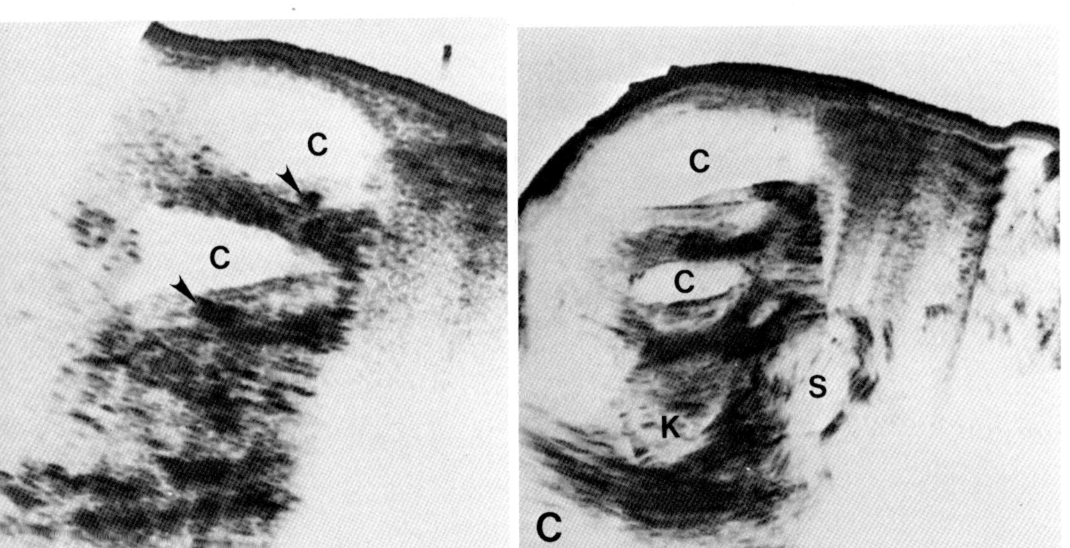

Figure 13.4 Cerebrospinal fluid (CSF) pseudocyst. Five-year-old boy with brainstem glioma and ventriculoperitoneal shunt presented with 1-week history of fever and abdominal distension. (*A*) Plain film of abdomen shows displacement of stomach and transverse colon suggesting hepatomegaly or mass in right upper quadrant. Abdominal portion of ventriculoperitoneal shunt seen in right upper quadrant making 2 turns with tip pointing inferiorly. (*B*) Longitudinal scan 5 cm to right of midline. (*C*) Transverse scan 4 cm above umbilicus. Multiloculated cystic structures (*C*) seen in right upper abdomen with echogenic material layering out in dependent portion of cyst, representing pus. Ventriculoperitoneal shunt catheter (*arrows*) seen as highly echogenic structure within cyst with acoustic shadowing behind it. *K*, Right kidney; *S*, spine. Patient operated upon and infected CSF pseudocyst drained.

Index